D1479675

ELSEVIER'S INTEGRATED REVIEW
BIOCHEMISTRY

ELSEVIER'S INTEGRATED REVIEW
BIOCHEMISTRY
SECOND EDITION

John W. Pelley, PhD
Professor
Texas Tech University School of Medicine
Lubbock, Texas

ELSEVIER
SAUNDERS

1600 John F. Kennedy Blvd. Ste 1800
Philadelphia, PA 19103-2899

ELSEVIER'S INTEGRATED REVIEW BIOCHEMISTRY,　　　　　　ISBN: 978-0-323-07446-9
SECOND EDITION

Copyright © 2012 by Saunders, an imprint of Elsevier Inc.
Copyright © 2007 by Mosby, Inc., an affiliate of Elsevier Inc.

No part of this publication may be reproduced or transmitted in any form or by any means, electronic or mechanical, including photocopying, recording, or any information storage and retrieval system, without permission in writing from the publisher. Details on how to seek permission, further information about the Publisher's permissions policies and our arrangements with organizations such as the Copyright Clearance Center and the Copyright Licensing Agency, can be found at our website: www.elsevier.com/permissions.

This book and the individual contributions contained in it are protected under copyright by the Publisher (other than as may be noted herein).

Notices

Knowledge and best practice in this field are constantly changing. As new research and experience broaden our understanding, changes in research methods, professional practices, or medical treatment may become necessary.

Practitioners and researchers must always rely on their own experience and knowledge in evaluating and using any information, methods, compounds, or experiments described herein. In using such information or methods they should be mindful of their own safety and the safety of others, including parties for whom they have a professional responsibility.

With respect to any drug or pharmaceutical products identified, readers are advised to check the most current information provided (i) on procedures featured or (ii) by the manufacturer of each product to be administered, to verify the recommended dose or formula, the method and duration of administration, and contraindications. It is the responsibility of practitioners, relying on their own experience and knowledge of their patients, to make diagnoses, to determine dosages and the best treatment for each individual patient, and to take all appropriate safety precautions.

To the fullest extent of the law, neither the Publisher nor the authors, contributors, or editors, assume any liability for any injury and/or damage to persons or property as a matter of products liability, negligence or otherwise, or from any use or operation of any methods, products, instructions, or ideas contained in the material herein.

Library of Congress Cataloging-in-Publication Data

Pelley, John W.
　Elsevier's integrated review biochemistry / John W. Pelley. – 2nd ed.
　　p. ; cm.
　Integrated review biochemistry
　Rev. ed. of: Elsevier's integrated biochemistry / John W. Pelley. c2007.
　Includes index.
　ISBN 978-0-323-07446-9 (pbk. : alk. paper)
　I. Pelley, John W. Elsevier's integrated biochemistry II. Title. III. Title: Integrated review biochemistry.
　[DNLM: 1. Biochemical Phenomena. 2. Molecular Biology–methods. QU 4]

　612'.015–dc23　　　　　　　　　　　　　　　　　　　　　　　2011035525

Acquisitions Editor: Madelene Hyde
Developmental Editor: Andrew Hall
Publishing Services Manager: Patricia Tannian
Team Manager: Hemamalini Rajendrababu
Project Manager: Antony Prince
Designer: Steven Stave

Working together to grow
libraries in developing countries

www.elsevier.com | www.bookaid.org | www.sabre.org

ELSEVIER　　BOOK AID International　　Sabre Foundation

Printed in China

Last digit is the print number:　9　8　7　6　5　4　3　2　1

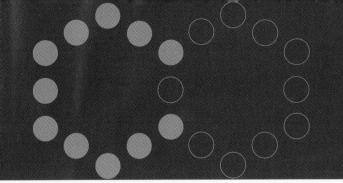

Preface

I wrote this book to make biochemistry easier to learn and easier to remember. Learning and remembering do not always go together, since any new material can be learned but forgotten quickly. It is only through integrative learning that long-term memory is built. Even if you have never had a biochemistry course or if you have taken biochemistry but forgotten much of it, you will find this innovative approach helpful.

To make learning easier, I have given careful attention to the sequence and organization of each chapter so that each topic builds on previous topics. Also, within each chapter, the material is presented in a way that suggests how it should be learned. For example, each metabolic pathway has five consistent organizing aspects: pathway components, regulation points, intersection with other pathways, unique features, and clinical features. Hence all chapters on metabolism, for example, have the same headings, allowing easy comparison and quicker integrative learning. An additional aid to easier learning is the minimal inclusion of chemical structures, thus shifting the learning emphasis in a more physiologic direction.

Information in biochemistry is easier to remember when it is integrated with information from other basic science disciplines. This approach can be seen in the clinical vignette case studies at the end of the text, which contain questions about other basic science disciplines in addition to biochemistry. Such integrative thinking will be needed in the clinic, where patients present with symptoms that cross the boundaries of traditional disciplines. Integration across disciplines is further enhanced throughout each chapter by the Integration Boxes.

This book is written as concisely, clearly, and completely as possible. I hope that it brings you the same helpful assistance that I try to bring to my students here at the Texas Tech School of Medicine.

John W. Pelley, PhD

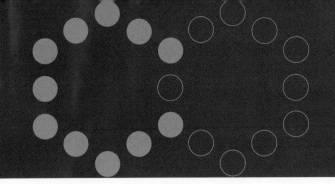

Editorial Review Board

Chief Series Advisor
J. Hurley Myers, PhD
Professor Emeritus of Physiology and Medicine
Southern Illinois University School of Medicine;
President and CEO
DxR Development Group, Inc.
Carbondale, Illinois

Anatomy and Embryology

Thomas R. Gest, PhD
University of Michigan Medical School
Division of Anatomical Sciences
Office of Medical Education
Ann Arbor, Michigan

Biochemistry

John W. Baynes, MS, PhD
Graduate Science Research Center
University of South Carolina
Columbia, South Carolina

Marek Dominiczak, MD, PhD, FRCPath, FRCP(Glas)
Clinical Biochemistry Service
NHS Greater Glasgow and Clyde
Gartnavel General Hospital
Glasgow, United Kingdom

Clinical Medicine

Ted O'Connell, MD
Clinical Instructor
David Geffen School of Medicine
UCLA;
Program Director
Woodland Hills Family Medicine Residency Program
Woodland Hills, California

Genetics

Neil E. Lamb, PhD
Director of Educational Outreach
Hudson Alpha Institute for Biotechnology
Huntsville, Alabama;
Adjunct Professor
Department of Human Genetics
Emory University
Atlanta, Georgia

Histology

Leslie P. Gartner, PhD
Professor of Anatomy
Department of Biomedical Sciences
Baltimore College of Dental Surgery
Dental School
University of Maryland at Baltimore
Baltimore, Maryland

James L. Hiatt, PhD
Professor Emeritus
Department of Biomedical Sciences
Baltimore College of Dental Surgery
Dental School
University of Maryland at Baltimore
Baltimore, Maryland

Immunology

Darren G. Woodside, PhD
Principal Scientist
Drug Discovery
Encysive Pharmaceuticals Inc.
Houston, Texas

Microbiology

Richard C. Hunt, MA, PhD
Professor of Pathology, Microbiology, and Immunology
Director of the Biomedical Sciences Graduate Program
Department of Pathology and Microbiology
University of South Carolina School of Medicine
Columbia, South Carolina

Neuroscience

Cristian Stefan, MD
Associate Professor
Department of Cell Biology
University of Massachusetts Medical School
Worcester, Massachusetts

Pathology

Peter G. Anderson, DVM, PhD
Professor and Director of Pathology Undergraduate
Education, Department of Pathology
University of Alabama at Birmingham
Birmingham, Alabama

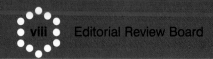
Pharmacology

Michael M. White, PhD
Professor Department of Pharmacology and Physiology
Drexel University College of Medicine
Philadelphia, Pennsylvania

Physiology

Joel Michael, PhD
Department of Molecular Biophysics and Physiology
Rush Medical College
Chicago, Illinois

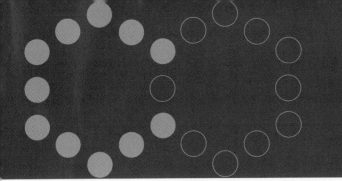

Acknowledgments

My wife, MJ, has always seen more in me than I have. Her love, encouragement, and patience were essential to the organization and composition of this book. It is also important to acknowledge the many intelligent students whom I have taught at Texas Tech. They probably do not realize how much their questions have taught me. Alex Stibbe deserves a substantial acknowledgment for her skill in bringing such a diverse group of authors together and creating the early integration between us that was so essential to the first edition of an innovative series such as this. Kate Dimock has been a tremendous help in continuing this integrative authorship, making the refinements that have led to a significant upgrade for this second edition. And, finally, a note of appreciation to Andy Hall, for his continuing support and perfect balance of professionalism and a great sense of humor.

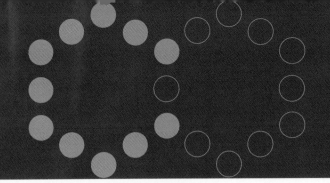

Contents

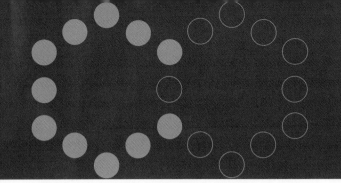

Series Preface

How to Use This Book

The idea for Elsevier's Integrated Series came about at a seminar on the USMLE Step 1 Exam at an American Medical Student Association (AMSA) meeting. We noticed that the discussion between faculty and students focused on how the exams were becoming increasingly integrated—with case scenarios and questions often combining two or three science disciplines. The students were clearly concerned about how they could best integrate their basic science knowledge.

One faculty member gave some interesting advice: "read through your textbook in, say, biochemistry, and every time you come across a section that mentions a concept or piece of information relating to another basic science—for example, immunology—highlight that section in the book. Then go to your immunology textbook and look up this information, and make sure you have a good understanding of it. When you have, go back to your biochemistry textbook and carry on reading."

This was a great suggestion—if only students had the time, and all of the books necessary at hand, to do it! At Elsevier we thought long and hard about a way of simplifying this process, and eventually the idea for Elsevier's Integrated Series was born.

The series centers on the concept of the integration box. These boxes occur throughout the text whenever a link to another basic science is relevant. They're easy to spot in the text—with their color-coded headings and logos. Each box contains a title for the integration topic and then a brief summary of the topic. The information is complete in itself—you probably won't have to go to any other sources—and you have the basic knowledge to use as a foundation if you want to expand your knowledge of the topic.

You can use this book in two ways. First, as a review book ...

When you are using the book for review, the integration boxes will jog your memory on topics you have already covered. You'll be able to reassure yourself that you can identify the link, and you can quickly compare your knowledge of the topic with the summary in the box. The integration boxes might highlight gaps in your knowledge, and then you can use them to determine what topics you need to cover in more detail.

Second, the book can be used as a short text to have at hand while you are taking your course ...

You may come across an integration box that deals with a topic you haven't covered yet, and this will ensure that you're one step ahead in identifying the links to other subjects (especially useful if you're working on a PBL exercise). On a simpler level, the links in the boxes to other sciences and to clinical medicine will help you see clearly the relevance of the basic science topic you are studying. You may already be confident in the subject matter of many of the integration boxes, so they will serve as helpful reminders.

At the back of the book we have included case study questions relating to each chapter so that you can test yourself as you work your way through the book.

Online Version

An online version of the book is available on our Student Consult site. Use of this site is free to anyone who has bought the printed book. Please see the inside front cover for full details on Student Consult and how to access the electronic version of this book.

In addition to containing USMLE test questions, fully searchable text, and an image bank, the Student Consult site offers additional integration links, both to the other books in Elsevier's Integrated Series and to other key Elsevier textbooks.

Books in Elsevier's Integrated Series

The nine books in the series cover all of the basic sciences. The more books you buy in the series, the more links that are made accessible across the series, both in print and online.

 Anatomy and Embryology

 Histology

 Neuroscience

 Biochemistry

 Physiology

 Pathology

 Immunology and Microbiology

 Pharmacology

 Genetics

Acid-Base Concepts 1

●●● WATER AND ELECTROLYTES

An understanding of the properties of water underlies an understanding of the properties of all biologic molecules. Water molecules have the ability to form hydrogen bonds with each other (intramolecular) and also with molecules that they solubilize (intermolecular). If water could not form extensive intramolecular hydrogen bonds, it would be a gas like other small molecules (e.g., CO_2, CH_4, NH_3, O_2, and N_2).

Hydrogen bonds are weak (and therefore reversible) chemical bonds that are formed between molecules that can either donate or accept a partially charged hydrogen atom (Fig. 1-1). Since water can serve both functions, its intramolecular bonds create tetrahedral structures that dynamically break and re-form. The hydrogen bonding forces that hold water molecules together also indirectly determine the shape of the biomolecules that they surround. Hydrogen bonds can also pull electrolytes apart to create charged ions and then can associate with those ions to neutralize their charges.

Hydrophobic and Hydrophilic Molecules

Hydrophilic molecules derive their solubility by forming hydrogen bonds with water. Molecules that can form many hydrogen bonds with water have higher solubility. Solubility decreases as size increases owing to the disruption of water structure. Therefore, large molecules such as proteins, polysaccharides, and nucleic acids are able to maintain their solubility by forming a very large number of hydrogen bonds with water.

Hydrophobic molecules have low solubility in water because they form few or no hydrogen bonds with water. This causes them to aggregate to minimize the disruption of water structure, as illustrated by the coalescence of oil droplets floating on a water surface. The process of forcing hydrophobic molecules together by water plays a major role in determining the three-dimensional structure of macromolecules and biologic membranes.

Electrolytes

Electrolytes dissociate into cations (positive charge) and anions (negative charge) when added to water; this permits water to conduct an electric current. Strong electrolytes such as HCl and NaCl dissociate completely in water. Weak electrolytes do not dissociate completely. Instead they establish an equilibrium between an undissociated form (the conjugate acid or protonated form, HA) and a dissociated form (conjugate base, A^-).

$$HA \leftrightarrow H^+ + A^-$$

Weak electrolytes are generally organic acids; phosphoric acid and carbonic acids are also in this category.

$$H_2CO_3 \rightleftharpoons H^+ + HCO_3^- \rightleftharpoons H^+ + CO_3^{--}$$
$$H_3PO_4 \rightleftharpoons H^+ + H_2PO_4^-$$
$$\rightleftharpoons H^+ + HPO_4^{--} \rightleftharpoons H^+ + PO_4^{---}$$

The hydrogen ion (proton) concentration in a solution of a weak acid is dependent on the equilibrium constant (K_{eq}) for the dissociation reaction:

$$HA \rightleftharpoons H^+ + A^-$$
$$K_{eq} = \frac{[H^+][A^-]}{[HA]}$$

The K_{eq} is unique for each conjugate pair (Table 1-1). Conjugate pairs make good buffers (i.e., solutes that act to resist change in pH), since they always try to reestablish equilibrium when adding either acid or base. Increasing acidity (adding protons) "pushes" the equilibrium toward the undissociated form (HA) to reduce the proton concentration. Similarly, decreasing acidity (adding base, or OH^-) "pulls" the equilibrium away from the HA form to restore the proton concentration.

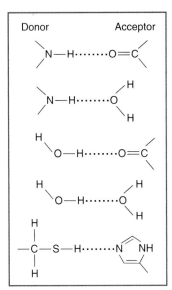

Figure 1-1. Hydrogen bonding between common donors and acceptors.

Water itself is also a weak electrolyte and is in a dissociation equilibrium, with one proton and one hydroxyl ion produced for each water molecule that dissociates (see Table 1-1).

PHARMACOLOGY

Aspirin Absorption

Aspirin must be in the uncharged protonated form on the left in order to diffuse through the cell membrane of the stomach mucosal lining. The stomach pH of around 2 is well below the carboxylic acid group pK of about 4, shifting the equilibrium to the necessary protonated form. The stomach mucosal intracellular pH around 6.8 to 7.1 is above the aspirin pK, shifting the equilibrium to the ionized form on the right, which then prevents the aspirin from crossing back into the stomach. The absorbed aspirin then crosses into the bloodstream, where it reaches its target.

TABLE 1-1. Conjugate Pairs and Their Equilibrium Constants

CONJUGATE PAIR	K_{eq}
$H_2O \rightleftharpoons H^+ + OH^-$	1.0×10^{-14}
$H_2PO_4^- \rightleftharpoons HPO_4^{--} + H^+$	2.0×10^{-7}
Acetic acid $\rightleftharpoons$ Acetate $+ H^+$	1.74×10^{-5}
Lactic acid $\rightleftharpoons$ Lactate $+ H^+$	1.38×10^{-4}

KEY POINTS ABOUT WATER AND ELECTROLYTES

■ Intermolecular hydrogen bonds confer a "structure" to water that is disrupted when it dissolves other molecules.

■ Hydrophilic molecules form many hydrogen bonds with water; hydrophobic molecules form few to no hydrogen bonds with water.

■ Weak electrolytes are generally weak acids that form a dissociation equilibrium.

●●● ACIDS AND BASES

Acidic solutions have more protons than are produced by the ionization of water. Likewise, alkaline (basic) solutions have fewer protons (and more hydroxide ions) than are produced by ionization of water. The ionization of water allows it to participate in the equilibria of weak acids. For example, when the strong electrolyte sodium acetate (reaction 1) is added to water, it dissociates completely. The acetate anion that is produced enters into equilibrium with the protons produced by water, thus reducing the proton concentration below that of pure water and producing a slightly alkaline solution (reactions 2 and 3).

1. $\underset{\text{Na acetate}}{CH_3COONa} \rightarrow CH_3COO^- + \underset{\text{Acetate ion}}{Na^+}$

2. $H_2O \rightleftharpoons H^+ + OH^-$

3. $H^+ + CH_3COO^- \rightleftharpoons \underset{\text{Acetic acid}}{CH_3COOH}$

● The functional group giving up (releasing) a free proton is "acting as" an acid.

● The functional group accepting (binding) a free proton is "acting as" a base.

● Thus acids are proton donors and bases are proton acceptors. In the above example, acetate is considered the conjugate base of acetic acid.

pH—An Expression of Acidity

pH is a convenient way to express proton concentration (i.e., representation as a positive whole number rather than a negative exponent of 10). pH is defined as the negative logarithm of the proton concentration.

$$pH = -\log[H^+]$$

This relationship produces pH units that are exponents of 10 and are, therefore, not directly but logarithmically related to acidity. This produces a reciprocal relationship between pH and acidity so that an increase in pH is equivalent to a decrease in acidity (Fig. 1-2).

The pK value for a reaction is the negative logarithm of the equilibrium constant. The pK of an electrolyte is always a constant, whereas pH can change with physiologic conditions.

The equilibrium constant for dissociation of a weak acid is often termed the Ka, and similarly the pK for an acid is defined as the pKa.

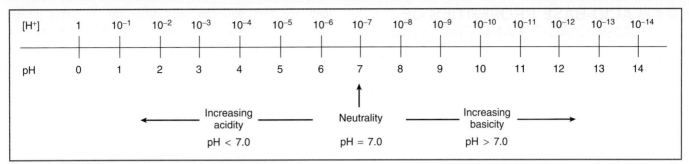

Figure 1-2. Relationship of pH to proton concentration.

- An acidic functional group is defined as having a pKa value less than 7.
- A basic functional group is defined as having a pKa value greater than 7.

Henderson-Hasselbalch Equation

When physiologic solutes, such as blood gases or metabolites, cause the pH of a solution to change, the new equilibrium changes the ratio of all conjugate acids (HA) to conjugate bases (A⁻). The quantitative relationship between the pH and the ratio of conjugate acid to conjugate base is described by the Henderson-Hasselbalch equation:

$$pH = \frac{pKa + \log(\text{conjugate base})}{(\text{conjugate acid})}$$

or

$$pH = \frac{pKa + \log(A^-)}{(HA)}$$

- Note: For pH problems, always set up the Henderson-Hasselbalch equation first, then fill in the known values and solve for the unknown value.
- Note: Remember that $\log(A^-)/(HA) = \log A^- - \log HA$.

Buffers and Titration Curves

Buffers are conjugate pairs that resist changes in pH. The effect of buffering on the change in pH is best illustrated by a titration curve (Fig. 1-3). The titration curve is a plot of the change in pH when a strong base, such as sodium hydroxide (NaOH), is added. pH is usually plotted from low to high pH values, and an inflection point is apparent in the region of effective buffering (resistance to pH change). The midpoint of the inflection in the curve (arrow in Fig. 1-3) is the point at which the pH equals the pKa. This part of the curve reveals the smallest change in pH for a given amount of base added. The best buffering range is at the pK ± 1 pH unit.

Carbonic Acid Conjugate Pair—A Special Case

Carbonic acid (H_2CO_3) is a major acid-base buffer in blood. It establishes an equilibrium with both a volatile gas, CO_2, and its conjugate base, bicarbonate ion (HCO_3^-).

$$H_2O + CO_2 \rightleftharpoons H_2CO_3 \rightleftharpoons H^+ + HCO_3^-$$

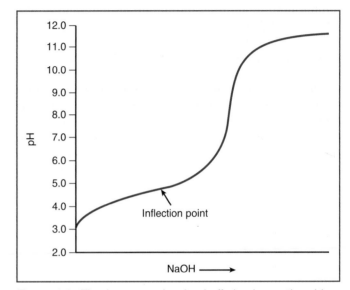

Figure 1-3. Titration curve showing buffering by acetic acid.

Because it is never present in significant amounts, carbonic acid is not included in the Henderson-Hasselbalch equation. It either rapidly breaks down to bicarbonate or is immediately converted to CO_2 by the enzyme carbonic anhydrase.

$$pH = pKa + \log$$

The overall equilibrium between bicarbonate and CO_2 is influenced by the rate of production of CO_2 in the tissues and its rate of elimination in the lungs. Thus the lungs play a major role in regulation of blood pH. Inability to eliminate CO_2 because of lung disease may lead to the acidification of blood, which is called respiratory acidosis.

KEY POINTS ABOUT ACIDS AND BASES

- Dissociation of a weak acid into a conjugate pair (acid plus anion) is at the midpoint when the pH equals the pK and provides maximum buffering.

- The Henderson-Hasselbalch equation relates the conjugate base-to-acid ratio to the pH.

- Titration curves have an inflection point for every ionizable functional group.

- The carbonic acid conjugate pair is in equilibrium with a volatile gas, CO_2.

●●● ACID-BASE PROPERTIES OF AMINO ACIDS AND PROTEINS

Proteins acquire their charge properties from the side chains of the amino acids that comprise them. Several of these side chains can ionize and act as weak acids. Depending on the pK of the functional group in the side chain, this ionization can produce a positive or a negative charge.

Ionized Forms of Amino Acids

Whether or not a given functional group is dissociated or protonated is determined by the pH of the solution. The Henderson-Hasselbalch equation describes the amount of ionization (ratio of dissociated to protonated) for each individual functional group, since each has its own pKa value and ionizes independently of the others.

The titration curve for alanine (Fig. 1-4) gives an illustration of the independent dissociation of both of its functional groups: the α-amino group and the α-carboxyl group. The titration curve from left to right illustrates the changing ionization state of alanine as depicted from left to right in Figure 1-5. As protons are removed from the molecule,

they are first removed only from the carboxyl group, since it has the lowest pK (pKa = 2.3). When the pH rises to the pK of the amino group (pK = 9.9), it then loses its protons. Each pKa represents the midpoints of the two equilibria, illustrating that amino acids (and proteins) have buffering power.

At pH 7.0, the ionizable amino acid side chains in proteins have characteristic charges:

- Positively charged: lysine, arginine.
- Negatively charged: aspartate, glutamate.
- Histidine becomes positively charged if pH drops below 6.0.
- Cysteine becomes negatively charged if pH rises above 8.0.

PHYSIOLOGY

Metabolic Acidosis

When acid accumulates in the blood (acidemia) and lowers the pH of blood (acidosis), it depletes serum bicarbonate by shifting the equilibrium toward carbonic acid. Carbonic anhydrase quickly converts the carbonic acid to CO_2 plus water, and the CO_2 is then exhaled by the lungs. If the acidosis is due to a metabolite (metabolic acidosis [e.g., ketoacidosis, lactic acidosis, or methylmalonic acidemia]), then the anion gap [$Na^+ - (Cl^- + HCO_3^-)$] is increased (normal anion gap, 10 to 16 mmol/L).

Note: Always check for bicarbonate depletion to diagnose metabolic acidosis.

Isoelectric pH

The net charge on an amino acid or a protein is equal to the sum of all charges on each amino acid side chain. The pH value that produces a net zero (neutral) charge on the molecule is the isoelectric pH, or pI.

- For pH > pI, the net charge on the amino acid (or protein) is negative.
- For pH < pI, the net charge on the amino acid (or protein) is positive.

Proteins do not migrate in an electrical field when the pH of the buffer is equal to their isoelectric point, since they have no net charge to attract them to either the cathode or the anode.

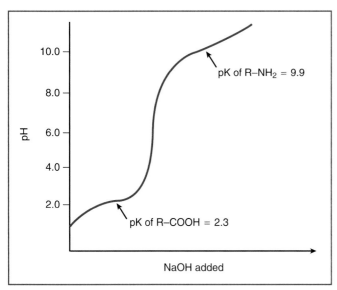

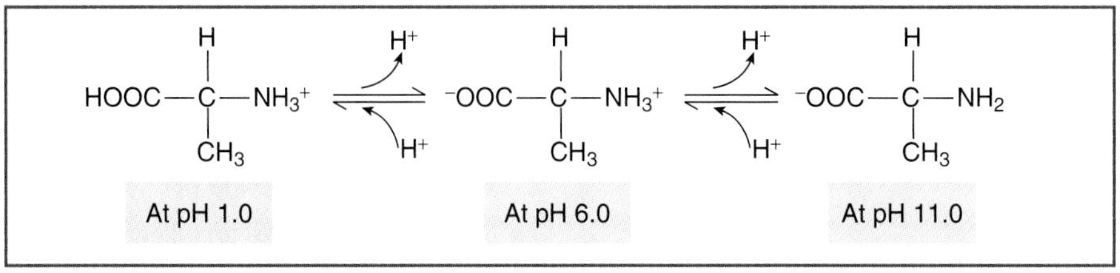

Figure 1-4. Titration curve for alanine.

Figure 1-5. Ionization states of alanine.

PHYSIOLOGY

Metabolic Alkalosis

When protons are lost from the blood, the carbonic acid equilibrium with CO_2 is shifted toward carbonic acid, which is then converted to bicarbonate and restores the lost protons. This results in the accumulation of bicarbonate in the blood. Metabolic alkalosis is less common than metabolic acidosis and is precipitated by persistent vomiting, diuretics, large intake of alkaline substances, Cushing syndrome, and primary aldosteronism.

Note: Always check for bicarbonate accumulation to diagnose metabolic alkalosis.

KEY POINTS ABOUT ACID-BASE PROPERTIES OF AMINO ACIDS AND PROTEINS

- The side chains of the amino acids asp, glu, lys, arg, cys, and his act as weak acids at physiologic pH and confer charge properties to proteins that contain them.
- The isoelectric point for either an amino acid or a protein is that pH where the net sum of all charges is zero.

Self-assessment questions can be accessed at www. StudentConsult.com.

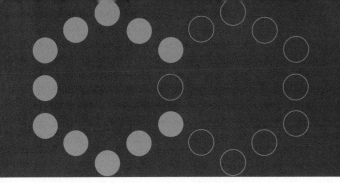

Structure and Properties of Biologic Molecules 2

●●● AMINO ACIDS

An amino acid contains four functional groups organized around the α-carbon: the α-amino group, the α-carboxyl group, a unique side chain (hydrogen in glycine), and hydrogen. The asymmetry of the α-carbon gives rise to two optically active (chiral) isomers termed L- and D-amino acids (Fig. 2-1). The L-form is unique to proteins, while the D-form appears in bacterial cell walls and some antibiotics.

The genetic code in DNA specifies 20 amino acids for the construction of polypeptides. The most useful method for grouping or classifying amino acids is by their hydrophobicity and charge properties in order to understand their location in proteins and their influence on protein structure.

Hydrophobic and Hydrophilic Amino Acids

Hydrophobic amino acids have nonpolar side chains and are usually found at the interior of a protein or where the surface interfaces with lipids (Table 2-1).

- Alanine and glycine have the smallest side chains. Glycine lacks a side chain, which makes it compatible with

hydrophobic environments. Alanine is prominent in the transport of nitrogen from muscle to liver during fasting (alanine cycle).

- Valine, leucine, and isoleucine are referred to as "branched-chain amino acids." Their metabolism is altered in maple syrup urine disease.
- Proline has a cyclized side chain joined back to its α-amino group to form an "imino" acid. It functions as a helix breaker in the secondary structure of proteins (see later discussion). It is also hydroxylated to hydroxyproline after incorporation into collagen (requires ascorbic acid).
- Phenylalanine, tyrosine, and tryptophan are aromatic amino acids. Phenylalanine is increased in the serum and tissues of patients with phenylalanine hydroxylase deficiency (phenylketonuria; PKU), characterized by an inability to synthesize tyrosine from phenylalanine. Tyrosine is a precursor to dopamine and the catecholamines and, in proteins, can be phosphorylated by the action of tyrosine kinases. Tryptophan serves as a precursor for serotonin and melatonin and can be converted to niacin. The aromatic amino acids are the primary sites of chymotrypsin cleavage in proteins.
- Methionine is a sulfur-containing amino acid. It is always the first amino acid incorporated into polypeptides, but it may be removed afterward. S-adenosyl methionine serves as a single carbon donor. Methionine is the site of cyanogen bromide cleavage in proteins.

Hydrophilic amino acids have side chains that form hydrogen bonds and are found where the surface interfaces with the water (Table 2-2).

- Serine and threonine are the hydroxyl-containing amino acids. Both can be phosphorylated by the action of various kinases. Serine serves as a single carbon donor to tetrahydrofolate (THF) to produce N^5,N^{10}-methylene THF and glycine.
- Cysteine, like its hydrophobic counterpart methionine, is a sulfur-containing amino acid. Its thiol group can undergo enzyme-catalyzed oxidation, but it is also sensitive to oxidation by air, forming cystine. Cysteine is a component of glutathione, a recyclable antioxidant in cells. It can form covalent disulfide crosslinks (Fig. 2-2) that stabilize the structure of proteins, especially secreted proteins.

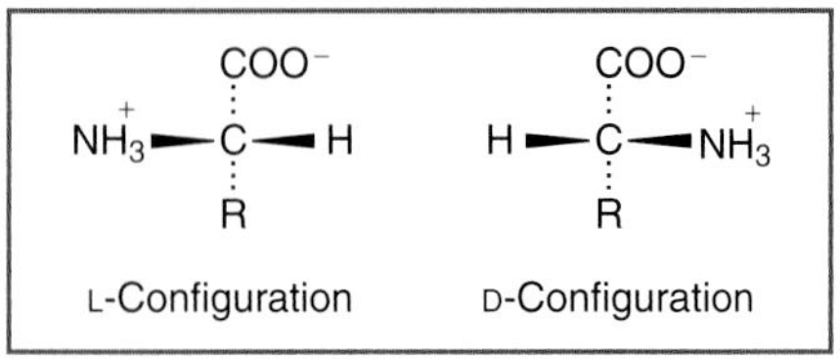

$$\begin{array}{cc}
\text{COO}^- & \text{COO}^- \\
\text{NH}_3^+ \blacksquare \overset{\vdots}{\text{C}} \blacksquare \text{H} & \text{H} \blacksquare \overset{\vdots}{\text{C}} \blacksquare \text{NH}_3^+ \\
\text{R} & \text{R} \\
\text{L-Configuration} & \text{D-Configuration}
\end{array}$$

Figure 2-1. General structure of amino acids.

- Aspartate, asparagine, glutamate, and glutamine are the acidic amino acids and their amides. Both aspartate and glutamate carry a negative charge at a pH of 7; aspartate is interconverted with oxaloacetate by aspartate aminotransferase (AST), and glutamate is interconverted with α-ketoglutarate by alanine aminotransferase (ALT). Asparagine and glutamine are polar, neutral amino acids. Glutamine is formed by glutamine synthetase action in the brain and liver to detoxify ammonia, and it also serves as a donor of amide nitrogen in the biosynthesis of purines and pyrimidines.

- Lysine, histidine, and arginine are the basic amino acids, and they carry a positive charge at a pH of 7. Lysine and arginine are the site of trypsin cleavage in proteins; both are present at high concentration in histones. Histidine is only weakly basic and is uncharged at a pH of 7. Histidine forms one of the six coordination bonds with Fe^{++} in the heme prosthetic group of hemoglobin and myoglobin. Arginine (pKa ~14) always has a positive charge at neutral pH; it has an important role in the binding of anionic molecules, such as nucleic acids.

TABLE 2-1. Amino Acids with Hydrophobic Side Chains

AMINO ACID	SIDE CHAIN
Glycine (Gly)*	HC—H
Alanine (Ala)	HC—CH₃
Valine (Val)	HC—C(CH₃)₂—H
Leucine (Leu)	HC—CH₂—CH(CH₃)—CH₃
Isoleucine (Ile)	HC—C(CH₃)(H)—CH₂—CH₃
Proline (Pro)	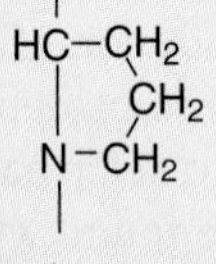 HC—CH₂—CH₂—N—CH₂ (ring)
Phenylalanine (Phe)	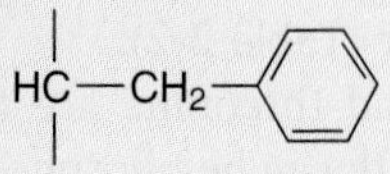 HC—CH₂—C₆H₅
Tyrosine (Tyr)	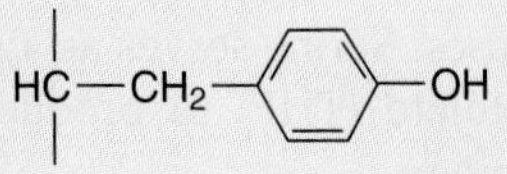 HC—CH₂—C₆H₄—OH
Tryptophan (Trp)	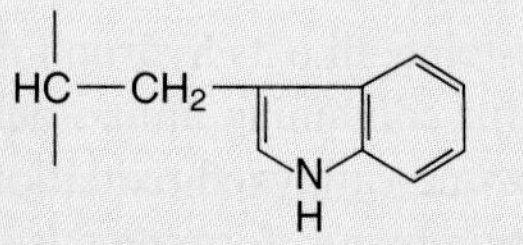 HC—CH₂—(indole)
Methionine (Met)	HC—CH₂—CH₂—S—CH₃

*Hydrophobic compatible.

TABLE 2-2. Amino Acids with Hydrophilic Side Chains

AMINO ACID	SIDE CHAIN
Serine (Ser)	HC—CH₂—OH
Threonine (Thr)	HC—C(CH₃)(H)—OH
Cysteine (Cys)	HC—CH₂—SH
Aspartate (Asp)	HC—CH₂—C(=O)—O
Asparagine (Asn)	HC—CH₂—C(=O)—NH₂
Glutamate (Glu)	HC—CH₂—CH₂—C(=O)—O
Glutamine (Gln)	HC—CH₂—CH₂—C(=O)—NH₂
Lysine (Lys)	HC—CH₂—CH₂—CH₂—CH₂—NH₃⁺
Histidine (His)	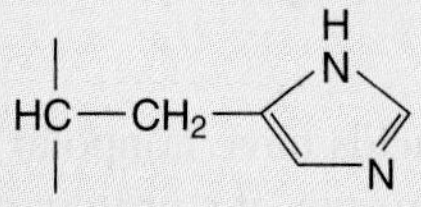 HC—CH₂—(imidazole)
Arginine (Arg)	HC—CH₂—CH₂—CH₂—NH—C(=NH₂⁺)—NH₂

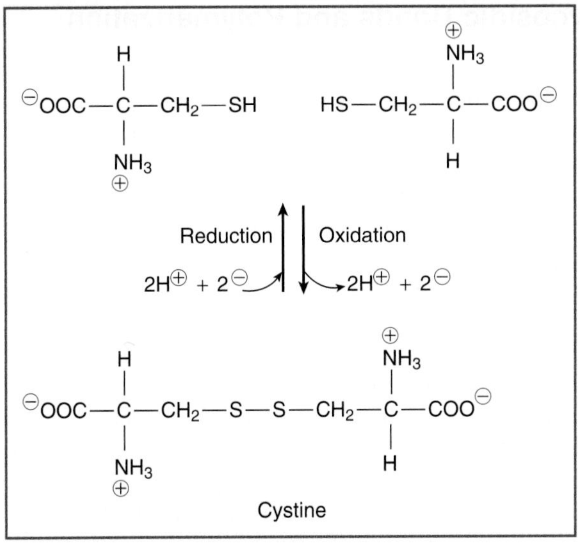

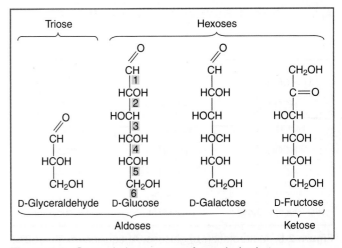

Figure 2-2. Equilibrium between cysteine and cystine. Cystine is only produced from total acid hydrolysis of proteins. Disulfide formation is enzyme-catalyzed in cells.

PHARMACOLOGY

Asparaginase Therapy

Asparagine is required in high amounts by some types of leukemia cells, making systemic administration of asparaginase (hydrolysis to aspartate and ammonia) an effective treatment.

KEY POINTS ABOUT AMINO ACIDS

- The amino acids that comprise polypeptides have a consistent structure and differ only by their side chain; they can be classified by their degree of hydrophobicity and the nature of the side chain functional groups.

- The sequence of amino acid side chains determines the native (tertiary) structure of the proteins that contain them.

- Free amino acids also have biologic functions in intermediary energy metabolism, in the endocrine system, and in neuronal function.

●●● CARBOHYDRATES

Carbohydrates (sugars) can be described as polyhydroxy aldehydes or ketones. The general molecular formula for carbohydrates is $C_x(H_2O)_x$ where $x = 6$ for a hexose. The hydroxyl, aldehyde, and ketone groups are all potential sites for reaction and modification that produce carbohydrate derivatives.

Carbohydrate Nomenclature

Carbohydrate length is denoted according to the number of monomers (Table 2-3). If the carbonyl is an aldehyde, the sugar is an aldose, and if the carbonyl is a ketone, the sugar is a ketose. The number of carbons is denoted by the relevant prefix (e.g., triose [3C], pentose [5C], and hexose [6C]).

Carbohydrate Structure

Carbohydrates can exist in open-chain (linear) or cyclized (ring) forms. The open-chain form (Fig. 2-3), termed the Fischer projection, has the most oxidized O_2 at or near the top. Physicochemical properties of carbohydrates include the following:

- At least one carbon is asymmetric, making the molecule optically active (rotates polarized light).
- The numbering of the carbons begins at the top of the Fischer projection (oxidized end).
- The D- or L- configuration is represented by the position of the hydroxyl group on the carbon farthest from the carbonyl (e.g., if it is on the right, it is a D-sugar).
- An equal mixture of D- and L- forms is called a racemic mixture.
- Sugars that differ at only one carbon atom are called epimers (e.g., glucose and galactose).

TABLE 2-3. Classification of Carbohydrates

CLASS	MONOMER COMPOSITION	EXAMPLES
Monosaccharides (simple sugars)	1	Glucose, fructose, ribose
Monosaccharide derivatives	1	Sugar acids, alcohols, amino sugars
Disaccharides	2	Lactose, sucrose, maltose
Oligosaccharides	2-10	Blood group antigens
Polysaccharides	10+	Starch, glycogen

Figure 2-3. Open-chain structures for carbohydrates.

Note: D- and L- refer to the configuration around the carbon, not the rotation of polarized light; the terms dextrorotatory and levorotatory refer to rotation of light to the right or the left, respectively.

The major features of the cyclic form are:
- Condensation of a hydroxyl with the carbonyl produces a cyclic structure referred to as a hemiacetal or a hemiketal.
- The flat, cyclic form, termed the Haworth projection, has the most oxidized O_2 at or near the right.
- Deoxyribose and fructose may form five- or six-membered furanose rings (Figs. 2-4, A and 2-4, B).
- Glucose (Figs. 2-4, C and 2-4, D) exists primarily as a six-membered pyranose ring.
- Cyclization creates a new asymmetric center at the carbonyl (anomeric) carbon.
- The cyclic form of glucose is in equilibrium with the open-chain form (mutarotation; Fig. 2-5) in a 40,000:1 ratio; this equilibrium creates a racemic mixture of α-anomers (α-hydroxyl pointing down) and β-anomers (α-hydroxyl pointing up). Anomers differ only in the configuration at the first anomeric carbon (see Figs. 2-4, C and 2-4, D).

Glycosidic Bonds and Polymerization

Glycosides are formed when the hydroxyl group on the anomeric carbon of a sugar and the hydroxyl group of another molecule condense to form an acetal or ketal linkage (Fig. 2-6), known as a glycosidic bond. Glycosides formed from glucose are glucosides; likewise, those from fructose are fructosides. If the second molecule forming the acetal is a sugar, then the glycoside is a disaccharide (Table 2-4).

Polymerization of glucose occurs by successive formation of glycosidic bonds between the anomeric carbon of the monomer and a hydroxyl group of the growing polysaccharide. Like polymerized amino acids and nucleic acids, the linkages in polysaccharides are read from left to right including specification of the anomeric form (e.g., α-1,4 linkages denoting the α-anomer pointing down from carbon 1 of the monomer condensed with carbon 4 of the second sugar).

Note: Glycosidic bonds stabilize the cyclic form, since they prevent formation of the linear structure and mutarotation.

Reducing sugars are oxidized by Fehling solution to produce color reaction. This includes those sugars whose rings can open to expose the reactive carbonyl groups.
- Reducing sugars include all monosaccharides and oligosaccharides: glucose, galactose, fructose, maltose, and lactose.
- Nonreducing sugars are sucrose and trehalose (ring structures cannot open) and polysaccharides. Large polysaccharides, such as amylose, glycogen, and starch, have one reducing end for each polymer chain—while they have one true reducing sugar group, they are generally considered nonreducing polysaccharides.

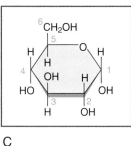
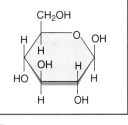

A   B

C   D

Figure 2-4. Cyclic structures for common carbohydrates. **A,** Deoxyribose. **B,** Fructose. **C,** α-D-Glucose. **D,** β-D-Glucose.

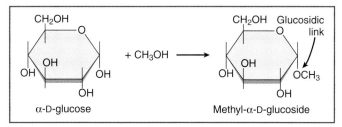

Figure 2-6. Formation of an acetal.

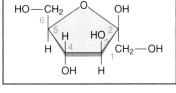

Figure 2-5. Mutarotation of glucose. At equilibrium, β = 62%; α = 38%.

TABLE 2-4. Various Glycosides Formed by Condensation Between a Sugar and Hydroxyl Group of Another Sugar		
SUGAR	**ALCOHOL**	**GLYCOSIDE**
Glucose	Any	Glucoside
Fructose	Any	Fructoside
Glucose	Sugar	Disaccharide
Glucose	Disaccharide	Trisaccharide
Glucose	Methyl alcohol	Methyl α-D-glucoside

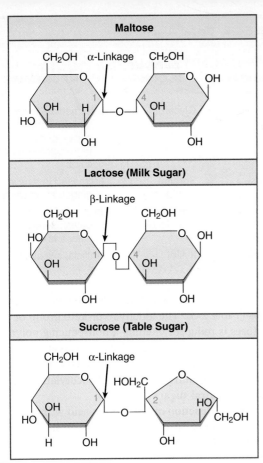

Figure 2-7. Nutritionally important disaccharides.

Disaccharides and Polysaccharides

Glucose forms glycosidic bonds with itself, fructose, and galactose to produce three nutritionally important disaccharides (Fig. 2-7):

Sucrose: glucose + fructose; table sugar

Lactose: glucose + galactose; milk sugar

Maltose: glucose + glucose; product of starch digestion

There are three nutritionally important polysaccharides, all of which are composed entirely of glucose:

- Starch (two major components):
  - Amylose (α-1,4 linkages) has only a linear structure.
  - Amylopectin (α-1,4 linkages + α-1,6 linkages) has a branched structure; a branch point occurs every 25 to 30 glucose residues (Fig. 2-8).
- Glycogen has a structure like amylopectin except that it is more highly branched (every 8 to 12 residues of glucose).
- Cellulose (β-1,4 linkages) has an unbranched structure.
  - Structural polysaccharide of plant cells.
  - Important source of fiber in the diet; not hydrolyzed by digestive enzymes; no caloric value.
  - Hyaluronic acid, heparin, and pectin are called hetero-polysaccharides, since they are formed from several different sugars, including sugar acids and amino sugars.

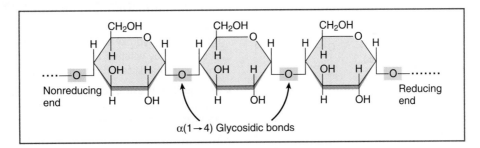

Figure 2-8. Polysaccharide structure. **A,** Linear amylose structure. **B,** Branched amylopectin structure (glycosidic bond with carbon 6).

PATHOLOGY

Protein Glycosylation

Sugars with aldehyde groups are also reactive with primary amino groups on proteins. The glycosylation reaction is nonreversible, forming advanced glycosylation end products, and if it occurs in excess, as in uncontrolled diabetes, it leads to microvascular disease. The extent of hyperglycemia in diabetics is also measured by determination of hemoglobin A_{1C}, which is formed from irreversible glycosylation of the terminal amino groups.

Carbohydrate Derivatives

Because of the abundance of hydroxyl groups, sugar molecules can form several types of carbohydrate derivatives.

- *Sugar acids*: Oxidation of glucose at carbon 1 produces "onic" acids, such as gluconic acid, and oxidation at carbon 6 produces "uronic" acids, such as glucuronic acid (Fig. 2-9). Uronic acids contribute a negative charge to polysaccharide chains, which promotes binding of cations. Glucuronic acid is conjugated with bilirubin in the liver. Ascorbic acid, or vitamin C, is a product of glucuronic acid metabolism, except in primates and guinea pigs.
- *Deoxy sugars*: Reduction of ribose at carbon 2 produces 2-deoxyribose.

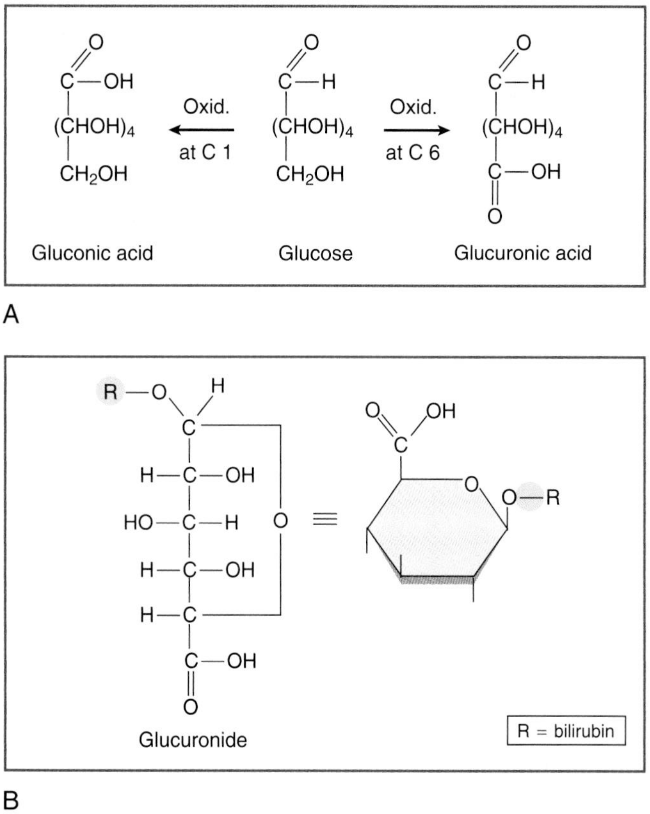

TABLE 2-5. Sugar Alcohols

SUGAR	DERIVED ALCOHOL	IMPORTANCE
Glyceraldehyde	Glycerol	Intermediate in fat metabolism; component of triglycerides and other lipids
Glucose	Sorbitol (glucitol)	Increased in lens in diabetes; cataracts
Galactose	Galactitol (dulcitol)	Increased in lens in galactosemia; cataracts
Xylulose	Xylitol	Artificial sweetener

- *Sugar alcohols*: Also called polyols, they have no carbonyl groups (Table 2-5). The aldehyde or keto group of aldoses or ketoses is reduced, yielding a nonreducing polyol.
- *Amino sugars*: Replacement of the hydroxyl group on carbon 2 by an amino group produces glucosamine and galactosamine. The amino group is usually acetylated (Fig. 2-10), yielding a neutral sugar.
- *Sugar esters*: Reaction of phosphoric acid with one or more hydroxyl groups produces sugar esters such as glucose 6-phosphate (see Fig. 2-10).

KEY POINTS ABOUT CARBOHYDRATES

- Carbohydrates (sugars) are a diverse group of polyhydroxy aldehydes or polyhydroxy ketones; they are classified by the number of carbons, by whether the carbonyl is an aldehyde or ketone, and by any modifications or attachments.
- An equilibrium exists for monosaccharides between an open-chain and a cyclized structure, with the open-chain structure reactive to Fehling solution (reducing sugar).
- The cyclized structure can react with other alcohol groups to form an acetal that prevents the ring from opening; polymerization occurs when the acetal is formed with another monosaccharide.
- Carbohydrate derivatives perform many functions in addition to intermediary energy metabolism, such as conjugation with lipid-soluble molecules and specialized modification of membrane components.

FATTY ACIDS

Lipid molecules are hydrophobic owing to the low number of functional groups that can hydrogen-bond with water. This hydrophobicity yields a special kind of behavior in an aqueous environment. Some fat-soluble molecules, such as triglycerides, form fat droplets that minimize the surface area interface with water. Others, such as fatty acids that contain various polar functional groups, are able to form an interface with water, producing membranes or micelles.

Figure 2-9. A, Formation of glucuronic acid and gluconic acid by oxidation (*Oxid*) of glucose. **B,** Bilirubin glucuronide.

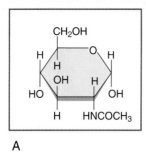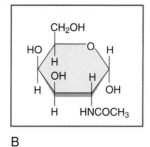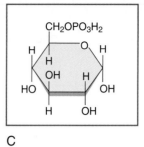

A   B   C

Figure 2-10. Structures of *N*-acetylglucosamine (A), *N*-acetylgalactosamine (B), and glucose 6-phosphate (C).

Fatty Acid Nomenclature

Fatty acids are monocarboxylic acids made up of unbranched aliphatic carbon chains. Most (>95%) have an even number of carbon atoms with a chain length of 16 to 20 carbons. Some odd-numbered carbon atom fatty acids are found in the diet. Fatty acid carbons are either saturated with hydrogens or are unsaturated when they contain one or more carbon-carbon double bonds. They are classified as short chain (2 to 4 carbons), medium chain (6 to 12 carbons), or long chain (14 to 26 carbons).

Fatty acids are named by either a common name or a systematic name (Table 2-6). Saturated fatty acids are named by their length, and unsaturated fatty acids are named by the position of the double bonds. Unsaturated fatty acids have two numbering systems to designate the position of the double bonds:

- Delta numbering system (Fig. 2-11), designated by three numbers: number of carbons, number of double bonds, and position of the double bonds (e.g., linoleic acid has systematic designation of $18:2:\Delta^9,\Delta^{12}$ for 18 carbons, two double bonds, double bond after carbons 9 and 12 from the carboxyl end).
- Omega numbering system (see Fig. 2-11), designated by distance from the most distal (methyl) carbon from the carboxylic acid, which is called the ω carbon (e.g., omega-3 fatty acids have one double bond between the third and fourth carbon from the end of the molecule).

Carbons 2 and 3 are also referred to as the α- and β-carbons; they are located at positions α and β to the carboxyl group.

The configuration around unsaturated bonds is designated as *cis* or *trans* (Fig. 2-12). Naturally occurring fatty acids always contain *cis* double bonds, while partially hydrogenated unsaturated fatty acids contain some of the *trans* form.

TABLE 2-6. Fatty Acid Nomenclature

COMMON NAME	SYSTEMATIC NAME	DOUBLE BONDS (NO.)	CARBON ATOMS (NO.)
Palmitic	Hexadecanoic	0	16
Stearic	Octadecanoic	0	18
Palmitoleic	*Cis*-Δ^9-hexadecanoic	1	16
Oleic	*Cis*-Δ^9-octadecanoic	1	18
Linoleic	All-*cis*-Δ^9,Δ^{12}-octadecadienoic	2	18
Linolenic	All-*cis*-$\Delta^9,\Delta^{12},\Delta^{15}$-octadecatrienoic	3	18
Arachidonic	All-*cis*-$\Delta^5,\Delta^8,\Delta^{11},\Delta^{14}$-eicosatetraenoic	4	20

Carboxyl terminus										ω-Terminus
COOH	CH₂	CH₂	CH₂	CH₂	CH₂	CH₂	CH₂	CH₂	CH₃	
Δ Numbering	1	2	3	4	5	6	7	8	9	10
ω Numbering	10	9	8	7	6	5	4	3	2	1
Letter designation		α	β	γ	δ					

Figure 2-11. Numbering of fatty acid carbons.

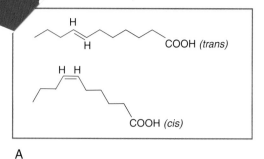

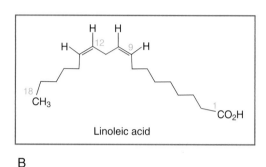

A

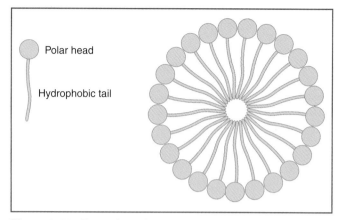

Figure 2-13. Formation of micelle by fatty acids.

triglyceride. When fatty acids are esterified to alcohols of 14 to 18 carbons, they are called waxes. Waxes are found in epidermal secretions, such as the outer ear canal.

B

Figure 2-12. A, *Cis* vs. *trans* configuration of a double bond. **B,** Linoleic acid.

Fatty Acid Properties

Fatty acids form spherical micelles in water due to their amphipathic properties (possession of both a polar end [carboxylate group] and a nonpolar end [hydrocarbon chain]). Fatty acids form the spherical micelles by orienting the hydrocarbon chains together at the center, thus positioning the polar carboxylate groups at the surface to hydrogen-bond with water (Fig. 2-13).

The melting point of fatty acids is determined by chain length and degree of unsaturation (Table 2-7).
- Increasing length increases melting point.
- Increasing unsaturation decreases melting point.
- *Cis*-unsaturation lowers melting point more than *trans*-unsaturation.

Triglycerides

The free carboxylate group on fatty acids can present both detergent and osmotic problems in cells that store fats. Esterification of the free carboxyl groups with glycerol solves this problem. Glycerol can be esterified with one, two, or three fatty acids to form a monoglyceride, diglyceride, or

KEY POINTS ABOUT FATTY ACIDS

- Fatty acids are monocarboxylic acids composed of unbranched hydrocarbon chains of from 3 to 26 carbons; they are classified by the number of carbons and the extent and position of any unsaturated bonds.
- Free fatty acids will form micelles through the association of the hydrocarbon chains toward the center and orientation of the carboxylic acid group toward the surface.
- Free fatty acids can esterify with glycerol to produce a molecule that does not present osmotic problems or unwanted side reactions.

●●● NUCLEIC ACIDS

Nucleic acids are composed of monomeric units called nucleotides that can join together to form polynucleotides. Nucleic acids have several levels of structure. As for proteins, primary structure is represented by the linear sequence of nucleotides, and secondary structure involves the regular extended helical structure stabilized by hydrogen bonds. The tertiary structure (which is described in the chapters on deoxyribonucleic acid [DNA] and ribonucleic acid [RNA] synthesis) involves the three-dimensional bending of the helix as seen in the formation of the compacted transfer RNA (tRNA) structure or in the formation of nucleosomes by DNA.

TABLE 2-7. Effect of Chain Length and Unsaturation Melting Point of Fatty Acids

CHAIN LENGTH	SATURATED	MELTING POINT (°C)	UNSATURATED	MELTING POINT (°C)
C_{16}	Palmitic	63	Palmitoleic (Δ^9)	0.5
C_{18}	Stearic	70	Oleic (Δ^9)	13.0
C_{18}	Linoleic ($\Delta^{9,12}$)	−5.0		
C_{18}	Linolenic ($\Delta^{9,12,15}$)	−10.0		

Nucleotide Structure

The nucleotide structure is organized around ribose or deoxyribose (Fig. 2-14).

- A purine or pyrimidine base is attached to the 1'-carbon.
- One or more phosphate groups are attached to the 5'-carbon.
- The 3'-carbon is reserved for linkage to the phosphate of another nucleotide during polymerization.
- The 2'-carbon determines whether the nucleotide is a deoxyribonucleotide (2'–H in place of OH) or a ribonucleotide (2'–OH).
- DNA and RNA are polymers of deoxyribose and ribose linked by phosphate diester linkages between the 3' and 5' hydroxyl groups of successive pentose units.

Five bases are found in RNA and DNA (Fig. 2-15):

- Uracil is found in RNA, and its methylated form (thymine) is found in DNA.
- Cytosine, adenine, and guanine are found in both DNA and RNA.
- Unusual bases, such as pseudouracil in tRNA and 5-methylcytosine in DNA, are produced by modification *after* transcription (posttranscriptional modifications).
- Pseudouracil contributes to the tertiary structure of tRNA.
- Methylation protects polynucleotides from nuclease digestion.

Nucleosides are nucleotides without the phosphate, and they are named for bases that comprise them (Table 2-8). The deoxynucleosides are shown in Figure 2-16.

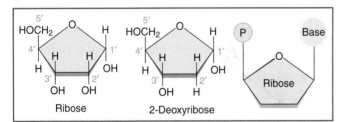

Figure 2-14. Relationship of base and phosphate to ribose in general nucleotide structure.

PHARMACOLOGY

Dideoxy Antiviral Drugs

The 3'-carbon site is blocked in drugs designed to prevent DNA synthesis by reverse transcriptase. Such drugs include azidothymidine (AZT) (now known as zidovudine, depicted below). The sugar phosphate backbone cannot be lengthened after incorporation of AZT into the growing DNA strand. This class of drugs is used as antiretroviral agents in the treatment of diseases such as AIDS.

Primary Structure of DNA and RNA

Both DNA and RNA are polynucleotides that are linked together by phosphodiester bonds between the ribose moiety of the nucleotides. This creates a "ribose-phosphate" backbone and a 5'-end that is phosphorylated; the 3'-end has a free 3'-hydroxyl (Fig. 2-17).

TABLE 2-8. Nucleotide Nomenclature

BASE	NUCLEOSIDE	NUCLEOTIDE
RNA		
Guanine	Guanosine	Guanylate (GMP)
Adenine	Adenosine	Adenylate (AMP)
Uracil	Uridine	Uridylate (UMP)
Cytosine	Cytidine	Cytidylate (CMP)
DNA		
Guanine	Deoxyguanosine	Deoxyguanylate (dGMP)
Adenine	Deoxyadenosine	Deoxyadenylate (dAMP)
Thymine	Thymidine	Thymidylate (dTMP)
Cytosine	Deoxycytidine	Deoxycytidylate (dCMP)

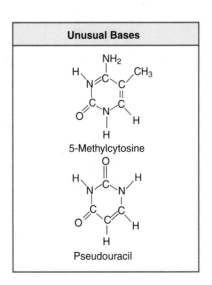

Figure 2-15. Common and unusual bases found in DNA and RNA.

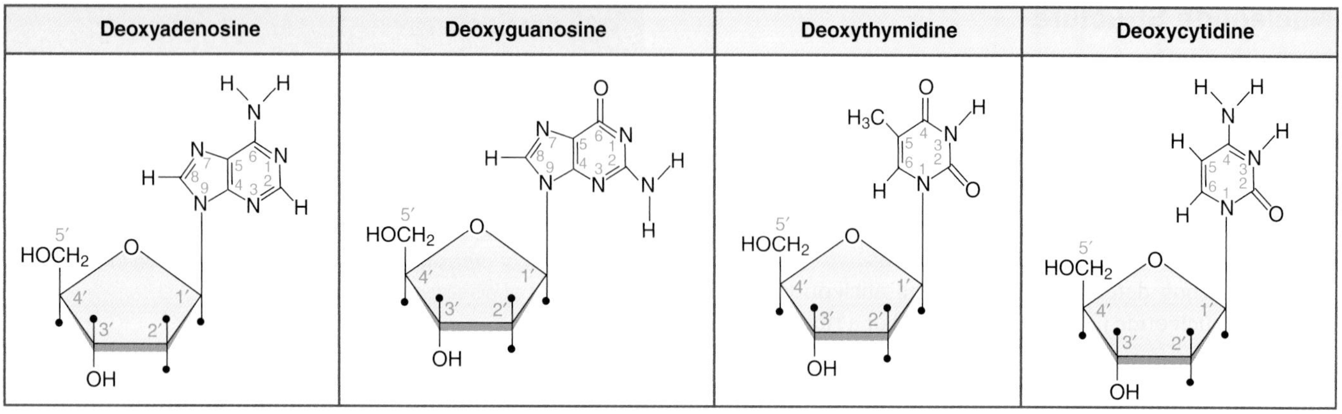

Deoxyadenosine	Deoxyguanosine	Deoxythymidine	Deoxycytidine

Figure 2-16. Deoxynucleoside structures.

- Like the primary structure of a polypeptide, polynucleotides have a sequence of side chains—in this case, the bases.
- Polynucleotide structure is always written left to right in the 5′ to 3′ direction. It is usually depicted as a sequence of bases with or without indicating the phosphates, such as pGpApC or guanyladenylcytosine (GAC).

Secondary Structure of DNA and RNA

The union of two complementary strands of DNA-DNA, RNA-RNA, or DNA-RNA occurs through precise complementary pairing of every purine and pyrimidine base. This generates an extended regular structure with the bases paired toward the center and alternating ribose-phosphate bonds toward the edge.

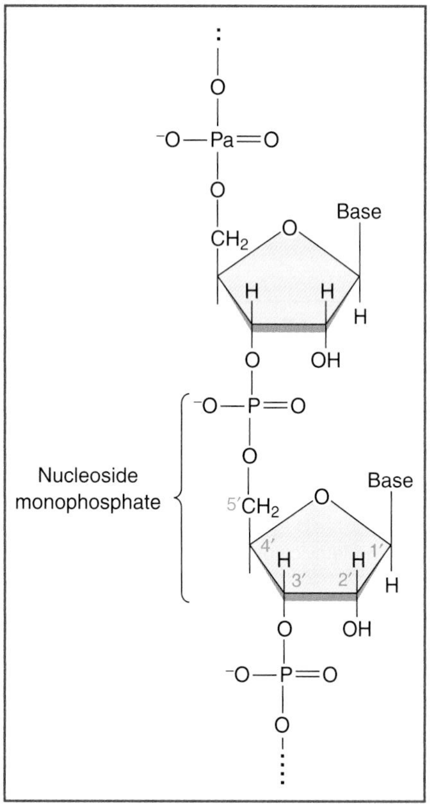

In addition to the hydrogen bonds formed during base-pairing, the DNA helix is stabilized by van der Waals and hydrophobic forces resulting from the stacking of adjacent bases. RNA-RNA helices are less stable, however, since the 2′-hydroxyl of ribose does not pack as well as deoxyribose in the double helical structure.

Pairing is permitted only between adenine/thymine (A-T pairs) and guanine/cytosine (G-C pairs), creating an isomorphic relationship between the strands (i.e., they specify each other's sequence) (Fig. 2-18).

- The DNA strands are oriented in opposite (antiparallel) directions.
- There are three major forms of DNA; all are antiparallel and maintain Watson-Crick base-pairing:
  - B-form DNA is the predominant, natural form; 10 base pairs per right turn and a periodicity of 34 Å per turn.
  - A-form DNA is produced by dehydrating purified DNA; 11 base pairs per right turn and a periodicity of 26 Å.
  - Z-form DNA is favored by long stretches of alternating C and G; 12 base pairs per left turn and a periodicity of 57 Å; also called Z-DNA.

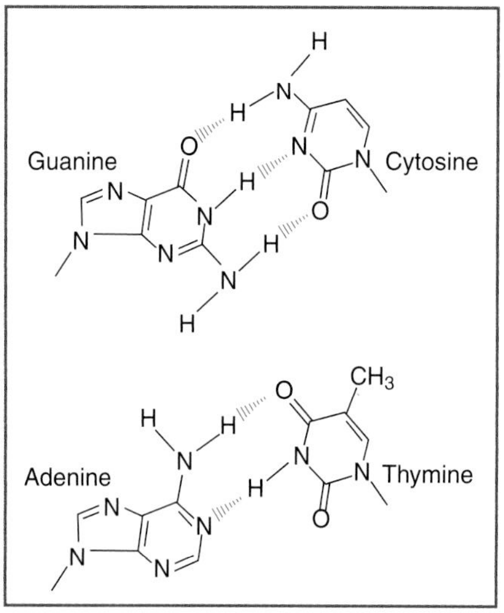

Figure 2-17. Ribose-phosphate backbone with bases attached.

Figure 2-18. Standard Watson-Crick base-pairing.

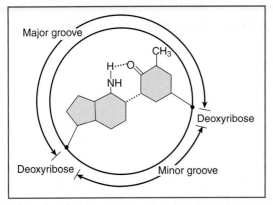

Figure 2-19. Cross-section of DNA double helix illustrating the major and minor grooves. Note the unique shape of the functional groups extending into the major groove.

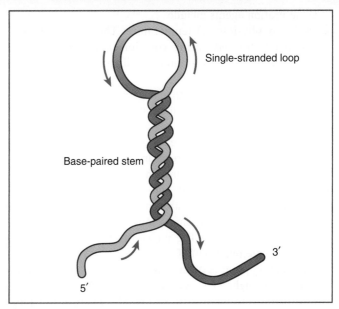

Figure 2-20. Stem-loop structure in RNA. Note antiparallel direction in base-paired stem.

- Since the bases pair at an angle, the two grooves in the helix are unequal in size (Fig. 2-19).
- The wider groove is called the major groove, and the narrower groove is called the minor groove.
- The purine and pyrimidine functional groups extend uniquely into both grooves; this includes the methyl groups on methylated cytosine and on thymine.
- Enzymes and structural proteins can interact with functional groups in both grooves, permitting them to recognize a sequence without unwinding the helix.

RNA structure reflects its role in gene expression. It is always produced in a single-strand form, called the sense strand (the antisense strand in the DNA is also called the template strand). Any single strand of RNA can fold back on itself to form a hairpin (completely paired) or stem-loop (partially paired) structure (Fig. 2-20) if it contains complementary sequences that can base-pair. Note that this maintains the antiparallel nature of base-pairing. Stem loops make up much of the structure of tRNA.

Denaturation of DNA

As for proteins, the structure of DNA can be denatured by physical and chemical agents. When the helix is denatured by raising the temperature, both strands separate, or "melt." This involves disruption both of complementary base-pairing and of the hydrophobic stacking forces. If the temperature is lowered gradually, the complementary strands renature (reanneal) into a double helix. During an initial slow nucleation step, short complementary sequences associate through random diffusion. This is followed by a rapid "zipping" step during which the remainder of the complementary sequences align. If the temperature is decreased too rapidly, the nucleation step is prevented.

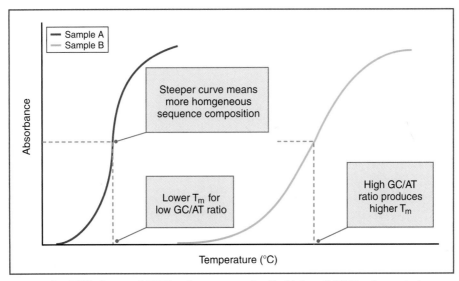

Figure 2-21. Melting curves for DNA. Lower GC/AT ratio compared with higher GC/AT ratio and steeper slope compared with broader slope.

Denaturation agents include:

- High (nonphysiologic) temperature: This disrupts hydrogen bonds formed during complementary base-pairing. It also reduces hydrophobic stabilization due to base-stacking.
- High pH: This creates a strong negative charge on the phosphodiester groups, producing a charge repulsion between strands.

Denaturation of DNA is measured through the property of hyperchromicity (i.e., an increase in absorbance of a DNA solution [at 260 nm] on denaturation). Increasing temperatures cause the helix to unwind and separate into the single-stranded form (greater UV absorption). If the absorbance is plotted against the increasing temperature, a melting curve is produced (Fig. 2-21). The midpoint of the melting curve is called the melting point (T_m):

- The melting point is higher for samples that contain more G-C pairs (higher GC/AT ratio). In the B-form of DNA, G-C pairs have three hydrogen bonds, whereas A-T pairs have only two.
- The melting curve is steeper for homogeneous samples (identical or similar sequences) of DNA molecules.

KEY POINTS ABOUT NUCLEIC ACIDS

- The nucleotides that compose nucleic acids have a consistent structure and differ primarily by the purine or pyrimidine base; they are classified according to the base, the oxidation state of the ribose, and whether they have one or more phosphate groups attached to the ribose.

- Both DNA and RNA have primary, secondary, and tertiary levels of structure that are similar to those of proteins; the sequence of bases provides primary structure, the formation of an extended helical structure provides secondary structure, and stem-loop structures and supercoiling provide tertiary structure.

- The DNA helix does not need to open up for the base sequence to be recognized, since the functional groups on the bases extend into the major and minor grooves in a unique pattern; enzymes and structural proteins can recognize the bases from their functional groups.

- Base-pairing requires that the strands of the helix be oriented in antiparallel fashion.

Self-assessment questions can be accessed at www.StudentConsult.com.

Protein Structure and Function

3

CONTENTS

The polymerization of amino acids produces a linear molecule referred to generically as a polypeptide (Fig. 3-2). More specific nomenclature can indicate the number of amino acids in the polypeptide (e.g., dipeptide [two amino acids] or oligopeptide [relatively few amino acids]). The properties of a polypeptide are determined by the side chains of their amino acids.

PATHOLOGY

Hemoglobin Mutations

Sickle cell hemoglobin (HbS) and hemoglobin C (HbC) both have single amino acid substitutions in residue 6 of the β-globin. Sickle cell globin has a nonpolar substitution (valine) for the normal polar residue (glutamate), whereas hemoglobin C has a polar substitution (lysine) for the polar glutamate. The resulting effect of these changes in primary structure on quaternary structure is the difference between serious sickling attacks with consequent hemolytic anemia (HbS) and a mild chronic hemolytic anemia (HbC) that requires little or no medical attention.

●●● LEVELS OF STRUCTURAL COMPLEXITY

Primary Structure

The primary structure of a protein is simply the linear sequence of amino acids held together by peptide bonds. The higher orders of structure, including any disulfide bonds, are determined in part by the primary structure. Since the primary structure correlates directly with the sequence of triplet bases in the corresponding gene, the genetic code contains a specification for all levels of protein structure.

The linear sequence of amino acids is read from left to right, with the amino terminal on the left. The following tetrapeptide is called alanylaspartylglycylleucine:

$$^{+}H_3N\text{-ala-asp-gly-leu-COO}^{-} \text{ or }$$
$$^{+}H_3N\text{-Ala-Asp-Gly-Leu-COO}^{-}$$

Peptide bonds are amide bonds between the α-carboxyl group of one amino acid and the α-amino group of another (Fig. 3-1). The result is a planar structure that is stabilized by resonance between the α-carboxyl and α-amino groups. The side chains are able to extend out from the peptide chain and interact with each other or with other molecules.

Secondary Structure

Secondary structure is a regular extended structure stabilized by hydrogen bonding between peptide bonds (Fig. 3-3). Although the side chains are not involved in the hydrogen bonding that forms the extended structure, they can determine the type of secondary structure and its stability. The two main types of structure produced by this type of bonding are the α-helix conformation and the β-pleated sheet structure.

α-Helix Conformation

The α-helix is a right-handed helix with the peptide bonds located on the inside and the side chains extending outward. It is stabilized by the regular formation of hydrogen bonds parallel to the axis of the helix; they are formed between the amino and carbonyl groups of every fourth peptide bond. Since proline has no free hydrogen to contribute to helix stability, it is

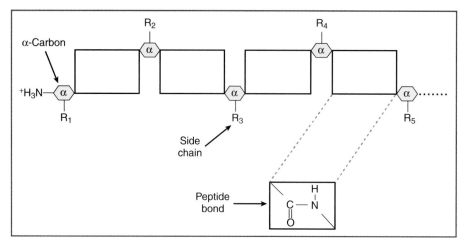

Figure 3-1. The peptide bond linking α-carbons and their side chains together into a polypeptide. The *trans* conformation is favored, producing a rigid structure that restricts freedom of movement except for rotation around bonds that join to the α-carbons.

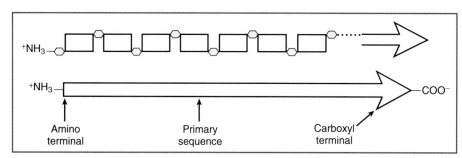

Figure 3-2. Polarity in a polypeptide.

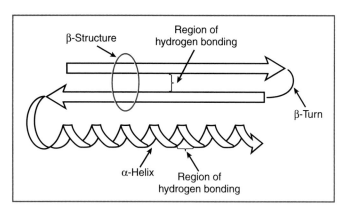

Figure 3-3. Secondary structure includes α-helix and β-pleated sheet (β-sheet).

MICROBIOLOGY

Prion Diseases

Prions (PrP^{Sc}) are formed from otherwise normal neurologic proteins (PrP) and are responsible for encephalopathies in humans (Creutzfeldt-Jakob disease, kuru), scrapie in sheep, and bovine spongiform encephalopathy. Contact between the normal PrP and PrP^{Sc} results in conversion of the secondary structure of PrP from predominantly α-helical to predominantly β-pleated sheet. The altered structure of the protein forms long, filamentous aggregates that gradually damage neuronal tissue. The harmful PrP^{Sc} form is highly resistant to heat, ultraviolet irradiation, and protease enzymes.

referred to as a "helix breaker." The α-helix is found in most globular proteins and in some fibrous proteins (e.g., α-keratin).

β-Pleated Sheet Structure Conformation

β-Pleated sheet structure (also called β-structure) consists of extended regions of adjacent side-by-side polypeptide sequences (see Fig. 3-3). It is likewise stabilized by hydrogen bonding between the peptide bonds of adjacent sequences. The orientation of the adjacent chains can be the same (parallel) or opposite (antiparallel) direction. β-Structures are found in 80% of all globular proteins and in silk fibroin.

Supersecondary Structure and Domains

Supersecondary structures, or motifs, are characteristic combinations of a secondary structure 10 to 40 residues in length that recur in different proteins. They bridge the gap between the less specific regularity of a secondary structure and the highly specific folding of a tertiary structure. The same motif can perform similar functions in different proteins.

- The four-helix bundle motif provides a cavity for enzymes to bind prosthetic groups or cofactors.
- The β-barrel motif can bind hydrophobic molecules such as retinol in the interior of the barrel.
- Motifs may also be mixtures of both α and β conformations.

- Motifs can have a specific ligand binding function, or they can contribute to the structure of a domain.

Primary structure is generally subdivided into domains of about 25 to 300 residues in length. Within each polypeptide, the individual domains can fold independently into a stable configuration. The region within the structural gene that codes for a domain is called an exon. A domain can consist of one or more secondary structure motifs, and although domains contribute to the three-dimensional (3-D) structure of protein, they do not describe complete (tertiary) structure of the protein. Interruption of a regular structure in domains is achieved through polypeptide bending.

- α-Helices bend at proline residues.
- β-Structure bends at β-turns (loops back into domain structure; see Fig. 3-3).

Tertiary Structure

Tertiary structure is the complete 3-D structure of a polypeptide. It is formed spontaneously and stabilized both by side chain interactions and, in extracellular proteins, by disulfide bonds. This folding brings distant sequences in a linear polypeptide together into a stable structure (Fig. 3-4). In soluble proteins, hydrophobic side chains are found in the interior of a protein; thus domains pack together so as to minimize the exposure of hydrophobic side chains to a water interface. Hydrophilic amino acids that can form hydrogen bonds to water are at the surface of soluble proteins. Since cellular membranes are a hydrophobic environment, integral membrane proteins are more likely to have hydrophobic groups spanning the membrane and hydrophilic groups on the surface.

The most stable structure under any given physiologic condition is called the native conformation of a protein. There are four side chain interactions that stabilize the native conformation.

- *Hydrophobic interactions*: Hydrophobic side chains are repelled by water and forced together at the interior of proteins to escape the aqueous environment.
- *Van der Waals forces*: A nonspecific attraction develops based on the proximity of interacting atoms; if the shape of the side chain allows a good fit between surfaces, an attractive force develops. A poor fit gives either repulsion or no force. Note: Both hydrophobic interactions and the shape of side chains are major factors in determining tertiary structure.
- *Electrostatic bonds*: Oppositely charged side chains can attract each other, forming salt bridges. They also play a role in the binding of substrates and allosteric effectors and in the association of the protein with other protein molecules (see later Quaternary Structure discussion). In addition, they can bind large amounts of water to solubilize the protein when located on the surface.
- *Hydrogen bonds*: Polar groups can share a partial positive charge between a hydrogen donor and a hydrogen acceptor to form a weak bond (see also Chapter 1).

To become functional, some proteins require the incorporation of a nonprotein molecule, a prosthetic group, into the tertiary structure. The apoprotein lacks the prosthetic group; the holoprotein includes the prosthetic group. The attachment can be either covalent or noncovalent (weak) bonds:

- *Biotin*: covalent attachment to lysine side chain
- *Heme*: noncovalent attachment in hydrophobic heme binding site

The tertiary structure of both fibrous proteins and globular proteins is adapted to their biologic role. For example, α-keratin is a multiunit elastic fibrous protein with protofibrils as the basic unit. The protofibrils consist of four right-handed α-helices wound in a left-handed supercoil. The protofibrils are coiled into microfibrils, which in turn are coiled into macrofibrils. Microfibrils are also cross-linked by disulfide bonds (fewer in flexible hair and skin, more in rigid fingernails). In contrast to α-keratin, the inelastic fibrous protein, silk fibroin, is composed of antiparallel β-pleated sheets. The β-structure is highly resistant to protease digestion.

Disulfide bonds serve to stabilize the native conformation in the extracellular space where physiologic conditions are more variable. Disulfide bonds are formed by the action of protein disulfide isomerase (located in the lumen of the endoplasmic reticulum) during folding of the polypeptide into its tertiary structure.

Quaternary Structure

Quaternary structure refers to the subunit composition of a protein (Fig. 3-5). Polypeptide subunits associate in a highly specific fashion to form a functional oligomer (oligo = several; mer = body). The most common number of subunits is either 2 (dimer) or 4 (tetramer), but trimers, pentamers, and hexadecamers and higher order structures also occur.

- *Heteromeric*: composed of different subunits, each produced by a different gene
- *Homomeric*: composed of the same monomer unit, produced by the same gene

Quaternary structure is held together by noncovalent bonds between complementary surface hydrophobic and hydrophilic regions on the polypeptide subunits. Additionally, acidic and basic side chains can form salt linkages. Since the same weak forces that stabilize tertiary structure are involved in stabilizing quaternary structure, the subunits can be dissociated from

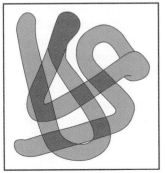
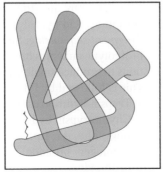

A   B

Figure 3-4. Tertiary structure of myoglobin (A) and β-globin (B).

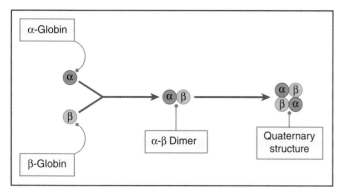

Figure 3-5. Quaternary structure of hemoglobin.

each other. It is also possible to have covalent stabilization by interchain disulfide bonds.

Contact between subunits permits an interaction that allows a change in the shape of one subunit to induce a change in the shape—and function—of an adjacent subunit. Thus multiple subunits can be affected by the binding of a single ligand.

NEUROSCIENCE

β-Amyloid Protein

Neurodegenerative diseases, such as Alzheimer disease (AD), are central nervous system disorders characterized by loss of function and death of neurons in the brain, leading to progressive loss of cognitive function and memory. Pathologic changes associated with AD include the formation of neuritic (also called senile) plaques and neurofibrillary tangles. The neuritic plaques contain β-amyloid protein derived from a proteolytic conversion of the neuronal β-amyloid precursor protein (APP). β-Amyloid deposits in neurons are neurotoxic.

Denaturation

The disruption and loss of native conformation is called denaturation; it is accompanied by a loss of biologic activity. Denaturation is caused by nonphysiologic conditions:
- Extreme changes in pH
- Extremes in ionic strength
- Detergents
- Increase in temperature
- Reaction with heavy metals (arsenic, mercury, lead)

As the physiologic conditions that stabilize higher order structure gradually change, there is a corresponding gradual disruption of secondary, tertiary, and quaternary structure leading to an opening up of the protein; primary structure is not affected. The denatured polypeptide becomes randomized and aggregates with other denatured polypeptides to form an insoluble precipitate. Because of their open conformation, denatured proteins are more susceptible to digestion by proteolytic enzymes. Indeed, stomach acid denatures dietary protein so that the digestive enzymes—pepsin, trypsin, and chymotrypsin—can hydrolyze dietary proteins to amino acids.

Some proteins are capable of spontaneous refolding after denaturation. For example, ribonuclease A renatures with gradual removal of denaturant. Other proteins retain varying capacities for renaturation depending on the extent to which they have denatured.

PATHOLOGY

Heinz Bodies

Heinz bodies are composed of denatured hemoglobin that has become oxidized in RBCs. The denatured hemoglobin forms visible aggregates on the RBC membrane. Heinz bodies will form under conditions of high oxidative stress, such as that caused by the antimalarial drug primaquine, or in patients with an unstable hemoglobin variant.

KEY POINTS ABOUT LEVELS OF STRUCTURAL COMPLEXITY

- Protein function is dependent on its stable native conformation, which is in turn determined by its primary structure or sequence.
- Primary structure is the simple linear sequence of amino acids connected by planar, covalent peptide bonds.
- Secondary structure is a regular extended structure that is limited to two forms: α-helix and β-structure.
- Supersecondary structure motifs are characteristic associations of secondary structure that recur in proteins that perform similar functions.
- Domains are independent 3-D structures composed of supersecondary structure motifs that perform specific functions within a protein; they are not the final structure of the protein.

●●● ANALYSIS OF PROTEIN STRUCTURE

Methods for Studying Primary Structure

The analysis of primary structure, or sequence analysis, reveals the effects of genetic mutations and shows homologies within families of proteins (e.g., the globin family). There are three major steps in the analysis of primary structure:
1. *Amino acid composition*: The amino acid composition is determined by quantitative analysis following protein digestion by acid hydrolysis (breaks all peptide bonds).
2. *Fragment sequencing*: Specific hydrolysis by chemicals or proteolytic enzymes breaks peptide bonds at specific locations to produce small, easy-to-manage peptide fragments. This is followed by Edman degradation of each fragment.
   - Trypsin hydrolyzes the carbonyl side of lys and arg.
   - Chymotrypsin hydrolyzes the carbonyl side of aromatic rings (phe, tyr, trp).
   - Cyanogen bromide cleaves on the carbonyl side of methionine.
   - Edman degradation involves the sequential removal and identification of N-terminal amino acid by reaction with

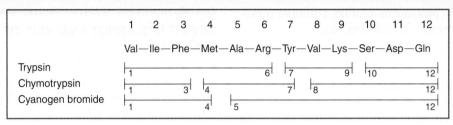

	1	2	3	4	5	6	7	8	9	10	11	12
	Val	Ile	Phe	Met	Ala	Arg	Tyr	Val	Lys	Ser	Asp	Gln

Figure 3-6. Overlapping fragments used in polypeptide sequence determination.

phenylisothiocyanate; it is used for peptide sequences up to 50 to 60 residues long.

3. *Fragment linking*: Cleavage of the protein at different points produces overlapping fragments (Fig. 3-6). The overall primary structure is then deduced by linking each fragment together.

   - The disulfide bond is stable to acid hydrolysis; a di-amino acid representing both cysteine residues is released as cystine. The disulfide bond may be cleaved by reaction with a reducing agent, such as mercaptoethanol, then prevented from re-forming by reaction with a sulfhydryl reagent, such as iodoacetate.

Methods for Studying Higher Order Structure

Methods for the purification and characterization of proteins take advantage of tertiary and quaternary structure.

Protein Precipitation

Increasing the salt concentration of a protein solution leads to dehydration of the proteins by progressively binding water in hydration shells. The dehydrated proteins aggregate and precipitate at a salting-out point that is unique for each protein. Thus proteins can be separated based on differential solubility.

Chromatography

A protein mixture when applied to a stationary matrix, usually in a column, will separate each protein if it has a different interaction with the matrix (gel exclusion does not depend on affinity for the matrix); the individual proteins can be collected in separate fractions upon elution. The interaction with the solid matrix can be based on physical or chemical characteristics:

- *Gel exclusion*: A porous matrix excludes molecules above a defined molecular weight; the volume accessible to large molecules is restricted, so that larger molecules elute first, followed by smaller molecules.
- *Ion exchange*: A positively or negatively charged matrix binds proteins of opposite charge; the proteins are removed separately with a salt (ionic strength) or pH gradient. Cation exchange chromatography is frequently used for separation and analysis of amino acids from protein hydrolysates.
- *Affinity*: Ligands covalently bound to a matrix resemble coenzymes, substrates, or other small molecules; the protein being purified binds tightly to the ligand and then elutes with either unbound ligand or pH gradients. This method is frequently used for purification of enzymes or receptors. Immunoaffinity chromatography uses immobilized antibodies for binding of specific molecules.

- *Reverse-phase or hydrophobic chromatography*: Molecules adsorbed to a nonpolar matrix are desorbed by a gradient of increasing concentration of water-miscible, nonpolar solvent.
- *High-performance liquid chromatography*: Microparticulate resins require high pressure for elution but yield separations of higher resolution.

Centrifugation

When a protein sample is subjected to a centrifugal field, individual proteins separate on the basis of sedimentation rate (size and shape). The units of sedimentation are expressed as Svedberg units (S).

Dialysis

When a protein sample is placed in a bag or other container composed of semipermeable membrane and immersed in buffer solution (Fig. 3-7), the smaller molecules diffuse through the membrane pores; the larger molecules (i.e., proteins) are retarded. Dialysis is commonly used to remove salt (e.g., following salt precipitation) or reversibly bound cofactors or inhibitors. Semipermeable filters, with specific molecular weight cut-offs, are used to separate molecules based on

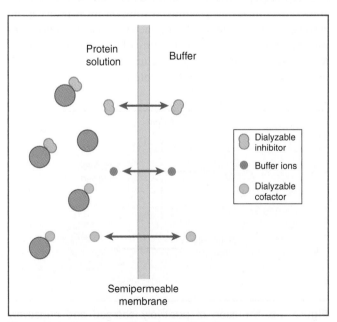

Figure 3-7. Protein purification by dialysis.

size or to concentrate proteins in solution. Filtration is promoted by positive pressure or centrifugation.

Electrophoresis

Protein samples applied to a porous gel (or cellulose acetate strip) in buffer solution and subjected to an electrical field will migrate toward the oppositely charged electrode. The rate of migration depends on the size, shape, and charge of each protein (Fig. 3-8). Electrophoresis is used for both purification and characterization of proteins. The migration pattern is usually visualized by direct staining with a dye or by blotting on nitrocellulose; visualization can be achieved by staining, an enzyme color reaction, or labeled antibodies.

Fingerprinting

A distinct and specific pattern is obtained when proteins are subjected to selective proteolytic digestion and then separated in two dimensions, first by chromatography and then by electrophoresis. Two-dimensional electrophoresis can also be used. Staining produces a pattern of spots that represents a unique protein fingerprint. Since most peptides migrate to a unique spot, this method can detect differences of only one amino acid between proteins. Every protein will have a unique fingerprint based on its unique primary structure.

X-Ray Diffraction

Since proteins have a single stable tertiary structure, they can form a crystal lattice that diffracts x-rays to produce electron density maps. The x-ray diffraction pattern can then be converted to an electronic form and processed by a computer to provide a precise 3-D picture of the protein's structure.

Nuclear Magnetic Resonance

Nuclear magnetic resonance (NMR), also called magnetic resonance imaging (MRI) when applied to organs and tissues, derives a 3-D image of proteins in solution by measuring the resonance frequencies of atomic nuclei. This method provides information on the solution structure of a protein but requires knowledge of the primary structure of the protein and is applicable primarily to smaller proteins.

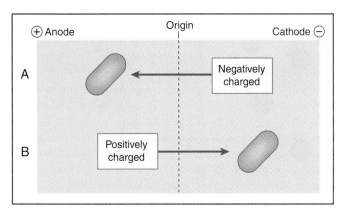

Figure 3-8. Migration of positively charged and negatively charged protein samples on electrophoresis.

KEY POINTS ABOUT ANALYSIS OF PROTEIN STRUCTURE

- Tertiary structure is the complete 3-D structure of a protein; it is composed of all the domain structures, with hydrophobic side chains found toward the center and hydrophilic side chains toward the water interface.
- Quaternary structure describes the subunit composition of a functional protein.
- The higher orders of protein structure are stabilized by weak chemical bonds that permit the small changes in conformation necessary when binding ligands or catalyzing reactions; disulfide bonds further stabilize secreted proteins.
- Breaking of weak chemical bonds by extremes of temperature, pH, ionic strength, and heavy metals results in loss of higher order structure and loss of function.
- Purification of proteins allows an analysis of tertiary and quaternary structure; further analysis of amino acid sequence permits comparison of homologous proteins.

●●● MODEL PROTEINS: HEMOGLOBIN AND MYOGLOBIN

Hemoglobin and Myoglobin Comparison

Hemoglobin and myoglobin are both well-studied and clinically relevant proteins. They serve as model proteins, since they help illustrate basic principles of structure and function. Both similarities and differences in function correlate with their structural characteristics. It will be seen that small differences in primary structure can produce large differences in function (Table 3-1).

Cellular Roles

Hemoglobin transports O_2 from the lungs to the tissues. It is found only in the erythrocyte (red blood cell; RBC) and, therefore, only in the blood. It binds oxygen reversibly, becoming

TABLE 3-1. Characteristics of Hemoglobin and Myoglobin

	HEMOGLOBIN	MYOGLOBIN
Function	O_2 transport	O_2 storage
Location	Only in the erythrocyte	Only in skeletal muscle
O_2 affinity in tissues	Low	High
O_2 affinity in lungs	High	High
O_2 affinity change with Po_2	Yes	No
Allosteric regulation	Yes	No
Quaternary structure	Yes—tetramer	No—monomer

saturated with oxygen at high oxygen concentration in the lungs. The oxygen is released at the lower oxygen tension in tissues where oxygen is used for aerobic metabolism. The oxygen affinity of hemoglobin is regulated (see later discussion), with higher affinity for oxygen in the lung, promoting binding for transport, and lower affinity in tissues, promoting release of oxygen for metabolism.

Myoglobin is found in heart and skeletal muscle but not in the blood. It binds oxygen more tightly than hemoglobin and serves as an oxygen buffer in tissues, releasing O_2 as the tissue becomes hypoxic. Unlike hemoglobin, myoglobin does not change its affinity for O_2 as it binds increasing amounts of O_2.

Quaternary Structure

Hemoglobin has a tetrameric quaternary structure composed of two different globin monomers, the specific monomer units depending on the developmental stage of the individual (Table 3-2). Each of the globins is produced by different genes that are active during different stages of human development. Hemoglobin F, composed of α and γ chains, is the predominant form in the fetus. Hemoglobin A, composed of α and β chains, is the predominant form in adults. One form of hemoglobin, hemoglobin A_{1C} (HbA_{1C}), is not determined genetically. It is a subclass of hemoglobin A that is formed from a spontaneous reaction between blood glucose and the amino terminal valine residue of the β-globin chain. Since the reaction rate is dependent on glucose concentration, a patient with uncontrolled diabetes mellitus (elevated blood glucose) has higher than normal concentrations of HbA_{1C}.

Myoglobin is always in monomeric form; therefore, it has no quaternary structure.

Tertiary Structure

Hemoglobin and myoglobin have similar tertiary structures:
- Both are all α-helical with connecting regions between helices (see Fig. 3-4).
- Both are highly compact with hydrophilic residues toward the outside and hydrophobic residues toward the inside.
- Both have a hydrophobic pocket for the association of one heme prosthetic group.

The formation of the tetrameric quaternary structure of hemoglobin, but not of myoglobin, is determined by hydrophobic and hydrogen-bonding interactions and salt bridges between amino acid residues on the surface of hemoglobin

monomers. In myoglobin, the surface amino acids are primarily polar and promote the solubility of the protein.

Heme Structure and Function

Heme is a planar iron-containing porphyrin ring with the iron held in the center of four pyrrole rings by coordination bonds (Fig. 3-9); there are six coordination bonds in all: four occupied by the pyrrole nitrogens, the fifth occupied by the proximal histidine (His-F8), and the sixth either occupied by O_2 or unoccupied. Although the heme iron binds O_2, it is not oxidized (i.e., it remains in the Fe^{++} form to bind O_2). Methemoglobin is hemoglobin in which the iron has been oxidized to Fe^{+++} and can no longer bind O_2.

Cooperativity

Cooperativity occurs when the binding of a ligand to one monomer of a multimeric protein affects the binding of that ligand to an adjacent monomer. Hemoglobin demonstrates

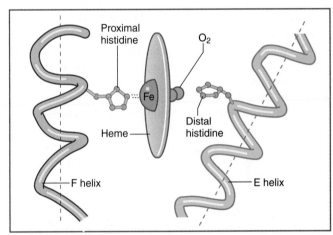

Figure 3-9. Structure of heme. The porphyrin ring is planar in structure, and the four coordination bonds it forms with iron lie within the plane. The fifth coordination bond with the proximal histidine is shown above the plane of the porphyrin ring, and the sixth coordination bond formed when oxygen binds is shown below the plane of the porphyrin ring. Oxygen binding on one side of the plane pulls the proximal histidine closer to the plane. This leads to a shift in conformation of the globin chain, breaking of the salt bridges, and a shift from the T-form to the R-form.

TABLE 3-2. Tetrameric Quaternary Structures of Hemoglobin			
DEVELOPMENTAL STAGE	ABBREVIATION	QUATERNARY STRUCTURE	FRACTION OF TOTAL HEMOGLOBIN IN ADULT
Embryo	Hb Gower-2	$\alpha_2\varepsilon_2$	0
Fetus	HbF	$\alpha_2\gamma_2$	~1%
Adult	HbA	$\alpha_2\beta_2$	90%
Adult	HbA$_2$	$\alpha_2\delta_2$	~2%
Adult	HbA$_1$	$\alpha_2\beta_2$-Glucose	~5%

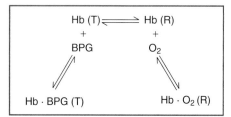

Figure 3-10. Equilibrium between the tense (*T*) and relaxed (*R*) forms of hemoglobin.

positive cooperativity by increasing its O_2 affinity as it binds increasing amounts of O_2. This is due to the ability of the globin monomers to switch between a high-affinity "relaxed" conformation (R-form) and a low-affinity "tense" conformation (T-form) (Fig. 3-10). The signal for switching between these forms is communicated through ionic bonds, or salt bridges, at the interface between the monomeric subunits. If a salt bridge is intact, the adjacent globin remains in the T-form; the breaking of a salt bridge induces a change in the adjacent globin to the R-form.

- Salt bridges are intact at a low O_2 concentration (partial pressure of O_2 [Po_2] and are broken when O_2 is bound to the heme.
- O_2 binding causes a change in the position of the heme iron and results in a pull on the proximal histidine in the fifth coordination position.
- Movement of the histidine produces a corresponding movement in the local structure of the globin, which includes the area containing the salt bridges.
- Breaking of the salt bridge does not lead to dissociation of the monomers but instead allows the adjacent monomer to adopt the R-form (i.e., to "relax").

The effect of the progressive increase in affinity as increasing amounts of O_2 are bound is illustrated in an O_2-binding plot. When the percent O_2 saturation of the O_2-binding protein is plotted against the Po_2, a significant difference is seen between hemoglobin and myoglobin (Fig. 3-11).

- Hemoglobin has a sigmoid, or S-shaped, curve. This type of curve is also demonstrated for substrate binding by enzymes that have a multimeric structure and indicates that the monomers can influence, or induce, each other's level of enzymatic activity.
- Myoglobin has a hyperbolic curve. This is expected in monomeric proteins that bind one ligand in a reversible equilibrium. Hyperbolic substrate versus velocity curves are also seen for monomeric enzymes that demonstrate classic Michaelis-Menten kinetics (see Chapter 4).

Allosterism

Allosterism describes the change in the affinity for binding of a ligand or substrate that is caused by the binding of another ligand away from the active site (allosteric = other site).
- Allosterism is not the same as cooperativity.
- Cooperativity creates the sigmoid curve.
- Allosterism shifts the curve to the right or left.
- Allosterism, therefore, affects cooperativity.

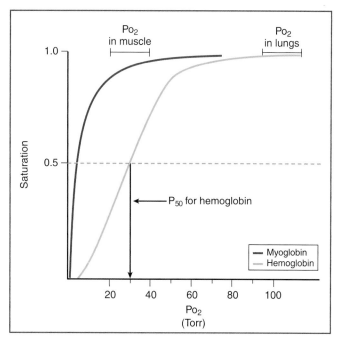

Figure 3-11. O_2 binding curve for hemoglobin and myoglobin. P_{50}, Po_2 at one-half saturation.

Higher affinities for the ligand are seen in curves more to the left (positive allosteric effect), and lower affinities produce curves shifted to the right (negative allosteric effect). There are several allosteric effectors for hemoglobin, all of which shift the curve to the right (negative allosteric effectors), that is, decreasing the affinity of hemoglobin for oxygen.

2,3-Bisphosphoglycerate (2,3-BPG)

2,3-Bisphosphoglycerate (2,3-BPG) is a metabolite present in high concentrations in RBCs and is the principal allosteric effector for hemoglobin. One BPG molecule binds reversibly to a tetramer with the monomers all in the T-form; it stabilizes the T-form, shifting the T $\rightleftharpoons$ R equilibrium toward the T-form (see Fig. 3-10). 2,3-BPG has little effect on the binding of oxygen to hemoglobin at high Po_2 but promotes release of O_2 from hemoglobin at low Po_2. It is formed in the RBC from the glycolytic intermediate, 1,3-BPG, by bisphosphoglycerate mutase.

Carbon Dioxide

Reaction of CO_2 with N-terminal amino groups of globin polypeptide chains forms carbamate:

$$CO_2 + Hb\text{-}NH_3^+ \rightarrow Hb\text{-}NH\text{-}COO^-$$

In this form, hemoglobin transports about 15% of the CO_2 carried in blood. Carbamate formation favors salt bridge formation and lowers the O_2 affinity of hemoglobin.

Protons

The Bohr effect refers to the loss of affinity for O_2 with decreasing pH (increased acidity), as occurs in the microcirculation as oxygen is consumed and CO_2 (carbonic acid) is released by tissues. Protons shift the equilibrium toward the

T-form by binding to surface amino acids. Through this equilibrium with protons, hemoglobin also contributes significantly to the buffering capacity of the blood.

A negative allosteric effect is seen with increased body temperature. This reduces hemoglobin O_2 affinity in a febrile patient, allowing increased unloading of O_2 during accelerated metabolism in tissues.

PHARMACOLOGY AND PHYSIOLOGY

Carbon Monoxide Poisoning

Carbon monoxide (CO) exerts its toxic effect by stabilizing the R-form of hemoglobin. Although toxic CO concentrations are well below the normal oxygen concentration, CO binds to Fe^{++} heme with a 200-fold greater affinity. CO binding shifts the subunit into the R-form and facilitates the loading of the rest of the molecule with the more plentiful oxygen (one of the symptoms of severe CO poisoning is a cherry-red skin color). The physiologic crisis occurs when the CO-hemoglobin cannot unload its oxygen in the tissues as a result of a left shift in its O_2 dissociation curve. When CO is bound to the Hb tetramer, it behaves more like myoglobin. Hyperbaric oxygen is the most effective treatment.

Fetal Hemoglobin

2,3-BPG has weaker binding to fetal hemoglobin (HbF) than to adult hemoglobin (HbA) because of the different amino acid composition at the allosteric site. This reduces the negative allosteric effect of 2,3-BPG, leading to a small increase in O_2 affinity of HbF relative to HbA. This is a molecular adaptation to the low P_{O_2} of the placental circulation; O_2 flows from HbA (maternal circulation, lower O_2 affinity) to HbF (fetal circulation, higher O_2 affinity).

Hemoglobinopathies

Hemoglobinopathies are genetic diseases caused by structural alterations in the globin chains or by altered rates of globin synthesis. Several hundred structurally altered forms of hemoglobin have been identified and illustrate that a small change in structure can produce a large change in function. Hemoglobinopathies resulting from a change in the rate of synthesis of hemoglobin monomers illustrate the importance of producing monomer subunits in the correct proportion.

Structural Alterations in Hemoglobin

Sickle cell hemoglobin (HbS) is caused by a mutation that replaces glutamic acid at residue 6 in β-globin with valine (β6 Glu → Val). This amino acid substitution leads to the formation of linear polymers of deoxygenated HbS. Removal of O_2 from HbS in the tissues exposes a complementary site that is also on the surface. The valine residue on the surface of HbS binds to the complementary site, linking the two tetramers together (Fig. 3-12). As more tetramers become linked, linear polymers are formed that convert the normally flexible RBCs into stiff, sickle-shaped cells. The inelastic, sickle-shaped cells plug the capillary beds and precipitate the sickling crisis. Note that the complementary site is not exposed in oxygenated blood, so the sickling is initiated in the peripheral tissues and joints.

HbS is the most common hemoglobin variant worldwide, since the heterozygous form confers a resistance to malaria. It occurs primarily in the black population of the United States, affecting 1 in 500 newborns. When the mutation occurs on both chromosomes (chromosome 11), it produces sickle cell disease; this has the most severe symptoms, since the RBC has no source of normal β-globin. With a mutation only on one chromosome (in heterozygotes), it produces sickle cell trait (1 in 10 newborns); the production of nearly equal amounts of normal β-globin and $β^s$-globin reduces the severity of the symptoms by lowering the degree of sickling that occurs.

Hemoglobin C is caused by a mutation at the same site (position 6) as sickle cell hemoglobin, except the alteration is glutamate to lysine (β6 Glu → Lys). Since lysine has little or no tendency to bind the complementary site, no sickling occurs.

Hb Boston is caused by a tyrosine substitution (β58 His → Tyr) close to the heme iron; this stabilizes the heme iron in the oxidized form, preventing the binding of O_2. Hb Boston is one

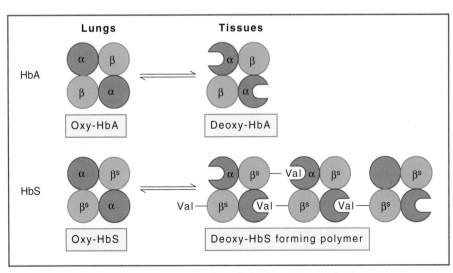

Figure 3-12. Formation of linear aggregates between molecules of sickle cell hemoglobin.

of several hereditary methemoglobinemias that are characterized by cyanosis.

Hb Chesapeake is caused by a leucine substitution (α92 Arg $\rightarrow$ Leu) that weakens the salt bridges, causing them to break more easily. The resulting increase in O_2 affinity, resulting from decreased sensitivity to negative allosteric effectors, makes it more difficult for RBCs to unload O_2 in the tissues, creating hypoxia. This signals an increase in RBC production and leads to polycythemia.

Hb Köln is caused by a methionine substitution (β98 Val $\rightarrow$ Met) that produces an unstable β-globin. The denaturation of the hemoglobin eventually leads to RBC fragility and hemolytic anemia.

Altered Rates of Globin Synthesis

Unbalanced production of either α-globin or β-globin leads to a class of diseases called thalassemias. These are primarily hemolytic anemias due to the production of altered tetramers. They can be caused by the following:
- Complete deletion of globin genes
- Impaired RNA synthesis
- Impaired primary mRNA splicing
- Frameshift or nonsense mutations producing quickly degraded globins

The β-thalassemias include thalassemia major (two mutated β-globin genes; chromosome 11) and thalassemia minor (heterozygote). Thalassemia major is lethal by adulthood, whereas thalassemia minor produces only a mild anemia.

The α-thalassemias are more complicated, since the α-globin is present before and after birth and there are two copies of the α-globin gene on chromosome 16. The progressive loss of α-globin genes results in more severe anemias, which affect the fetus.

KEY POINTS ABOUT MODEL PROTEINS—HEMOGLOBIN AND MYOGLOBIN

- Hemoglobin structure matches its physiologic role by increasing its affinity for oxygen in the lungs and decreasing its affinity for O_2 in the tissues.
- Myoglobin has no quaternary structure, since its localization in muscle cells does not require that it change affinity for O_2.
- The different quaternary structures for hemoglobin throughout development reflect specialized needs for O_2 transport.
- Cooperativity refers to the interaction of the subunit structure of a protein to change its activity when binding its primary ligand; hemoglobin changes its affinity for O_2 as it binds oxygen.
- Allosterism is the change in cooperativity that results from binding a ligand, or effector, at a site other than the primary site; negative allosteric effectors for hemoglobin are 2,3-BPG, CO_2, and protons.
- Hemoglobinopathies are diseases caused by alteration either in hemoglobin structure or in its rate of synthesis.

Self-assessment questions can be accessed at www.StudentConsult.com.

Enzymes and Energetics

4

●●● BIOLOGIC CATALYSTS

Enzymes are biologic catalysts that can increase the rate of noncatalyzed reactions by 10^6 to 10^{11}. Except for a class of catalytic ribonucleic acids (RNAs) called ribozymes, all enzymes are proteins. Their high specificity for a substrate ensures catalysis of the desired reaction while reducing side reactions. Enzymes are not changed by the reaction they catalyze, although they may become temporarily altered during the reaction.

Enzyme Energetics

Every chemical reaction (or physical process) in the body is accompanied by a change in free energy, ΔG. In order for a reaction to proceed in a given direction (i.e., to be spontaneous),

it must be accompanied by a negative ΔG (i.e., a decrease in G). Reactions proceed downhill from a thermodynamic or energetic point of view. The following equation shows that ΔG depends on both the change in enthalpy (where H = heat) and the change in entropy (where S = disorder):

$$\Delta G = \Delta H - T\Delta S$$

In simpler terms, a release of heat and an increase in disorder both contribute to the spontaneity of a reaction. Spontaneity is different from rate. The ΔG of a reaction tells whether it will proceed forward from the equilibrium state; it says nothing about the rate. The reaction of O_2 with H_2 to form H_2O has a large negative ΔG. Although this reaction is "spontaneous" and will proceed with a large increase in enthalpy (heat) and entropy (gas formation), these gases can be mixed at room temperature without a detectable rate of combustion.

The free energy change is the difference in the free energy of the initial state minus that of the final state. To reach the final state, a reaction must first reach an activation energy. While the initial and final state determine spontaneity, it is the activation energy that determines rate (Fig. 4-1). Thus even a spontaneous reaction will proceed slowly if the activation energy is very high. This is the case for the reaction of O_2 with H_2. In this case, the reaction can be initiated by addition of heat and raising the temperature of the molecules—something that cannot be done in the body. In biologic systems, the rate of reactions is increased when a catalyst such as an enzyme acts to decrease the activation energy. Since an enzyme cannot change the equilibrium of a reaction, the reaction rate increases in both directions but proceeds farthest in the direction of negative ΔG. In simpler terms, enzymes cannot force a reaction that is not spontaneous.

Common Intermediates and Coupling

Although enzymes cannot force a reaction in a nonspontaneous direction, such a reaction can be carried out when it is coupled through a common intermediate to a reaction with a negative ΔG. When a product of one reaction serves as a reactant in a second reaction, it is referred to as a common intermediate and the reactions are coupled. In the two following coupled reactions, D is the common intermediate:

$$A + B \rightarrow C + D$$
$$D + E \rightarrow F + G$$

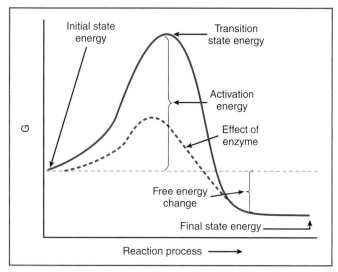

Figure 4-1. Free energy change during a reaction. Lowering the energy of activation increases the rate of reaction.

The free energy changes for both reactions are additive, and a negative value for the combined free energy change indicates a spontaneous overall forward direction for the coupled reactions.

Spontaneity and Product Removal

Free energy changes may be expressed as standard free energy changes when they are measured under reproducible standard conditions: 1 mol/L for all reactants in solution, 25° C, 1 atm, and pH 7. Although chemical reactions in biologic systems occur under conditions far from standard, the standard free energy makes a contribution to the overall actual free energy change. For the general chemical reaction

$$A + B \rightarrow C + D$$

the actual free energy change is given by the following equation:

$$\Delta G = \Delta G^{\circ\prime} + RT \ln[C][D]/[A][B]$$

This equation recognizes the concentrations of reactants and products that exist at any given moment at a given temperature (where R = the gas constant and T = degrees Kelvin). In simpler terms, the tendency of a reaction to proceed is dependent on both its normal (standard) tendency to proceed under standard conditions and a mass action effect that depends on actual conditions. This equation is important to the spontaneity of metabolic pathways because fuel is constantly added and waste is constantly removed from biologic systems.

Metabolic Pathways

A metabolic pathway is a series of two or more reactions that are coupled together by common intermediates. Since free energy changes are summative for all coupled pathway reactions, the continual addition of fuel to a catabolic pathway (extraction of energy) and the continual removal of pathway products (CO_2 and H_2O) result in a large negative ΔG.

Pathways are designed to achieve several major types of objectives:

- Catabolism: The pathways that extract from fuels and store energy as adenosine triphosphate (ATP). The complex fuel molecules are degraded into simpler products in systematic energy-releasing reactions.
- Anabolism: The pathways that couple energy-releasing (from ATP) reactions to energy-requiring synthesis reactions to produce complex molecules from simpler precursors.
- Digestion: The pathways that degrade complex molecules to produce simpler molecules, suitable for catabolism, but without extracting and storing energy.

Enzyme Nomenclature

Enzymes are classified according to the type of reaction they catalyze.

- *Oxidoreductases* transfer electrons from donors to acceptors (oxidation/reduction reactions); dehydrogenases transfer electrons that remain attached to hydrogen atoms.
- *Transferases* transfer functional groups between donors and acceptors; transaminases transfer amino groups, and kinases transfer phosphoryl groups.
- *Hydrolases* catalyze cleavage of bonds by addition of water, producing two products (e.g., peptidases cleave peptide (C–N) bonds).
- *Lyases* add water, ammonia, or CO_2 to double bonds, or remove them to create double bonds (e.g., ATP-citrate lyase produces acetyl-coenzyme A and oxaloacetate from citrate).
- *Isomerases* interconvert isomeric forms by transferring groups within the same molecule (e.g., phosphoglucose isomerase interconverts hexose aldehyde [glucose 6-phosphate] and ketone [fructose 6-phosphate] forms.
- *Ligases*, also called synthetases, use ATP to form new covalent bonds (e.g., DNA ligase creates a new phosphodiester bond in a gap between two adjacent nucleotides in the DNA helix).

Coenzymes

Many enzymes require nonprotein cofactors, or coenzymes, for their action. If they are tightly bound to the enzyme, they are referred to as a prosthetic group. The apoenzyme is the form that lacks the prosthetic group, and the holoenzyme is the fully functional form. Many coenzymes enter the reaction as a substrate but are regenerated through coupling with other pathways. Thus the concentration of a coenzyme may be much smaller than that of the metabolites in the reaction. Coenzymes can be vitamins that have been converted into an active form (e.g., thiamine is activated to thiamine pyrophosphate). In addition, metal ions can serve as cofactors (e.g., magnesium ions are required by kinases and zinc ions are required by carbonic anhydrase).

KEY POINTS ABOUT BIOLOGIC CATALYSTS

- Except for ribozymes (catalytic RNA), all biologic catalysts are proteins called enzymes.
- Enzymes are highly specific for the substrates they act on and they are not changed by the reaction.
- For a reaction to proceed in a given direction (i.e., to be spontaneous), it must be accompanied by a negative ΔG; spontaneity is different from rate.
- Enzymes cannot force a reaction that is not spontaneous.
- When a product of one reaction serves as a reactant in a second reaction, it is referred to as a common intermediate and the reactions are coupled.
- The tendency of a reaction to proceed is dependent on both its normal (standard) tendency to proceed under standard conditions and a mass action effect that depends on actual conditions.
- A metabolic pathway is a series of two or more reactions that are coupled together by common intermediates.
- Enzymes are classified according to the type of reaction they catalyze.
- Coenzymes are nonprotein cofactors required for enzyme action; they are often derived from vitamins or minerals.

⬤⬤⬤ ACTIVE SITE PROPERTIES

Enzymes lower the activation energy by binding the substrates in a specific configuration and in a protected environment within the enzyme. Active sites are often found in a "cleft" in the enzyme tertiary structure, requiring that the substrates diffuse in and the products diffuse out. The amino acid residues of the active site may be far apart in the primary structure owing to the folding required for tertiary structure.

PATHOLOGY

Hydroxyproline Formation

Vitamin deficiency symptoms correlate with their enzyme cofactor function. Scurvy, a vitamin C deficiency, is characterized by bleeding gums, loose teeth, and poor wound healing, all due to weak connective tissue. The collagen in these tissues is deficient in hydroxyproline since vitamin C, ascorbic acid, is required to hydroxylate proline residues in procollagen. Without hydroxyproline, the collagen triple helix denatures at body temperature.

Induced Fit

Although the binding site is a three-dimensional catalytic center, it is not rigid as would be found with a lock-and-key relationship. Instead, it is induced to undergo a change in conformation when the substrates bind (Fig. 4-2). The new conformation is formed by an induced fit and is necessary before the substrates can be converted to the transition state.

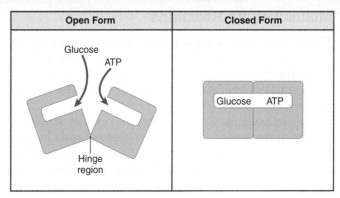

Figure 4-2. Induced fit (i.e., change from open form to closed form) during binding of substrate to the enzyme.

An induced fit is needed for reactions that must exclude water to avoid side reactions such as hydrolysis.

Amino Acid Composition

Active site amino acids form ionic and hydrogen bonds, and hydrophobic interactions with the substrate. This explains the dependence of enzyme activity on conditions that affect these types of bonds, such as pH, temperature, and ionic strength. The requirements for substrate binding are so specific that the amino acids forming the active site for the same enzyme are highly conserved between different species. Thus the optimal conditions for pH, temperature, and ionic strength will be conserved between species as well.

Transition State

Binding to an active site causes bonding rearrangements, and the substrate adopts an intermediate "transition" state. The transition state represents a rearranged form of substrate that is activated or "strained" immediately preceding the formation of products. Transition state analogs, synthesized to closely resemble the transition state rather than the substrates, are highly effective enzyme inhibitors. Since they are chemically stable and do not react to form products, they bind at the active site in place of the substrates and block the reaction. They are characterized by having an affinity several orders of magnitude greater than that of the substrate.

Analytic Methods

Methods used to study active sites allow the development of highly specific drugs.
- *Affinity labels* are substrate analogs that react with one or more of the amino acids that make up the active site; sequence determination of the labeled enzyme allows identification of active site amino acids.
- *X-ray diffraction* analysis with either the substrate or a transition state analog bound to an active site reveals spatial relationships within the active site.
- *Site-directed mutagenesis* creates mutant enzymes with amino acid substitutions at active sites; substitutions that alter normal activity help identify amino acids crucial to the active site.

Multisubstrate Reactions

When two or more substrates are involved in a reaction, the order in which they bind may be random or sequential. For a sequential mechanism, both substrates must bind before the reaction takes place; they may bind either in random order or in a specific order.

The ping-pong mechanism is a special case of sequential binding. It requires each substrate to bind and react in turn. This creates an intermediate form of the enzyme in which one product is formed and diffuses off of the enzyme before the next substrate binds to complete the reaction. This mechanism is used by transaminases.

KEY POINTS ABOUT ACTIVE SITE PROPERTIES

- Amino acid residues of the active site may be far apart in the primary structure owing to the folding required for tertiary structure.

- The active site is induced to undergo a change in conformation when the substrates bind.

- The requirements for substrate binding are so specific that the amino acids forming the active site for the same enzyme are highly conserved between different species.

- Transition state analogs, synthesized to closely resemble the transition state rather than the substrates, are highly effective enzyme inhibitors.

- Affinity labels, x-ray diffraction analysis, and site-directed mutagenesis are methods used to analyze the active site.

- When two or more substrates are involved in a reaction, the order in which they bind may be random or sequential.

●●● KINETICS

For study of the kinetic properties of enzymes, the reaction velocity is measured under initial conditions (initial rate) to assure that there is no interference with the reverse reaction. Also, the molar concentration of substrate is much higher than that of the enzyme. Enzyme amounts are reported in units; 1 unit = μmol/min means that the enzyme will convert one micromole of substrate to product under specific reaction conditions (pH, buffer, temperature). The concentration of enzyme is expressed either as units per liter (U/L) or international units per liter (IU/L).

Reaction Order

The number of substrates that affect the rate of reaction determines the order of the reaction.

- *Zero order*: Enzyme is saturated with substrates; no more will bind. Increasing substrate concentration has no effect on rate of reaction.
- *First order*: Reaction rate is directly (linearly) proportional to the substrate added.
- *Second order*: Reaction rate is proportional to the concentration of two substrates.

Michaelis-Menten Kinetics

The most common way to express the kinetic properties of enzymes is the Michaelis-Menten model. Several simplifying assumptions govern Michaelis-Menten kinetics.

- A single substrate (S) binds reversibly to form the enzyme substrate complex, ES.

$$E + S \rightleftharpoons ES \rightarrow E + P$$

- ES can complete the reaction to form product (P).
- ES can also break down to enzyme and substrate without reacting.

Enzyme activity is plotted as the change in velocity as a function of increasing substrate concentration; this always produces a rectangular hyperbola (Fig. 4-3).

- The activity is linearly proportional (first order) to substrate concentration at low concentrations of substrate.
- The activity is not dependent on substrate concentration (zero order) at saturating concentrations of substrate; the maximal velocity is expressed as V_{max}.
- The substrate concentration required to produce a reaction rate equal to one half of V_{max} is called the Michaelis constant, or K_m. K_m is a concentration term with units, typically micromoles or millimoles.
- The K_m is an inverse measure of affinity of the enzyme for the substrate; a low K_m corresponds to a high affinity and vice versa.
- The V_{max} is directly proportional to the enzyme concentration; decreasing the enzyme concentration decreases the V_{max}.

A linear plot of Michaelis-Menten kinetics is obtained in the Lineweaver-Burk plot.

- Plotted as a double reciprocal plot of $1/v \times 1/S$
- Intersection with $1/S$ axis is equal to $1/K_m$
- Intersection with $1/v$ axis is equal to $1/V_{max}$

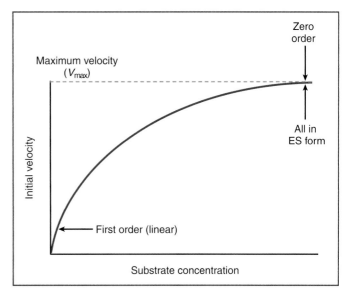

Figure 4-3. Substrate vs. velocity curve for an enzyme-catalyzed reaction.

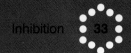

KEY POINTS ABOUT KINETICS

- The reaction velocity is measured under initial conditions (initial rate) to ensure that there is no interference with the reverse reaction.
- The number of substrates that affect the rate of reaction determines the order of the reaction.
- Michaelis-Menten kinetics assume that a single substrate (S) binds reversibly to form the enzyme substrate complex, ES.
- Enzyme activity is plotted as the change in velocity as a function of increasing substrate concentration.
- The substrate concentration required to produce a reaction rate equal to one half of V_{max} is called the Michaelis constant, or K_m.
- A linear plot of Michaelis-Menten kinetics is obtained in the Lineweaver-Burk plot.

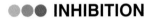 **INHIBITION**

Inhibition, either reversible or irreversible, of an enzyme molecule by a nonphysiologic agent (e.g., drugs and toxins) occurs by complete inactivation of the enzyme. In contrast, inhibition by metabolites, called allosteric inhibitors (see Regulation section), occurs by a gradual reduction in the enzyme activity.

Competitive Inhibitors

A competitive inhibitor competes with substrate for binding to an active site. When the inhibitor occupies the active site, it forms an enzyme-inhibitor complex and the enzyme cannot react (Fig. 4-4) until the inhibitor dissociates. Such inhibitors are commonly substrate analogs, since they have a structure similar to the substrate but are unreactive. An example of a competitive inhibitor is the antineoplastic drug methotrexate. Methotrexate has a structure similar to that of the vitamin folic acid (Fig. 4-5). It acts by inhibiting the enzyme dihydrofolate

Figure 4-4. Equilibrium between a competitive inhibitor (*EI*) and an enzyme (*E*). The inhibitor creates a competing equilibrium to that of the substrate (*S*), removing a fraction of the enzyme to an inactive form. Adding more substrate will yield more of the active enzyme substrate (*ES*) form. *P*, product.

reductase, preventing the regeneration of dihydrofolate from tetrahydrofolate. This interferes with DNA synthesis and blocks cell division in rapidly dividing cancer cells.

Competitive inhibition is proportional to the amount of inhibitor bound in the active site and is therefore proportional to inhibitor concentration. Because the inhibitor binds reversibly, the substrate can compete with it at high substrate concentrations. Thus a competitive inhibitor does not change the V_{max} of an enzyme. On the other hand, competitive inhibitors do raise the K_m of an enzyme since higher concentrations of substrate would be required to achieve half-maximal activity. This is seen in the Lineweaver-Burk plot as changing the 1/S intercept but not affecting the 1/v intercept (Fig. 4-6). In simpler terms, competitive inhibitors raise the K_m but do not change the V_{max}.

Noncompetitive Inhibitors

A noncompetitive inhibitor binds reversibly to the enzyme at a site away from the active site; this allows the substrate to bind normally (Fig. 4-7). However, the enzyme is completely inactivated when the inhibitor is bound and the substrate cannot be converted to the product. There is no competition for the active site (or for the inhibitor binding site).

Since the effective concentration of active enzyme is reduced as the noncompetitive inhibitor is bound, the V_{max}

Figure 4-5. Structure for methotrexate (A) and tetrahydrofolate (B).

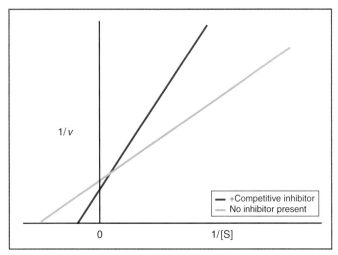

Figure 4-6. Lineweaver-Burk double reciprocal plot with and without a competitive inhibitor.

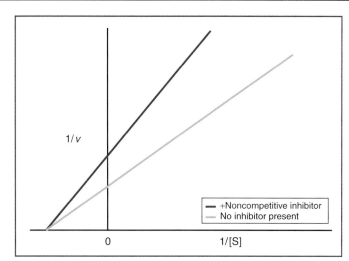

Figure 4-8. Lineweaver-Burk double reciprocal plot with and without a noncompetitive inhibitor.

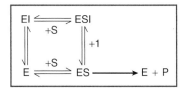

Figure 4-7. Equilibrium between a noncompetitive inhibitor (*EI*) and an enzyme (*E*). The inhibitor allows binding of substrate (*S*) to inactive enzyme (*ESI*) but prevents formation of product (*P*).

is reduced. However, the K_m is not affected, since the non-competitive inhibitor does not block the active site (which would reduce affinity). This is seen in the Lineweaver-Burk plot as changing the 1/*v* intercept without affecting the 1/*S* intercept (Fig. 4-8).

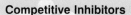

PHARMACOLOGY

Competitive Inhibitors

Many drugs are competitive inhibitors. Propranolol, a competitive inhibitor of β-adrenergic receptors, is used in the treatment of hypertension. Although it binds to the receptor, it does not cause an increase in cellular cyclic adenosine monophosphate. Therefore, propranolol inhibits the β-adrenergic (epinephrine) receptor by blocking the binding of epinephrine.

Irreversible Inhibitors

Irreversible inhibitors permanently inactivate enzymes. The only means for reversing the inhibition is the synthesis of new enzyme protein by the cell.

Optimal Conditions

Enzymes demonstrate a temperature optimum that is determined by an initial rate increase that is eventually slowed and then reversed as denaturation destroys the tertiary structure.

Enzymes demonstrate a pH optimum resulting from effects on both overall enzyme structure and optimal ionization at an active site. Denaturation of the tertiary structure takes place at extreme pH values, while variations in ionization of amino acid side chains in the active site change the affinity of the enzyme for the substrate; at the optimum pH, the affinity for the substrate is maximal.

The same enzyme from different sources (e.g., the bovine and human forms of the digestive enzymes pepsin and trypsin) can have different temperature optima, cellular location, V_{max}, K_m, and amino acid composition, but they will have the same pH optimum; most of the molecule can vary, but the active site is conserved (i.e., displays the same strict spatial arrangement of functional groups).

PHARMACOLOGY

Irreversible Inactivation

Aspirin and ibuprofen are both inhibitors of cyclooxygenase I, the enzyme that mediates the pathways for synthesis of prostaglandins (potent inflammatory agents) and thromboxanes (potent platelet aggregating agents). However, the effect of ibuprofen is reversible, whereas the effect of aspirin is irreversible. This is due to the acetyl group on aspirin that is not on ibuprofen. This acetyl group is transferred to the active site of cyclooxygenase, irreversibly blocking the reaction. This inhibition can be overcome only by synthesis of a new enzyme.

KEY POINTS ABOUT INHIBITION

■ Inhibition, either reversible or irreversible, of an enzyme molecule by a nonphysiologic agent (e.g., drugs and toxins) occurs by complete inactivation of the enzyme.

■ Inhibition is not regulation, which occurs under the influence of normal cellular metabolites.

- A competitive inhibitor competes with substrate for binding to an active site; its effect is to raise the K_m but not change the V_{max} of an enzyme.
- A noncompetitive inhibitor binds reversibly to the enzyme at a site away from the active site; the V_{max} is reduced but the K_m is not affected.
- Irreversible inhibitors permanently inactivate enzymes.
- The same enzyme from different sources can have different temperature optima, cellular location, V_{max}, K_m, and amino acid composition, but they will have the same pH optimum.

●●● REGULATION

Regulation is the response of enzyme activity to changing physiologic conditions. It is programmed into the structure of the enzyme molecule in the form of specialized sites that recognize both external and internal signals.

- External signals are transmitted as second messengers generated from the binding of hormones to their receptors.
- Internal signals are generally metabolic intermediates.

External signals are transmitted primarily through the mechanism of covalent modification, and internal signals are transmitted primarily through allosteric regulation.

Covalent Modification

Regulation by covalent modification occurs primarily through the action of a protein kinase that phosphorylates a specific serine, threonine, or tyrosine in the regulated enzyme (Fig. 4-9). The nonphosphorylated form can be restored by a protein phosphatase that dephosphorylates the regulated enzyme. The phosphorylated state may either be active or inactive, but in all cases the effect of the regulation matches the function of the hormone that generated the signal (e.g., gluconeogenic enzymes are turned on by phosphorylation, and glycolytic enzymes are turned off by phosphorylation during fasting).

The intracellular signaling pathway occurs through a cascade mechanism that is designed to amplify the hormonal signal. A cascade involves a series of enzymes that sequentially activate each other (Fig. 4-10). Since the product of each activation is a catalyst, each step results in a geometric increase in signal. The last enzyme in the cascade controls a target metabolic pathway or other cellular process.

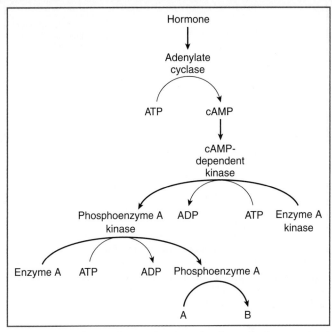

Figure 4-10. Cascade mechanism for hormonal control of enzyme activity. As hormone increases cyclic adenosine monophospate (*cAMP*) concentrations, the cAMP-dependent kinase is activated. This leads to activation of enzyme A kinase, which in turn activates enzyme A. Each step is an amplification, since the product is a catalyst. *ATP*, adenosine triphosphate; *ADP*, adenosine monophosphate.

Allosteric Regulation

Allosterism is a response to an effector molecule by an enzyme that results in an increase or decrease in its activity. To be regulated by an allosteric effector, the enzyme must first demonstrate cooperativity, an interactive property of multimeric enzymes. Cooperativity involves an interconversion of the monomer subunits between a tense form (less active subunits) and a relaxed form (more active subunits).

As seen with hemoglobin, cooperativity is a result of communication between subunits (monomers) of the enzyme quaternary structure. The binding of a ligand induces a change in conformation in adjacent subunits.

- *Positive cooperativity*: Binding of a ligand to one subunit increases the binding of the ligand on the adjacent subunit; this produces S-shaped substrate versus velocity plot (Fig. 4-11).

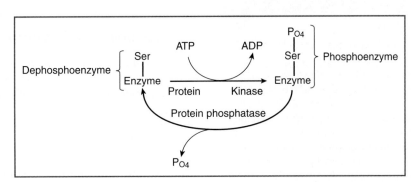

Figure 4-9. Regulation by covalent modification. *ATP*, adenosine triphosphate; *ADP*, adenosine monophosphate.

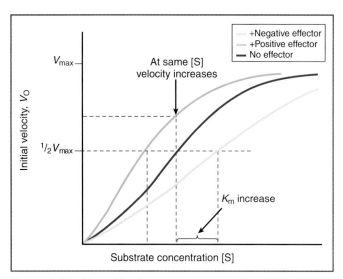

Figure 4-11. Sigmoid substrate vs. velocity plot. Effectors can move the plot left (rate increase) or right (rate decrease) by shifting the K_m for substrate.

- *Sequential mechanism*: Change in activity occurs one subunit at a time; this produces enzyme molecules containing both tense and relaxed forms.
- *Concerted mechanism*: A change in activity occurs simultaneously in all subunits; this produces enzyme molecules that contain either tense or relaxed forms, but not both.

Allosterism involves the binding of a ligand (effector) at an allosteric (allosteric = other shape) site. Note that allosteric effectors induce a change in shape (stereochemistry) of the enzyme before the binding of substrates. This is in contrast to the induced fit model of the active site in which the change in active site geometry occurs after the binding of substrates.

- *Positive effectors*: Ligands stabilize the relaxed (more active) form; activation is seen as sigmoidal curve displaced to the left (see Fig. 4-11).
- *Negative effectors*: Ligands stabilize the tense (less active) form; inactivation is seen as sigmoidal curve displaced to the right (see Fig. 4-11).
- Curves for nonallosteric enzymes are hyperbolic.

Some allosteric enzymes have specialized regulatory subunits. These are noncatalytic and serve only to bind effectors, leading to changes in the catalytic subunits.

PATHOLOGY

Creatine Kinase Isoenzymes

The distribution of the creatine kinase isoenzymes in different tissues allows it to serve as a diagnostic tool for myocardial infarction. The isoenzymes are composed of two subunits: B from brain and M from skeletal muscle. Skeletal muscle has a predominantly MM dimer, and muscle trauma will elevate the serum creatine kinase, but mainly the MM form. Brain damage would likewise mainly elevate the BB form. Heart muscle has a characteristic MB isoenzyme form that indicates myocardial damage when it appears in the serum, usually within hours of the event.

KEY POINTS ABOUT REGULATION

- Regulation is the response of enzyme activity to changing physiologic conditions; this is programmed into the structure of the enzyme molecule in the form of specialized sites.
- Regulation by covalent modification occurs primarily through the action of a protein kinase that phosphorylates a specific serine, threonine, or tyrosine in the regulated enzyme.
- Allosterism is a response to an effector molecule by an enzyme that results in an increase or decrease in its activity; however, the enzyme must first demonstrate cooperativity, an interactive property of multimeric enzymes.
- Allosterism involves the binding of a ligand (effector) at an allosteric (other shape) site.

●●● CELLULAR REGULATORY STRATEGIES

Multiple regulatory strategies reflect the wide variety of adaptations that must be made within cells and within the entire body.

Metabolic Pathway Regulation

Humans have the need to regulate processes over a span of time intervals from immediate to long term. There are four primary mechanisms by which cells regulate their metabolic pathways:

1. *Compartmentation*: This is permanent regulation achieved through physical separation of competing metabolic pathways within cellular compartments. It provides controlled access of substrates to their enzymes.
2. *Gene regulation*: This is long-term regulation of metabolism; the response is slow, requiring hours to days. The genes for multiple enzymes in a metabolic pathway are often regulated together.
3. *Covalent modification*: This is rapid regulation, taking only seconds to minutes. Enzymes in opposing pathways are reciprocally regulated to prevent futile cycles.
4. *Allosteric regulation*: This is instantaneous regulation. Allosteric effectors are usually end products of the regulated pathway and, therefore, do not resemble the substrate for the enzyme. The regulated enzymes catalyze rate-limiting, often irreversible, steps at the beginning of metabolic pathways.

Proenzymes (and Prohormones)

Inactive storage forms of enzymes (or hormones) are activated as needed by proteolytic removal of a portion of the proenzyme. This contrasts with interconversion between an active and inactive form by covalent modification and allosterism. Examples of proenzymes are the complement pathway in innate immunity and the clotting (coagulation) pathway, both of which are found in blood. An example of a prohormone is insulin that is stored as proinsulin so that large quantities can be activated and released on demand.

Isoenzymes

Isoenzymes (also called isozymes) are alternative forms of the same enzyme activity that exist in different proportions in different tissues. Isoenzymes differ in amino acid composition and sequence and multimeric quaternary structure; mostly, but not always, they have similar (conserved) structures. Their expression in a given tissue is a function of the regulation of the gene for the respective subunits. Each isoenzyme form will have different kinetic and/or regulatory properties that reflect its role in that tissue. Isoenzymes are generally identified in the clinical laboratory by electrophoresis.

Diagnostic Enzymology

In normal patients, only a few active enzymes (e.g., clotting factors) are found in the serum. However, tissue damage causes a tissue-specific release of enzymes into the serum; their amounts are proportional to the extent of tissue damage. These released enzymes are often isoenzyme forms that are specific for a given tissue.

- The creatine kinase isoenzyme, MB form, is released from damaged heart tissue.
- Alanine aminotransferase is diagnostic for liver damage when it is elevated in the serum.

KEY POINTS ABOUT CELLULAR REGULATORY STRATEGIES

- There are four primary mechanisms by which cells regulate their metabolic pathways: compartmentation, gene regulation, covalent modification, and allosteric regulation.
- Proenzymes (and prohormones) are inactive storage forms of enzymes (or hormones) that are activated as needed by proteolytic removal of a portion of the proenzyme.
- Isoenzymes (isozymes) are alternative forms of the same enzyme activity that exist in different proportions in different tissues.
- Tissue damage causes a tissue-specific release of enzymes into the serum; their amounts are proportional to the extent of tissue damage.

Self-assessment questions can be accessed at www. StudentConsult.com.

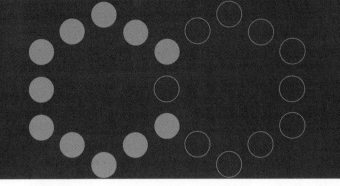

Membranes and Intracellular Signal Transduction

5

●●● MEMBRANE STRUCTURE AND COMPOSITION

Membranes are composed of various lipids, proteins, and carbohydrates that determine several important biologic functions. Their selective permeability affords both a physical and chemical compartmentation of intracellular enzyme systems. Membranes also contain enzymes and receptors that allow cells to respond selectively to external signals, as well as to generate chemical and electrical signals. Their selective permeability is regulated by molecular channels and pumps that extend between the two surfaces. Their external surface composition determines cell-to-cell recognition processes mediating cell adhesion and immune responses.

Membrane Components

The membrane lipids include phospholipids, sphingolipids, and cholesterol (see Chapter 11).

The phospholipids contain two fatty acids (usually 16 to 18 carbons) attached to glycerol in addition to a phosphate group. The fatty acids may be either unsaturated or saturated. Most phospholipids have ethanolamine, choline, inositol, or serine esterified to the phosphate.

The sphingolipids include sphingomyelin, cerebrosides, and gangliosides. The cerebrosides and gangliosides, sugar-containing lipids called glycosphingolipids, are located primarily in the plasma membrane. Sphingomyelin is prominent in myelin sheaths.

Cholesterol is primarily found in the plasma membrane with its hydroxyl group on the surface at the water interface.

Membranes are generally 40% to 50% protein but can range from extremes such as 20% protein in the myelin membrane to 80% protein in the inner mitochondrial membrane. Protein and lipid composition is unique for each membrane, and their distribution is asymmetric.

Integral Membrane Proteins
Integral membrane proteins may penetrate the membrane partially or may exist as transmembrane proteins interfacing with both the cytosol and external environment.

They interact strongly with the membrane lipids through hydrophobic side chains of amino acids and can only be removed by destroying membrane structure with detergent or solvent. They are usually composed of multiple α-helices with hydrophobic side chains; cylindrical arrays form pores for transport of polar molecules.

Peripheral Membrane Proteins
Peripheral membrane proteins are loosely associated with the surface of either side of the membrane; they interact with the membrane through hydrogen bonding or salt-bridging with membrane proteins or lipids and can be removed without disrupting the structure of the membrane.

Membrane carbohydrates exist only as extracellular covalent attachments to lipids and proteins (e.g., glycoproteins or glycolipids). Carbohydrate structures are highly variable and may be highly antigenic, thereby contributing to the immune recognition of cells.

Membrane Structure

Membranes achieve their selective permeability by separation of the internal and external aqueous compartments with a phospholipid bilayer. The bilayer is formed from two mono-layers, or leaflets, composed of phospholipids with the hydro-philic phosphate head groups oriented toward the aqueous solution and the hydrophobic fatty acid tails oriented toward the center of the bilayer (Fig. 5-1). The bilayers form sheetlike structures measuring between 60 and 100 Å in thickness and are held together entirely by noncovalent forces.

Although the bilayer structure is symmetric with respect to orientation of the amphipathic lipids (containing both hydro-philic and hydrophobic regions), the composition is asymmet-ric. For example, the red blood cell plasma membrane has the following phospholipid composition:

- *Exterior monolayer*: mostly sphingomyelin and phosphati-dylcholine
- *Interior monolayer*: mostly phosphatidylserine and phos-phatidylethanolamine

Cholesterol is more evenly distributed, with the precise composition determined by the function of the membrane.

Membrane proteins are distributed asymmetrically to pro-vide localization of enzyme activity, energy transduction through ion pumps, facilitated transport, and receptors for extracellular signals. Peripheral proteins often contain a lipid anchor that extends into the membrane.

Membrane composition and asymmetry are maintained by addition of new membrane structure to preexisting membrane structure. Self-assembly permits self-sealing of damage to the phospholipid bilayer.

Fluid Properties of Membranes

The assembly of proteins and lipids into a membrane creates a fluid mosaic, named for the fluid properties of its constituents. Both the proteins and lipids undergo two-dimensional lateral diffusion in membrane. Transverse diffusion is energetically very unfavorable; neither proteins nor lipids "flip-flop" from one side to the other, except when the process is catalyzed by enzymes called flippases.

Fluidity is affected by several factors:
- Long-chain saturated fatty acids interact strongly and reduce fluidity.
- Double bonds increase fluidity, greater with *cis*-configuration than with *trans*-configuration.
- Cholesterol prevents movement of fatty acid chains and reduces fluidity.
- Fluidity increases with temperature.

KEY POINTS ABOUT MEMBRANE STRUCTURE AND COMPOSITION

- Membranes serve several important functions: compartmenta-tion of enzyme systems, receptor recognition of hormone signals, generation of chemical and electrical signals, selective transport of molecules, and cell-to-cell recognition and adhesion.

- Membranes contain lipid, protein, and carbohydrate arranged in a fluid mosaic bilayer leaflet.

- Membrane lipids include phospholipids, sphingolipids, and cholesterol.

- Membrane proteins make up between 20% and 80% of a given membrane, but typically 40% to 50%.

- Integral membrane proteins are hydrophobic and cannot be iso-lated without destroying the membrane; peripheral membrane proteins are associated only with the surface and can be removed easily.

- Membrane carbohydrate is found on the external surface attached to proteins and lipids and helps determine immune recognition of cells.

- Membrane proteins and lipids are distributed asymmetrically and undergo lateral diffusion only.

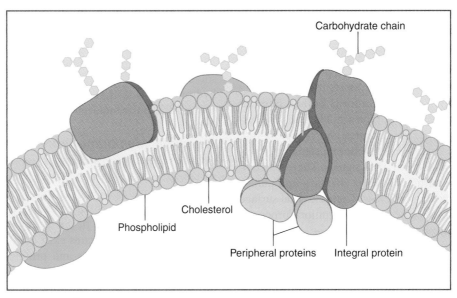

Figure 5-1. Membrane components.

●●● MEMBRANE TRANSPORT

The hydrophobic property of membranes effectively blocks the movement of hydrophilic molecules across the membrane. Furthermore, the structural integrity of the membrane restricts diffusion through the lipid bilayer. Thus movement of molecules across the membrane is governed by several forms of transport: simple diffusion, facilitated diffusion, and active transport.

Simple Diffusion

Water, gases (O_2, CO_2, NO), and lipophilic molecules (small fatty acids, steroids, urea, ethanol) cross membranes by simple diffusion. Simple diffusion always occurs down a concentration gradient and may be in either direction, depending only on the direction of the gradient. A steep concentration gradient produces faster diffusion than a shallow gradient, and smaller molecules diffuse faster than larger molecules. Simple diffusion is not saturable (i.e., the rate of diffusion increases linearly with the increase in substrate concentration gradient across the membrane).

Facilitated Diffusion

When molecules are excluded from simple diffusion owing to size or charge, facilitated diffusion mechanisms exist. Specialized carrier proteins in the membrane either diffuse across the membrane with their substrate or extend across the membrane, forming a channel.

Similarities to simple diffusion:
- Diffusion occurs down a concentration gradient.
- Energy is supplied by the gradient, not by cellular energy.
  Differences from simple diffusion:
- Facilitated diffusion is faster than simple diffusion.
- The carrier has specificity for the transported substance.
- Facilitated diffusion displays saturation (hyperbolic) kinetics (Fig. 5-2).

Carrier proteins are variously called translocases, porters, and permeases; their similarity to enzymes is shown by the following:
- Structural specificity for transported molecules.

- Dissociation constant for the transported molecule, Tm, analogous to K_m for enzymes.
- Inhibition by agents that block the transport of specific molecules.
- Exhibited saturation kinetics (V_{max}).

Facilitated diffusion has three primary modes: ion channels, uniporters, and cotransporters.

Ion channels are protein-lined channels that selectively allow ions to flow at a high rate when they are open. The ion channel is formed by multiple transmembrane domains of the specific ion channel protein. Some channels are referred to as "gated," since they are only opened transiently in response to specific signals. The signal for a ligand-gated channel is the binding of the specific ligand to a receptor. Voltage-gated channels respond to changes in the membrane potential.

Uniporters (Fig. 5-3) facilitate diffusion of single substances, such as glucose or a specific amino acid. The GLUT family of sodium-independent glucose transporters are uniporters that passively transport glucose (and/or galactose and fructose) into most cells. Alternative conformations of the transporter allow binding at the exterior surface (high glucose concentration) and release at the interior surface (low glucose concentration). Also, the discovery of aquaporins shows that water can also enter by facilitated diffusion.

Cotransporters transport more than one molecule simultaneously (see Fig. 5-3). Symporters carry two different molecules in the same direction at the same time, whereas antiporters carry two different molecules in opposite directions at the same time.

An example of a symporter is found in the kidney and intestine, where glucose must be transported from the lumen into the cell against a concentration gradient. The sodium-dependent glucose symporter relies on a gradient generated by active transport of sodium out of the cell (Fig. 5-4), then the downhill transport of sodium is coupled to the uphill transport of glucose.

An example of an antiporter is the chloride-bicarbonate transporter in erythrocyte membranes. Bicarbonate must undergo compensating transport with CO_2 (i.e., CO_2 in, HCO_3^- out). This is mediated by the chloride-bicarbonate exchanger (Fig. 5-5). Bicarbonate transport is accompanied by

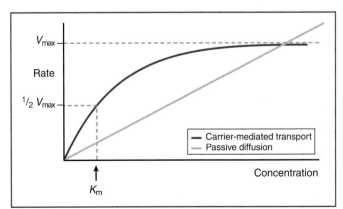

Figure 5-2. Comparison of carrier-mediated transport with passive diffusion. Carrier-mediated transport can reach saturation kinetics.

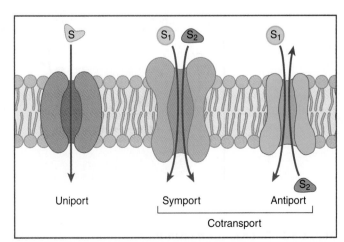

Figure 5-3. Uniport vs. cotransport.

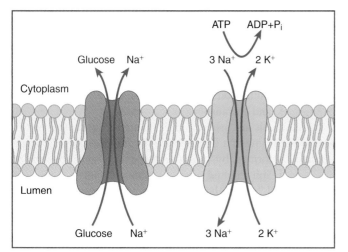

Figure 5-4. Sodium-dependent glucose transporter. The Na^+/K^+ adenosine triphosphate (*ATP*) pump maintains an Na^+ gradient for cotransport with glucose. *ADP*, adenosine diphosphate.

Cl^- transport in the opposite direction (antiport) to maintain electrical neutrality. Like other antiporters, the chloride-bicarbonate transporter works in either direction as determined by the concentration gradient (lungs or tissues).

Active Transport

Carrier proteins that transport molecules against a gradient can be directly coupled to hydrolysis of adenosine triphosphate (ATP) (i.e., hydrolysis of ATP provides the energy to drive the uphill transport process). This process is called active transport and is unidirectional. Like facilitated diffusion it is specific for the molecules being transported, it demonstrates saturation kinetics, and it can be specifically inhibited. Since it is tightly coupled to the hydrolysis of ATP, there is no ATP hydrolysis without transport.

The sodium/potassium ATPase (Na^+/K^+-ATPase) antiporter is an example of active transport. This active transport pump is located in the plasma membrane of every cell. It maintains low intracellular Na^+ and high intracellular K^+. This antiporter pumps 3 Na^+ out and 2 K^+ in for every ATP hydrolyzed (see Fig. 5-5).

KEY POINTS ABOUT MEMBRANE TRANSPORT

- Lipophilic molecules, including small, uncharged molecules such as water and oxygen, diffuse through membranes by simple diffusion down a concentration gradient.

- Specialized carrier proteins facilitate the diffusion of many molecules; they are specific for the molecule transported and move down a concentration gradient.

- Facilitated diffusion may involve more than one molecule in one direction (uniport), so that two molecules are exchanged (antiport) or transported together (symport).

- Active transport against a gradient is accomplished by coupling transport with ATP hydrolysis.

●●● INTRACELLULAR SIGNAL TRANSDUCTION

Hormones are physiologic signals that influence cellular metabolism by triggering a sequence of coordinated intracellular responses. The conversion of the signal from the hormone molecule to the final change in activity of the target enzymes is transmitted (transduced) through a signal transduction cascade. Since each reaction step in the cascade produces a catalyst as its product, each step in the cascade serves to amplify the signal. The signal can be lipophilic or hydrophilic (Table 5-1).

Plasma Membrane Receptors

Plasma membrane receptors are transmembrane proteins that generate an intracellular response following binding of hormones, cytokines, and other signals on the exterior surface of the cell. They share several characteristics with enzymes:

- Hormone binding induces a conformational change in the receptor protein (such as allosteric regulation).
- Hormone binding demonstrates reversibility (such as the enzyme-substrate complex).
- Hormone binding demonstrates inhibition (by antagonists; competitive or noncompetitive kinetics).

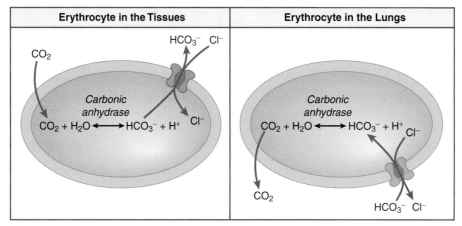

Figure 5-5. Chloride-bicarbonate transporter. Chloride is exchanged for bicarbonate to "pull" CO_2 from the tissues into the red blood cell. Reversal in the lungs allows for expiration of CO_2.

TABLE 5-1. Hormone Signals

CHARACTERISTIC	HYDROPHILIC	LIPOPHILIC
Intracellular messenger	cAMP, cGMP, phosphoinositides, diacylglycerol, Ca^{++}	Hormone-receptor complex
Duration of action	Minutes	Hours to days
Location of receptor	Plasma membrane	Intracellular
Type of hormone	Polypeptide hormones, growth factors, cytokines	Steroids, retinoids, calcitriol, thyroxine

The response to a given hormone can be positive or negative depending on which receptors are present. Receptor-hormone dissociation constants correlate with the physiologic concentrations of the hormones. Only a small fraction of the receptors needs to be occupied to provide an effective response.

PHARMACOLOGY

Cardiotonic Steroids

Digoxin and digitoxin (cardiotonic steroids) affect heart contractility by inhibiting Na^+/K^+-ATPase. This inhibits the calcium-sodium transporter, causing intracellular calcium to increase. The increased intracellular calcium augments myocardial contractility, producing a cardiotonic effect.

Cyclic Adenosine Monophosphate System—Epinephrine and Glucagon

When epinephrine and glucagon bind to their receptors, they send a wave of phosphorylation through the cell that leads to coordinated changes in metabolism. The initial signal that is generated in this pathway is the second messenger molecule, cyclic adenosine monophosphate (cAMP). cAMP is synthesized by a membrane-bound adenylate cyclase when the hormone binds to the receptor (Fig. 5-6). The concentration of cAMP is determined by the balance between adenylate cyclase and cAMP phosphodiesterase activity that degrades the cAMP to AMP.

The increased concentration of cAMP, in turn, allosterically converts more protein kinase A to its active form (Fig. 5-7). Protein kinase A regulates a variety of target proteins and enzymes by phosphorylation with ATP.

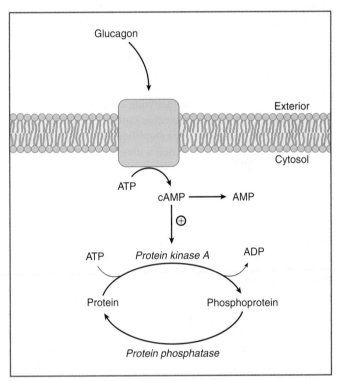

Figure 5-7. Activation of protein kinase A by cyclic adenosine monophosphate (*cAMP*). *ATP*, adenosine triphosphate; *ADP*, adenosine diphosphate.

PATHOLOGY

Cystic Fibrosis

Cystic fibrosis is due to a defective chloride ATPase pump in the epithelial cells of the lungs, intestines, skin, and pancreas. This leads to very high concentrations of Na^+ and Cl^- in sweat and the production of highly viscous mucus that obstructs the pancreatic and bile ducts and the airways in the lungs.

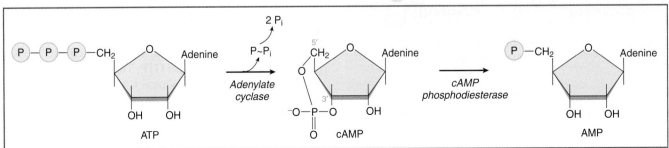

Figure 5-6. Synthesis and degradation of cyclic adenosine monophosphate (*cAMP*).

G-Protein–Mediated Signal Transduction

The epinephrine and glucagon receptors do not affect adenylate kinase directly. Instead they activate a G-protein complex that interacts with the adenylate cyclase. G-protein–coupled receptors contain seven α-helical domains (seven-helix motif) extending across the membrane. An extracellular domain contains the hormone-binding site, and an intracellular domain interacts with the G-proteins. The hormone receptor activates either stimulatory or inhibitory G-proteins (Table 5-2). The process for activation of adenylate cyclase (Fig. 5-8) follows:

1. Hormone binding causes a change in intracellular domain, allowing interaction with the heterotrimeric G_s protein.
2. The α-subunit of the G_s protein releases bound guanosine diphosphate (GDP) and binds guanosine triphosphate (GTP).
3. The α-subunit–GTP complex dissociates from the β-γ dimer and interacts with adenylate cyclase.
4. Binding one hormone molecule causes the formation of many active α-subunits; this amplifies the hormonal signal.
5. The α-subunit deactivates itself within minutes by hydrolyzing GTP to GDP (GTPase activity); the GDP remains bound.
6. The α-subunit–GDP complex reassociates with the β-γ dimer to form an inactive complex. (Note: Spontaneous GTP hydrolysis gives G-proteins an automatic deactivating mechanism.)

KEY POINTS ABOUT INTRACELLULAR SIGNAL TRANSDUCTION

- Plasma membrane receptors have a hormone recognition domain, one or more transmembrane domains, and an intracellular domain that generates the intracellular signal.

- cAMP is generated by adenylate cyclase and stimulates phosphorylation throughout the cell by allosteric activation of protein kinase A.

- The epinephrine and glucagon receptors act by causing the dissociation of the G_s subunit from its parent G-protein; the G_s subunit then stimulates adenylate cyclase.

- G-proteins have an automatic GTPase deactivating mechanism, since they are active only when GTP is bound.

- Inactivation of the active epinephrine hormone-receptor complex by phosphorylation desensitizes the receptor.

TABLE 5-2. Function of G-Proteins

G-PROTEIN	FUNCTION
G_s	Stimulates adenylate cyclase (cAMP pathway)
G_i	Inhibits adenylate cyclase
G_q	Stimulates phospholipase C (phosphoinositide pathway)
Transducin	Stimulates cGMP phosphodiesterase

cAMP, cyclic adenosine monophosphate; *cGMP,* cyclic guanosine monophosphate.

Desensitization to Epinephrine

The epinephrine receptor (β-adrenergic receptor) undergoes accommodation (physiologic response reduced upon repeated stimulation) to sustained, but unchanging, concentrations of epinephrine. As the G_s subunits dissociate from the receptor, the β-adrenergic receptor kinase phosphorylates the cytoplasmic domain of the receptor (see Fig. 5-8). The phosphorylated domain will not interact with G_s protein even with epinephrine bound to the receptor. Since the kinase phosphorylates only the hormone-receptor complex and not the free receptor, the concentration of epinephrine must increase to generate a new active hormone-receptor complex. If epinephrine levels remain constant, no active receptor is available, even if it binds epinephrine. In this way, the epinephrine sensitivity of the cell will decrease with constant stimulation, yielding a refractory state.

Phosphoinositide Cascade

Some hormones such as angiotensin II, epinephrine ($α_1$-receptors), vasopressin, and oxytocin stimulate the action of phospholipase C in the plasma membrane. Phospholipase C hydrolyzes phosphatidylinositol 4,5-bisphosphate (PIP_2) to produce two messenger molecules: inositol 1,4,5-trisphosphate (IP_3) and diacylglycerol (Fig. 5-9).

Inositol 1,4,5-Trisphosphate

IP_3 causes a rapid release of Ca^{++} from the endoplasmic reticulum by opening Ca^{++} channels. Cytosolic Ca^{++} then binds to the regulator protein, calmodulin. The Ca^{++}-calmodulin complex then activates Ca^{++}-calmodulin–dependent protein kinases. The Ca^{++}-calmodulin–complex also activates a Ca^{++}-ATPase pump, quickly restoring low intracellular $[Ca^{++}]$. Calcium is a potent enzyme activator, and its access to the cytoplasm is tightly regulated. The response is normally rapid and transient, paralleling the rate of muscle contraction. Free $[Ca^{++}]$ in the cytosol is normally around 100 nmol, whereas extracellular $[Ca^{++}]$ is 10,000-fold higher.

Smooth muscle contraction is activated by Ca^{++} through this signaling mechanism (see Fig. 5-9). Uncomplexed Ca^{++} also activates protein kinase C, which plays a role in platelet activation and prostaglandin action.

Diacylglycerol

Diacylglycerol (DAG) increases the activity of protein kinase C by increasing its affinity for Ca^{++}. Protein kinase C regulates target proteins by serine and threonine phosphorylation. Note that both IP_3 and DAG activate protein kinase C, but by different mechanisms.

The phosphoinositide-related hormones activate the G_q protein by allowing it to bind GTP. The active GTP-G_q complex then activates phospholipase C until its concentrations are reduced. Like the other G-proteins the G_q protein automatically inactivates itself by hydrolyzing its bound GTP. As hormone concentrations drop, so does the renewal of active G_q-GTP complex. Phosphatases degrade IP_3 to inositol, and DAG is degraded to phosphatidic acid.

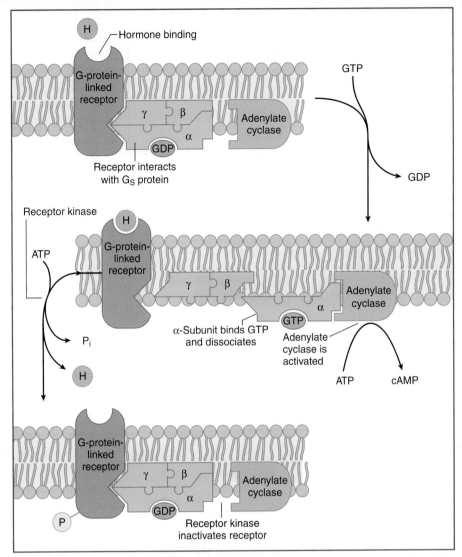

Figure 5-8. Epinephrine receptor activation of G_s protein. Dissociation of G_s protein permits guanosine triphosphate (*GTP*) binding followed by guanosine diphosphatase activity. Inactive guanosine diphosphate (*GDP*) G_s reassociates with G-protein and binds to receptor for next binding of hormone. Phosphorylation of intracellular domain of the hormone-receptor complex "desensitizes" response to constant levels of epinephrine. *ATP*, adenosine triphosphate; *cAMP*, cyclic adenosine monophosphate.

Tyrosine Kinase Receptors

Insulin and several other growth factors communicate their signal through tyrosine kinase receptors. Unlike the G-protein receptors, the tyrosine kinase receptors span the plasma membrane with only one α-helix. The intracellular domain has two types of tyrosine kinase catalytic activity:

1. The receptors phosphorylate themselves (autophosphorylation).
2. They phosphorylate tyrosine residues on target proteins that may, in turn, become signals themselves.

Insulin Receptor

The insulin receptor is a tetramer that is stabilized by internal disulfide bonds. Upon binding insulin to the external domain, the internal tyrosine kinase domain phosphorylates tyrosine residues on insulin receptor substrate 1 (IRS-1) to transduce the insulin signal by two pathways (Fig. 5-10):

1. IRS-1 converts phosphatidylinositol in the plasma membrane to PIP_2. Protein kinase B is then activated by binding to PIP_2. This route is used for short-term effects of insulin, such as increased glucose uptake and stimulation of glycogen synthase activity.
2. IRS-1 converts inactive ras (another type of G-protein) into its active GTP-bound form. Ras-GTP activates mitogen-activated protein (MAP) kinase, which then migrates to the nucleus to regulate gene expression. This route is used for the long-term effects of insulin such as increased glucokinase concentrations.

The insulin signal is terminated by endocytosis of the insulin-receptor complex in endosomes formed from clathrin-coated pits on the plasma membrane. (Clathrin is a membrane protein designed to form lattices around membranous vesicles.) The insulin is digested, leaving clathrin and the receptor intact; they then recycle to the plasma membrane.

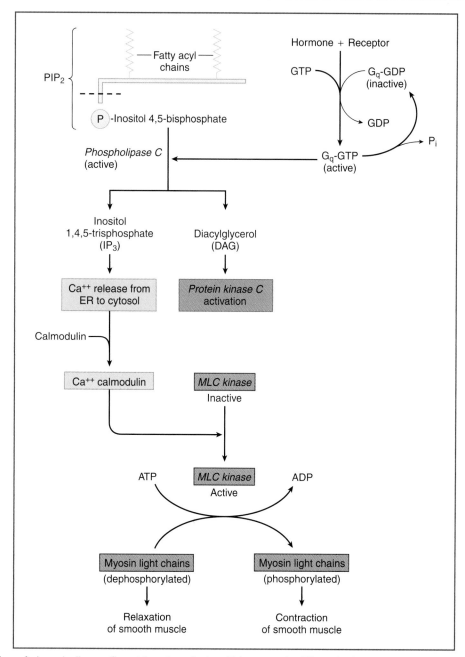

Figure 5-9. Activation of phospholipase C and the phosphoinositide cascade. *ER*, endoplasmic reticulum; *MLC*, myosin light chain; *PIP₂*, phosphatidylinositol 4,5-bisphosphate; *GTP*, guanosine triphosphate; *GDP*, guanosine diphosphate; *ATP*, adenosine triphosphate; *ADP*, adenosine diphosphate.

PHYSIOLOGY

Oxytocin and Vasopressin

Oxytocin and vasopressin act through the phosphoinositide pathway. Oxytocin stimulates smooth muscle contraction in the uterus and in the lactiferous ducts of the breast. Vasopressin (antidiuretic hormone) increases the permeability of the renal collecting cell duct membranes to water, permitting greater reabsorption.

Other Tyrosine Kinase Receptors

Monomeric tyrosine kinase receptors, like the epidermal growth factor receptor and platelet-derived growth factor receptor, aggregate on binding of the hormone. Their receptors also phosphorylate tyrosine residues and undergo autophosphorylation. Similar to insulin, they activate the MAP kinase pathway to regulate genes involved in cell division.

Nitric Oxide and Cyclic Guanosine Monophosphate

Nitric oxide (NO) activates the cytosolic form of guanylate cyclase, which increases the intracellular cyclic guanosine monophosphate (cGMP) concentration in vascular endothelial cells. cGMP relaxes smooth muscle and produces vasodilation. NO is synthesized by NO synthase from arginine and O_2, with reducing equivalents donated by reduced nicotinamide adenine dinucleotide phosphate. The short (10-second) life span of NO

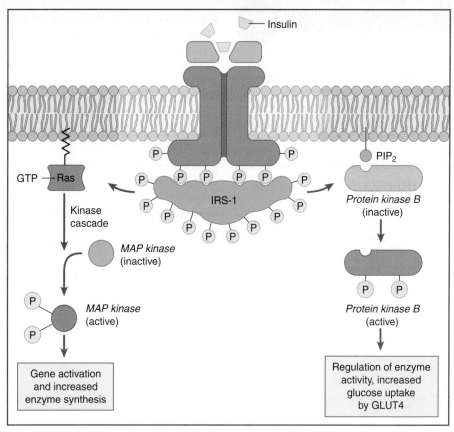

Figure 5-10. Insulin receptor with ras-dependent and ras-independent pathways. *MAP kinase*, mitogen-activated protein kinase.

confines its action close to its source of synthesis. However, it readily crosses membranes to enter target cells. Nitric oxide also stimulates bactericidal activity in macrophages, inhibits platelet aggregation, and serves as a neurotransmitter in that brain.

PATHOLOGY

***Ras* Oncogene**

Ras is a G-protein, and GTP-ras stimulates normal cell growth and differentiation. Its GTPase activity controls its action by spontaneously converting to its inactive GDP-ras form. This GTPase activity keeps cell growth under control. However, the oncogenic ras protein has very low GTPase activity and essentially adopts a constitutively active form. The cell responds as if high levels of growth factors were present, which leads to increased proliferation.

Intracellular Receptors of Lipophilic Hormones

Cytosolic receptors bind lipophilic hormones, such as the steroid hormones or retinoic acid (see Table 5-1). Cytosolic receptor-hormone complexes are transported to the nucleus, where they regulate gene expression. Their action is much slower than membrane receptor pathways, taking hours to days to reach full effect.

Clinical Aspects of Intracellular Signaling

Adenosine Diphosphate Ribosylation of G-Proteins

Several bacterial toxins catalyze the covalent attachment of adenosine diphosphate (ADP)-ribose to G-proteins:

- Cholera toxin ADP-ribosylates the G_s α-subunit. G_s is permanently activated and cannot hydrolyze GTP. This affects only intestinal mucosa; it produces excessive water and electrolyte secretion (i.e., diarrhea).
- Pertussis toxin ADP-ribosylates the G_i α-subunit. G_i is permanently inactivated and cannot inhibit adenylate cyclase; this produces whooping cough.
- Diphtheria toxin ADP-ribosylates eEF-2. This blocks polypeptide synthesis.

Erectile Dysfunction

The mechanism of erection of the penis involves release of NO in the corpus cavernosum as a result of sexual stimulation. The NO activates the enzyme guanylate cyclase, which results in increased levels of cGMP, producing smooth muscle relaxation in the corpus cavernosum and allowing inflow of blood. Drugs for treatment of erectile dysfunction enhance the effect of NO by inhibiting phosphodiesterase type 5, which is responsible for degradation of cGMP in the corpus cavernosum. This results in smooth muscle relaxation and inflow of blood to the corpus cavernosum.

MICROBIOLOGY

Cholera Toxin

The cholera toxin is produced by *Vibrio cholerae*, pertussis toxin is produced by *Bordetella pertussis*, and diphtheria toxin is produced by *Corynebacterium diphtheriae*.

KEY POINTS ABOUT INTRACELLULAR SIGNAL RECEPTORS

- The phosphoinositide cascade results when phospholipase C is stimulated by the G_q-GTP complex to produce diacylglycerol and IP_3.

- IP_3 creates a rapid release of Ca^{++} into the cell, forming a Ca^{++}-calmodulin complex that activates protein kinases. DAG activates protein kinase C.

- Insulin and other growth factors act through tyrosine kinase receptors that undergo autophosphorylation in addition to phosphorylation of tyrosine residues on signal proteins in the cytoplasm.

- NO is generated from arginine and stimulates guanylate cyclase to produce cGMP; this leads to relaxation of smooth muscle in blood vessels and vasodilation.

- Cytosolic receptors bind lipophilic hormones and regulate gene expression in the nucleus.

- Clinical manifestations of abnormal intracellular signaling include the action of bacterial toxins, unregulated cell growth, and erectile dysfunction.

Self-assessment questions can be accessed at www.StudentConsult.com.

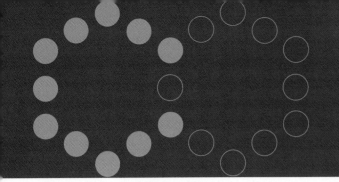

Glycolysis and Pyruvate Oxidation

6

●●● FIVE PERSPECTIVES FOR LEARNING METABOLISM

Intermediary metabolism is composed of interacting metabolic pathways involved in the extraction and/or storage of energy from fuel molecules. There are five perspectives that provide a consistent organization for reviewing these pathways:

1. Pathway reaction steps: Each reaction has unique characteristics with respect to substrates, products, enzymes, cofactors, and inhibitors.
2. Regulated reactions: Some steps in metabolism are regulated by hormones, metabolites, or both, so as to restrict or accelerate the flow of metabolites through a pathway.
3. Unique characteristics: Each pathway has features that describe unique aspects of its function and identify its general contribution to metabolism.

4. Interface with other pathways: Many metabolic intermediates are substrates for alternative pathways, providing a means for interfacing one pathway with another.
5. Related diseases: Reduced or absent activity of enzymes creates a buildup or reduced availability of metabolites, leading to imbalances in homeostasis.

●●● PATHWAY REACTION STEPS

Glycolysis—Glucose to Pyruvate

The glycolytic pathway is composed of two smaller pathways: (1) five reactions that require energy by converting glucose to triose phosphates, and (2) five reactions that produce energy by converting triose phosphates to pyruvate (Fig. 6-1).

Conversion of Glucose to Glyceraldehyde 3-Phosphate
Hexokinase (or glucokinase in liver)
Glucose is first phosphorylated with adenosine triphosphate (ATP), trapping glucose inside the cell. This is an irreversible step.

Phosphoglucose isomerase
Glucose 6-phosphate (G6P) is converted to its isomer, fructose 6-phosphate (F6P). This moves the carbonyl nearer to the middle of the molecule, preparing it to be divided into two triose (3-carbon) molecules.

Phosphofructokinase
Before F6P is cleaved, it acquires another phosphate from ATP, producing fructose 1,6-bisphosphate (F1,6-BP). Now the molecule can be split into two phosphorylated products, the triose phosphates.

Aldolase
Cleavage of F1,6-BP produces the triose phosphates: dihydroxyacetone phosphate (DHAP) and glyceraldehyde 3-phosphate (G3P).

Triose phosphate isomerase
DHAP is brought back into the glycolytic pathway by isomerization to G3P. In effect, this reaction allows two G3P molecules to be formed from one F1,6-BP.

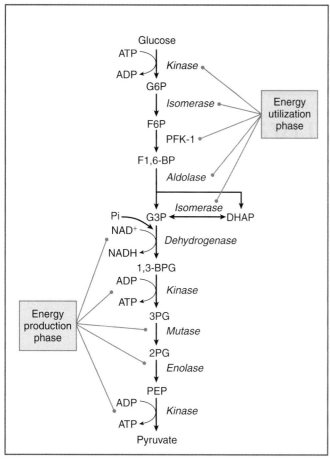

Figure 6-1. Glycolytic pathway reactions. See text for complete enzyme names and abbreviations.

Conversion of Glyceraldehyde 3-Phosphate to Pyruvate

Glyceraldehyde 3-phosphate dehydrogenase
Simultaneous oxidation and phosphorylation of G3P produces 1,3-bisphosphoglycerate (1,3-BPG) and nicotine adenine dinucleotide (NADH). Inorganic phosphate, rather than ATP, is used in this phosphorylation step.

Phosphoglycerate kinase
Transfer of a phosphate from 1,3-BPG to adenosine diphosphate (ADP) produces ATP and leaves 3-phosphoglycerate (3PG) to be metabolized further. This is one of three reactions that create ADP outside the oxidative phosphorylation process; it is known as substrate-level phosphorylation of ADP because an identifiable high-energy substrate, 1,3-BPG, donates a phosphate to ADP to make ATP.

Phosphoglyceromutase
The phosphate group is shifted to carbon 2 to produce 2-phosphoglycerate (2PG).

Enolase
Removal of a molecule of water produces phosphoenolpyruvate (PEP); fluoride inhibits enolase by combining with Mg^{++}. Fluoride is often included in blood collection tubes to prevent metabolism of glucose during blood transport and storage in the clinical laboratory.

Pyruvate kinase
Substrate-level phosphorylation of ADP with PEP produces ATP and pyruvate. (The third substrate level phosphorylation reaction occurs in the citric acid cycle.)

Pyruvate Oxidation—Pyruvate to Acetyl–Coenzyme A

After transport of pyruvate into the mitochondrial matrix, it is oxidized by a multienzyme complex, the pyruvate dehydrogenase complex (PDC). Pyruvate oxidation links glycolysis with the citric acid cycle. Three steps produce acetyl-coenzyme A (CoA) and NADH as the final products (Fig. 6-2).

Pyruvate Dehydrogenase
Pyruvate binds to thiamine pyrophosphate (TPP) on the pyruvate dehydrogenase (PDH) enzyme and undergoes decarboxylation. CO_2 is released, and two of the original carbons of pyruvate, in the form of a hydroxyethyl group, remain bound to TPP on the enzyme.

Dihydrolipoyl Transacetylase
The hydroxyethyl group is transferred from TPP to lipoic acid. During this transfer, the lipoic acid is reduced and the hydroxyethyl group is oxidized to an acetyl group, now attached to lipoic acid. The lipoyl group is attached to the dihydrolipoyl transacetylase, preventing the 2-carbon acetate intermediate from diffusing away. The acetate is subsequently transferred to CoA to produce acetyl-CoA. This leaves the lipoyl coenzyme in the reduced form, requiring reoxidation to its active form.

Dihydrolipoyl Dehydrogenase (Lipoamide Dehydrogenase)
The reduced lipoyl coenzyme is oxidized using flavin adenide dinucleotide (FAD) as a coenzyme. The electrons from the reduced form of FAD ($FADH_2$) are used to reduce NAD^+ to produce NADH as a reaction product.

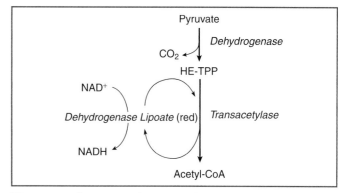

Figure 6-2. Sequence of reactions for the pyruvate dehydrogenase multienzyme complex. Lipoate alternates between a reduced form (*red*) and an oxidized form. The oxidized form has a disulfide bond. *HE-TPP*, hydroxyethyl thiamine pyrophosphate; *NADH*, nicotine adenine dinucleotide; *CoA*, coenzyme A.

KEY POINTS ABOUT PATHWAY REACTION STEPS

■ The first half of the glycolytic pathway uses energy, and the last half produces energy.

■ The enzymes in the PDH pathway are coordinated in a multienzyme complex.

●●● REGULATED REACTIONS

Regulation of Glycolysis

Glycolysis is regulated at three points, each serving a different function (Fig. 6-3). Hexokinase, present in all tissues except the liver, is allosterically inhibited by G6P. Hexokinase regulation ensures that cells do not take more glucose out of the blood, and away from the brain, than they really need. Liver contains glucokinase, an isoform of hexokinase that is not inhibited by G6P.

Phosphofructokinase (PFK-1) controls entry of G6P into glycolysis. When the rate of PFK-1 is slowed, G6P accumulates and is routed toward glycogen synthesis or the pentose phosphate pathway. PFK-1 is allosterically regulated by several effectors:

● *Fructose 2,6-bisphosphate (F2,6-BP)*: This effector is a "well-fed" signal that allosterically stimulates PFK-1 in the liver (Fig. 6-4). It is synthesized from F6P by PFK-2 when insulin (and glucose) levels are high. Elevated glucagon, a fasting hormone, inhibits PFK-2 and lowers F2,6-BP concentration.

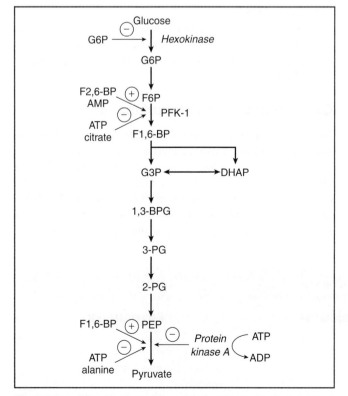

Figure 6-3. Regulated reactions in glycolysis. Each regulated step is irreversible. See text for expansion of all abbreviations.

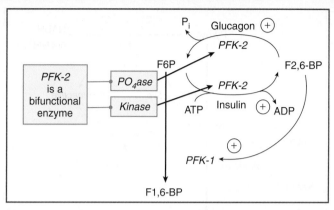

Figure 6-4. Regulation of phosphofructokinase (*PFK-1*) by fructose 2,6-bisphosphate (*F2,6-BP*). PFK-2 can act as either a kinase or a phosphatase. Glucagon increases the phosphatase activity by increasing the phosphorylated form of PFK-2. Insulin increases the kinase activity by increasing the dephosphorylated form. *PO₄ase*, phosphatase. See text for expansion of all abbreviations.

● Adenosine monophosphate (*AMP*): This effector is produced in increasing amounts from ATP during exercise. It allosterically stimulates PFK-1 in muscle, increasing glycolysis to restore the ATP concentrations to normal.
● *ATP and citrate*: These negative effectors slow glycolysis when energy is abundant.

Pyruvate kinase regulation controls the flow of PEP to pyruvate or to gluconeogenesis.

In well-fed conditions, pyruvate kinase is allosterically stimulated by F1,6-BP; this prevents a metabolic roadblock when PFK is active.

In fasting conditions, pyruvate kinase is allosterically inhibited by ATP and alanine (mobilized from muscle). This prevents PEP that is needed for gluconeogenesis from being converted directly back to pyruvate.

Regulation of Pyruvate Oxidation

The PDC is regulated by covalent modification of the first enzyme, pyruvate dehydrogenase (PDH). PDH kinase inactivates PDH by phosphorylation with ATP (Fig. 6-5). Reactivation is achieved by the action of PDH phosphatase. Both of these regulatory enzymes are regulated.
● PDH kinase is stimulated by NADH and acetyl-CoA. It is inhibited by pyruvate.
● PDH phosphatase is stimulated by Ca^{++} and insulin.

KEY POINTS ABOUT REGULATED REACTIONS

■ Glycolysis is regulated at the steps catalyzed by hexokinase, PFK-1, and pyruvate kinase.

■ The PDC is regulated by covalent modification through the action of a specific kinase and phosphatase; the kinase and phosphatase are regulated by changes in NADH, acetyl-CoA, pyruvate, and insulin.

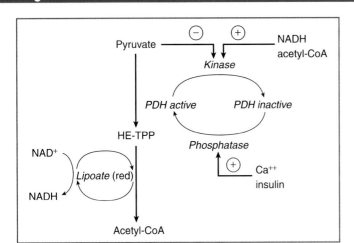

Figure 6-5. Regulation of the pyruvate dehydrogenase (*PDH*) complex. Only the first enzyme component, pyruvate dehydrogenase, is regulated. Both insulin and pyruvate stimulate production of the unphosphorylated, active form. The products of the reaction, nicotine adenine dinucleotide (*NAD*) and acetyl-coenzyme A (*CoA*), promote a lower percentage of the pyruvate dehydrogenase in the active form. *HE-TPP*, hydroxyethyl thiamine triphosphate.

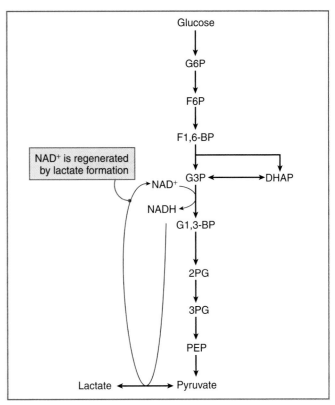

Figure 6-6. Formation of lactic acid from nicotine adenine dinucleotide (*NAD*$^+$) produced in glycolysis. See text for expansion of all abbreviations.

●●● UNIQUE CHARACTERISTICS

Anaerobic Glycolysis

The capacity to recycle NADH back to NAD$^+$ anaerobically (i.e., without mitochondrial involvement) serves important functions in several tissues.

Liver

Conversion of pyruvate to lactate to recycle NADH (Fig. 6-6) allows the liver to dispose of excess of either NADH (hypoxia, excessive alcohol consumption) or pyruvate (PDH deficiency) produced under conditions that alter normal physiology. The lactate can be either converted back to pyruvate when conditions return to normal or excreted in the urine. The net production of energy from anaerobic glycolysis is 2 ATP per glucose molecule; no CO_2 is produced.

Muscle

Fast-twitch muscle fibers possess a substantial capacity for glycolysis to supply energy rapidly. These muscle fibers contain high concentrations of lactate dehydrogenase to sustain high rates of glycolysis. Since these fibers are adapted to

anaerobic metabolism (the slow-twitch fibers are adapted to aerobic metabolism), they contain few mitochondria.

Red Blood Cells

The lack of mitochondria in red blood cells (RBCs) prevents oxidative phosphorylation as a source of ATP. Thus there is total reliance on anaerobic metabolism to provide energy for RBC functions.

Glucokinase Versus Hexokinase

Hexokinase exists in two different isoforms that have different kinetic and regulatory properties (Table 6-1).

Glucokinase, the isoform in liver, has kinetic properties that allow it to capture much of the dietary glucose that enters the liver from the intestines via the portal circulation. This high-capacity uptake provides glucose for conversion to glycogen or fatty acids. The high K$_m$ also minimizes the uptake of

TABLE 6-1. Comparison Between Glucokinase and Hexokinase		
CHARACTERISTIC	**GLUCOKINASE**	**HEXOKINASE**
Kinetic properties	K$_m$ = 5 mmol/L	K$_m$ = 0.1 mol/L
Substrate specificity	Glucose only	Glucose, fructose, and galactose
Inhibition by glucose 6-phosphate	Not inhibited	Inhibited
Insulin response	Induced by insulin	Constitutive

glucose by the liver during fasting, thereby preventing unnecessary synthesis of glycogen and the development of hypoglycemia. Glucokinase also is present in the pancreatic B cells that produce insulin so that the intracellular G6P increases only when the blood sugar is elevated following a meal. Insulin induces synthesis of glucokinase to help the liver adapt to repeated high-carbohydrate meals.

Hexokinase is the most widely distributed isoform. Its low K_m allows glucose to enter cells, especially brain cells and RBCs, under fasting conditions. Excess removal of glucose from the blood into tissues is prevented by the allosteric inhibition of hexokinase by its product, G6P.

HISTOLOGY

Cellular Compartmentation

The glycolytic pathway is compartmented in the cytoplasm, whereas the PDH pathway is compartmented within the mitochondrial matrix. These locations provide for more focused regulation of both pathways. Cells that rely on anaerobic glycolysis for their energy, such as fast-twitch muscle fibers and RBCs, have few to no mitochondria.

PHYSIOLOGY

Function of Glucokinase in B cells

The B cells in the pancreatic islets of Langerhans contain glucokinase instead of hexokinase to prevent the inappropriate secretion of insulin, which would lead to a persistent hypoglycemia. Since the elevated G6P serves as the insulin release signal, insulin is released only when blood glucose rises above the normal fasting levels.

Multienzyme Complexes

The PDC is an example of a large multienzyme unit that has a highly coordinated function. It is composed of multiple copies of three enzymes in a geometric arrangement that allows transfer of each reaction product to the next enzyme. This prevents intermediate products from diffusing, ensuring that the reaction goes to completion. Other examples of multienzyme complexes are α-ketoglutarate dehydrogenase, branched-chain ketoacid dehydrogenases, and fatty acid synthase.

Energy Production

The amount of ATP produced in the oxidation of glucose depends on the availability of O_2.

Under aerobic conditions, the complete conversion of glucose to CO_2 and water produces 36 to 38 ATP/glucose.

Under anaerobic conditions, the complete conversion of glucose to lactate (with regeneration of NAD^+) produces 2 ATP/glucose (see Fig. 6-6).

KEY POINTS ABOUT UNIQUE CHARACTERISTICS OF GLYCOLYSIS AND PYRUVATE OXIDATION

- When anaerobic conditions prevent the use of NADH produced in glycolysis, it is used by lactate dehydrogenase to form lactate; conditions that accelerate this reaction lead to lactic acidosis.
- Glucokinase is a specialized hexokinase in liver that allows for the rapid uptake of dietary glucose from the hepatic portal vein.

⬤⬤⬤⬤ INTERFACE WITH OTHER PATHWAYS

The metabolic pathway from glucose to acetyl-CoA has several branch points that connect with other metabolic pathways (Fig. 6-7).

Glucose 6-Phosphate

Since glucose 6-phosphate is also a product of gluconeogenesis, it serves as a substrate for glucose-6-phosphatase in the liver. The action of this enzyme releases free glucose into the bloodstream.

Conversion of glucose 6-phosphate to glucose 1-phosphate by phosphoglucomutase provides for interchange between

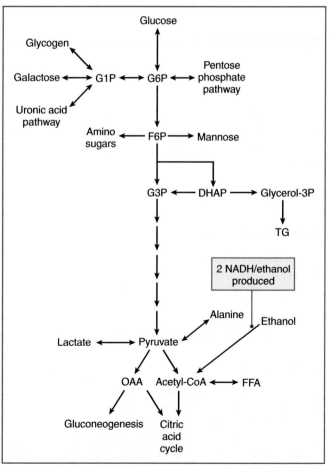

Figure 6-7. Intersection of glycolysis and pyruvate dehydrogenase reactions with other major metabolic pathways. *OAA*, oxaloacetate; *FFA*, free fatty acids. See text for expansion of other abbreviations.

glycogen, galactose, and uronic acid metabolism (see Chapters 8 and 9). First, glucose 1-phosphate is activated to the uridine diphosphate precursor, which then contributes to glycogen polymerization, to galactose metabolism, or to glucuronic acid formation.

If glucose 6-phosphate is oxidized by glucose 6-phosphate dehydrogenase, it enters the pentose phosphate pathway (see Chapter 9).

Fructose 6-Phosphate

F6P is the precursor for the synthesis of amino sugars, such as galactosamine and glucosamine. These amino sugars serve as precursors for glycoproteins and glycosaminoglycans (see Chapters 9 and 17).

In addition, F6P can be converted to mannose 6-phosphate, also a precursor for glycoprotein synthesis.

Dihydroxyacetone Phosphate

DHAP is converted to glycerol 3-phosphate by glycerol-3-phosphate dehydrogenase. This provides a source of glycerol 3-phosphate for triglyceride and phospholipid metabolism from the glycolytic pathway. It also provides a source of carbons for gluconeogenesis, since triglycerides are mobilized and the free glycerol is transported to the liver.

Pyruvate

When pyruvate is not being actively converted to acetyl-CoA, it is being converted to oxaloacetate by pyruvate carboxylase as a precursor for gluconeogenesis.

Pyruvate also is interconverted with alanine by alanine aminotransferase (see Chapter 12); when these processes are occurring between skeletal muscle and liver, the process is called the alanine cycle.

Pyruvate is interconverted with lactate in both skeletal muscle and liver during the Cori cycle.

Acetyl-Coenzyme A

Acetyl-CoA is both a precursor for fatty acid synthesis and the product of fatty acid β-oxidation.

Acetyl-CoA is also a product of ethanol catabolism and ketone body catabolism.

●●● RELATED DISEASES

Lactic Acidosis

Lactic acidosis is the result of an increase of lactate in the blood due to overproduction, generally occurring either in the liver or skeletal muscle. It is usually caused by an increase in the supply of NADH, but it may also be due to an increase in pyruvate. Lactic acidosis refers to the increased production of lactic acid, whereas lactic acidemia refers to the presence of excess lactate in the blood.

Increased NADH can result from hypoxia (e.g., as a result of exercise), acute respiratory distress syndrome, or shock (massive blood loss), since oxygen is required for oxidation of NADH in the mitochondrial electron transport chain (see Chapter 7). Slower electron transport also is accompanied by a drop in ATP production (thus an increase in AMP), causing an acceleration of glycolysis. This further increases the production of NADH.

Excess consumption of ethanol also will elevate NADH, since 2 NADH are produced for every molecule of ethanol that is catabolized to acetate.

An excess of pyruvate can result from PDH deficiency or pyruvate carboxylase deficiency (see Chapter 8). In addition, hypoxia-induced acceleration of glycolysis will produce pyruvate faster than it can be metabolized through the citric acid cycle.

Pyruvate Kinase Deficiency

Pyruvate kinase deficiency is the most common enzyme deficiency in the glycolytic pathway. Patients have only 5% to 25% of the normal level of the pyruvate kinase isoform found in erythrocytes. Since RBCs cannot use fats for metabolism, there is a severe reduction in the ability to produce ATP that leads to premature destruction of RBCs and a condition known as hemolytic anemia.

Pyruvate Dehydrogenase Deficiency

Deficiencies have been identified in each of the three enzyme components of the PDC. A deficiency in the conversion of pyruvate to acetyl-CoA leads to an increase in lactate (see previous discussion) and lactic acidosis. Since the amount of pyruvate entering the citric acid cycle is dramatically reduced, the overall energy supply to the cell is reduced, leading to myopathy (e.g., movement disorders) and neuropathy (e.g., encephalopathy).

GENETICS & PATHOLOGY

Pyruvate Kinase Deficiency

Pyruvate kinase deficiency is the most common glycolytic enzyme deficiency. Since the conversion of PEP to pyruvate is critical for the net production of ATP, a reduction in the energy needed for electrolyte balance leads to an osmotic imbalance and to RBC swelling and rupture and produces hemolytic anemia.

PHYSIOLOGY

Lactic Acidosis

PDH deficiency prevents the oxidation of pyruvate, leading to its accumulation in the cytoplasm. This increases the conversion of pyruvate to lactate and produces an increase in both blood lactate and pyruvate. The protons that accompany these anions are neutralized by the serum bicarbonate, creating a metabolic acidosis with an increased anion gap. Lactic acidosis is one of several metabolic acidosis conditions caused by the accumulation of organic acids in the blood (e.g., ketoacidosis, methylmalonic acidemia).

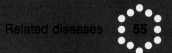

Arsenate and Arsenite Poisoning

Arsenate poisoning is due to the uncoupling of substrate level phosphorylation by G3P dehydrogenase. Arsenate is a structural analog of phosphate and is incorporated into 3PG to form an unstable mixed anhydride. The end result is the release of arsenate without the formation of ATP. This eliminates the net gain of ATP from anaerobic glycolysis and is therefore most damaging to the RBC. Aerobic cells are affected when arsenate is incorporated into ATP during oxidative phosphorylation with the subsequent spontaneous hydrolysis to produce ADP and free arsenate. In both cases, the heat associated with ATP hydrolysis is also released.

Arsenite poisoning is due to the covalent reaction of arsenite with lipoic acid, thus preventing it from transferring the hydroxyethyl group from thiamine to CoA.

KEY POINTS ABOUT METABOLIC PATHWAYS AND CLINICAL DISEASES

■ Interchange with other major pathways occurs with G6P, F6P, DHAP, pyruvate, and acetyl-CoA.

■ Pyruvate kinase deficiencies produce hemolytic anemia as a result of lower intracellular concentrations of ATP.

Self-assessment questions can be accessed at www.StudentConsult.com.

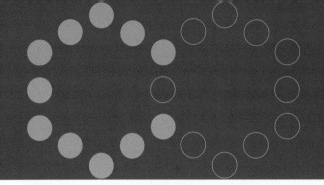

Citric Acid Cycle, Electron Transport Chain, and Oxidative Phosphorylation

7

●●● PATHWAY REACTION STEPS

Citric Acid Cycle—Acetyl–Coenzyme A to CO_2

The citric acid cycle (CAC) accepts the 2-carbon acetyl-coenzyme A (CoA) molecule and oxidizes it completely to CO_2 and H_2O. Energy is obtained in three forms: nicotine adenine dinucleotide (NADH), flavine adenine dinucleotide ($FADH_2$), and guanosine triphosphate (GTP). Note that in comparison with the glycolytic pathway, none of the CAC intermediates are phosphorylated. The CAC is composed of two smaller energy-capturing pathways (Fig. 7-1): (1) four reactions that assimilate acetyl-CoA and then remove both of its carbon atoms as CO_2 to produce succinate, and (2) four reactions that convert succinate back to oxalo-acetate (OAA).

Citrate to Succinyl–Coenzyme A
Citrate synthetase
Acetyl-CoA condenses with OAA to form citrate and free CoA.

Aconitase
Citrate is isomerized to isocitrate. Aconitase forms *cis*-aconitate as an enzyme-bound intermediate in this reversible reaction.

Isocitrate dehydrogenase
Isocitrate undergoes oxidative decarboxylation, producing the 5-carbon α-ketoglutarate. Oxidative decarboxylation produces free CO_2 and NADH.

α-Ketoglutarate dehydrogenase
The 5-carbon α-ketoglutarate undergoes oxidative decarboxylation to succinyl-CoA. This produces the second CO_2 and one more NADH.

Succinyl–Coenzyme A to Oxaloacetate
Succinate thiokinase
CoA is removed from succinyl-CoA, producing free succinate; this is coupled with substrate-level phosphorylation of guanosine diphosphate (GDP) to GTP.

Succinate dehydrogenase
Succinate is oxidized to fumarate, producing $FADH_2$; this enzyme is part of the succinate-Q reductase (complex II) in the electron transport chain (ETC).

Fumarase
The fumarate double bond is hydrated to form malate.

Malate dehydrogenase
Malate is oxidized to OAA with production of NADH; this returns the cycle to the beginning, with OAA available to condense with another molecule of acetyl-CoA.

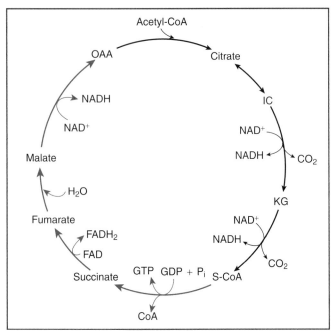

Figure 7-1. Steps in the citric acid cycle pathway. *IC*, isocitrate; *KG*, α-ketoglutarate; *S-CoA*, succinyl-coenzyme A; *OAA*, oxaloacetate. See text for expansion of other abbreviations.

HISTOLOGY

Mitochondria as Symbionts

Exchange between the mitochondrial matrix and the cytoplasm is highly selective and requires specific transporters. This is consistent with the concept of the mitochondrion as a highly specialized derivative of a symbiotic prokaryote. The DNA of mitochondria is circular, and its ribosomes also have prokaryotic characteristics. An increase in the number of mitochondria requires DNA replication and fission of the original mitochondrion into two daughter mitochondria. This process serves the purpose of allowing separate regulation for cytoplasmic and mitochondrial metabolism. The mitochondria are not true symbionts, however, since most of the mitochondrial proteins are specified by the nuclear DNA.

KEY POINTS ABOUT THE CITRIC ACID CYCLE

- The CAC releases both carbons from acetyl-CoA as CO_2 and produces NADH, $FADH_2$, and GTP.

- The CAC has three points of regulation—the most important of which is IDH—that are controlled by the supply of adenosine triphosphate (ATP) and NADH.

- The CAC serves as a metabolic traffic circle that receives carbon skeletons from amino acids and fatty acids and donates carbon skeletons to amino acids and porphyrins.

- An increase in flow of acetyl-CoA into the CAC is made possible by pyruvate carboxylase conversion of pyruvate to OAA, thus providing substrate to combine with the increased amount of acetyl-CoA.

Electron Transport Chain and Oxidative Phosphorylation—NADH/H$^+$/FADH$_2$ and O$_2$ to H$_2$O

The concept of a metabolic pathway for electron transport and oxidative phosphorylation is not very different from that of other metabolic pathways except that the products and reactants are almost entirely electrons and protons rather than metabolites. Instead of an occasional reduction/oxidation step, this mechanism applies to every step in the ETC. Another difference regarding the production of protons is that protons in other metabolic pathways are simply buffered. However, the protons produced during electron transport are pumped from the mitochondrial matrix to the inner membrane space, where they form a proton gradient across the inner mitochondrial membrane.

Electron Transport Chain

All enzyme complexes involved in the ETC and oxidative phosphorylation (ATP synthesis) are embedded in the inner mitochondrial membrane (Fig. 7-2). Therefore the ETC and ATP synthesis are isolated from the cytoplasm but exposed to the metabolites in the matrix, such as adenosine diphosphate (ADP) and NADH.

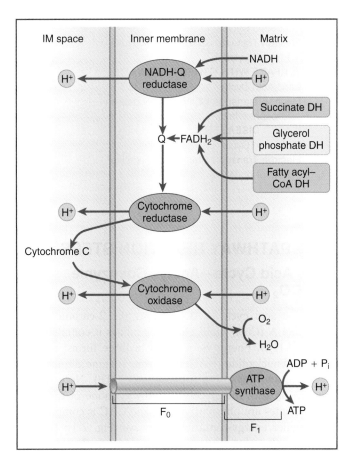

Figure 7-2. Steps in the electron transport chain. The entire pathway is a sequence of oxidation and reduction steps. *IM*, intermembrane. See text for expansion of other abbreviations.

NADH-Q reductase (also known as NADH dehydrogenase or complex I)

This multisubunit complex transfers electrons from NADH in the mitochondrial matrix (and not from NADH in the cytoplasm) to coenzyme Q through its riboflavin coenzyme, flavin mononucleotide (FMN).

Succinate-Q reductase (complex II)

Similar to complex I, this multisubunit complex donates electrons from a riboflavin coenzyme, $FADH_2$, to coenzyme Q. This complex contains three enzymes, all of which have FAD as a prosthetic group:
- Succinate dehydrogenase, from the CAC
- Glycerol-3-phosphate dehydrogenase, from the glycerol phosphate shuttle
- Fatty acyl–CoA dehydrogenase, from the first step in β-oxidation of fatty acids

Coenzyme Q

Coenzyme Q, a lipid-soluble quinone (Fig. 7-3), also known as ubiquinone, accepts electrons from $FMNH_2$ in complex I and $FADH_2$ in complex II and carries them rapidly by diffusion through the inner mitochondrial membrane to cytochrome c reductase (complex III).

Cytochrome c reductase (complex III)

This multisubunit complex accepts electrons from coenzyme Q and donates them to cytochrome c. Two of the protein components of complex III are cytochrome b and cytochrome c_1.

Cytochrome c

This water-soluble protein diffuses along the surface of the inner membrane facing the intermembrane space (between the outer and inner mitochondrial membranes) to transfer electrons from complex III to complex IV.

Cytochrome oxidase (complex IV)

This multisubunit protein transfers electrons from cytochrome c to O_2. Two of the protein components of complex IV are cytochromes a and a_3. This complex is unique in the ETC in having copper as a component. However, copper is a common component in other oxidase enzymes that also react with O_2. The product of O_2 reduction by the ETC is a water molecule. One molecule of water is produced for each molecule of NADH or $FADH_2$ oxidized in the ETC.

PHARMACOLOGY

Zidovudine and Fat Metabolism

Mitochondrial DNA replication enzymes are sensitive to nucleoside analogs, such as zidovudine (AZT), that are used in HIV therapy. This causes a reduction in the mitochondrial population and a reduced ability to metabolize fats. The CAC, which is contained only in the mitochondria, is an absolute necessity for fat metabolism, since the main product of fat oxidation is acetyl-CoA.

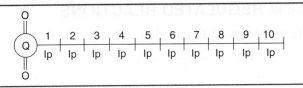

Figure 7-3. Structure of coenzyme Q. This quinone (Q) is made very hydrophobic by adding 10 isoprene units (*lp*) as a "tail." Isoprene is formed in the pathway for cholesterol synthesis.

Proton Pumping and Adenosine Triphosphate Synthesis

Complex I, complex III, and complex IV pump several protons into the intermembrane space for every pair of electrons that they transport to O_2. A sufficient number of protons are pumped to maintain a 10:1 concentration gradient (one pH unit) between the intermembrane space and the matrix.

Adenosine triphosphate synthase complex

The ATP synthase complex (F_oF_1-ATP synthase) allows protons to flow back into the matrix and uses the free energy change from this process to synthesize ATP from ADP and inorganic phosphate P_i. It is located in knob-shaped structures embedded in the cristae (invaginations of the inner mitochondrial membrane) and extending into the matrix.
- The F_o protein (the "o" in F_o refers to its sensitivity to oligomycin, a poison that blocks the flow of protons) extends through the inner mitochondrial membrane and serves as the proton channel between the intermembrane space and the matrix.

  The ATP synthase (F_1-ATPase) is attached to the F_o protein on the inside of the matrix. F_1-ATPase uses the protons flowing into the matrix to bind ADP and P_i and release ATP. The F_1-ATPase is named by the reverse reaction it catalyzes when it is isolated from mitochondria and thus uncoupled from the proton gradient.

KEY POINTS ABOUT THE ELECTRON TRANSPORT CHAIN

- The ETC is located in the mitochondrial inner membrane and contains several different kinds of electron carriers: FMN, iron-sulfur proteins, coenzyme Q, heme-containing cytochromes, and copper ions.

- Three large multiprotein complexes serve as proton pumps by harnessing the energy from electron flow through the ETC to oxygen; in turn, the chemiosmotic energy in the proton gradient that is created by the pumps is coupled to the synthesis of ATP by the (F_1-ATPase) complex.

- ATP regulates its own synthesis and the flow of electrons through respiratory control; if ATP synthesis slows down, electron transport slows down and vice versa.

- Cytosolic NADH cannot pass through the mitochondrial membrane, so it shuttles its electrons through the glycerol phosphate shuttle and the malate-aspartate shuttle.

- ATP and ADP are transported in exchange for each other by the ATP/ADP translocase.

●●● REGULATED REACTIONS

Regulation of Citric Acid Cycle

There are three main regulatory points for the CAC (Fig. 7-4). More than one site of regulation is needed to allow shunting of carbons into gluconeogenesis (OAA) during fasting or into fat (citrate) after feeding. Note that acetyl-CoA input into the cycle is substantial in both fasting (from β-oxidation) and feeding (from glycolysis).

Isocitrate dehydrogenase (IDH) is the primary regulation point, the "pacemaker," for the CAC. It is the only allosteric enzyme in the cycle and is stimulated by ADP; ATP and NADH allosterically inhibit this enzyme. Thus, when energy needs are met, isocitrate levels increase and shift the equilibrium to increase citrate. Citrate can then be transported out of the mitochondrion as an acetyl carrier for fat synthesis, or it can inhibit citrate synthase (CS), to redirect OAA into gluconeogenesis.

CS is inhibited by an increase in its product, citrate, or a decrease in the substrate, OAA. Thus an increase in citrate will prevent the entry of acetyl-CoA into the CAC, causing acetyl-CoA to be shunted toward the pathway that forms ketone bodies (see Chapter 10).

α-Ketoglutarate dehydrogenase complex (KGDC) is inhibited by its products, NADH and succinyl-CoA.

Regulation of Electron Transport Chain and Oxidative Phosphorylation

An isolated ETC that is uncoupled from ATP synthesis will transport electrons and pump protons as fast as O_2 can diffuse to the cytochrome oxidase and be reduced to water. However, in the cell, the ETC is tightly coupled to ATP synthesis, exerting a regulatory effect on the flow of electrons. Tight coupling prevents unnecessary O_2 consumption when the ATP supply is adequate. This is termed respiratory control. Oxygen is not consumed unless energy is needed, and the rate of oxygen consumption increases with energy needs (e.g., during exercise).

- Electron transport and O_2 consumption increase when ADP becomes plentiful.
- Electron transport and O_2 consumption decrease when ADP becomes limiting.
- Likewise, any condition that slows or blocks electron transport will slow the synthesis of ATP (see Related Diseases section).

●●● UNIQUE CHARACTERISTICS

Citric Acid Cycle

Anaplerosis

As the concentration of acetyl-CoA entering the CAC increases, a proportional increase in OAA is required for the formation of citrate. To provide the additional OAA, pyruvate is converted directly to OAA by pyruvate carboxylase (Fig. 7-5). This process of replenishment is referred to as anaplerosis. Pyruvate carboxylase is allosterically stimulated by acetyl-CoA, ensuring that increased formation of acetyl-CoA stimulates increased formation of OAA by pyruvate carboxylase.

Energy Production

Each molecule of acetyl-CoA that enters the CAC produces the equivalent of 12 ATP. Although substrate-level phosphorylation produces GTP, it is readily converted to ATP. The total energy produced by oxidation of one mole of glucose through the CAC is 36 to 38 moles of ATP.

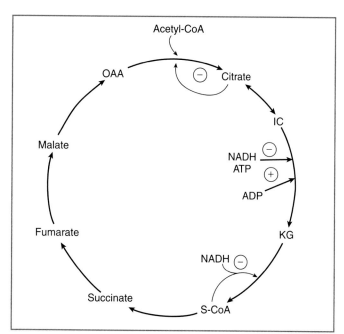

Figure 7-4. Regulated reactions in the citric acid cycle. Each regulated step is irreversible. See text for expansion of all abbreviations.

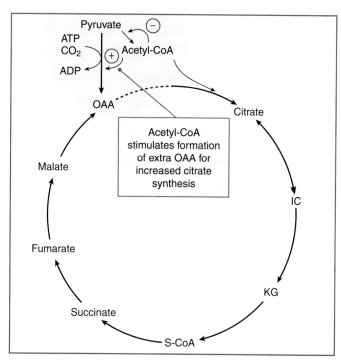

Figure 7-5. Anaplerosis: pyruvate carboxylase catalysis of pyruvate conversion to oxaloacetate. See text for expansion of all abbreviations.

Multien...

Both pyr
KGDC i
to the p
bind an
followed
is then t
behind
lipoic ac
ponents
function
identica

Electr
Phosp

Iron-S

Iron-su
(Fig. 7-
bound
in the
transpo
tion an

Heme

The cy
partici

The
the sa
ever,
the he
dized

The
slightl
long

Cher

The
ATP
chem
wher

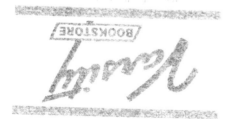

Fig
elemental and cysteine (...)... ing
with iron (*Fe*).

---

free energy state is used to pump protons and create the proton gradient, thus transforming electrochemical energy into chemiosmotic energy.

There are three sites where the free energy change is sufficient to do work in the form of proton pumping—complexes I, III, and IV:

- 3 ATP are generated for every electron pair donated by NADH.
- 2 ATP are generated for every electron pair donated by $FADH_2$.
- Complete oxidation of glucose to CO_2 yields between 36 and 38 ATP. The difference is determined by the shuttle mechanism used to transport NADH-reducing equivalents from the cytoplasm (see Interface with Other Pathways section).

P/O Ratio

The P/O ratio is a calculation of the moles of ATP synthesized per mole of O_2 consumed.

- NADH produces 3 ATP for each pair of electrons and therefore has a P/O ratio of 3.
- $FADH_2$ produces 2 ATP for each pair of electrons and therefore has a P/O ratio of 2.
- Leaky membranes (i.e., those in which electron transport and phosphorylation of ATP are uncoupled) have a low P/O ratio because many of the protons reenter the mitochondrial matrix by pathways independent of the ATPase.

●●● INTERFACE WITH OTHER PATHWAYS

Citric Acid Cycle

The CAC interfaces with several other pathways (Fig. 7-7). It serves not only as a destination for the oxidation of carbon skeletons from amino acids but also as a source of precursors for biosynthesis pathways.

If the citrate concentration increases beyond that needed for energy generation by the CAC, then it is transported to the cytoplasm, where it is converted to acetyl-CoA and OAA by citrate lyase (see Chapter 10).

Carbon skeletons from deamination of amino acids enter at acetyl-CoA, α-ketoglutarate, succinyl-CoA, fumarate, or OAA. Carbons entering the CAC at succinyl-CoA, fumarate, or OAA can contribute their carbon skeletons to gluconeogenesis; they are termed glucogenic (see Chapter 12).

α-Ketoglutarate and OAA can leave the cycle, also through transamination, to be used for the synthesis of the carbon skeletons of the nonessential amino acids.

Succinyl-CoA can leave the cycle to serve as a precursor in the synthesis of porphyrins (see Chapter 12). It can also contribute to the use of ketone bodies in peripheral tissues by donating its CoA group to acetoacetate. Succinyl-CoA is formed from propionyl-CoA, a product of odd-chain fatty acid oxidation and the catabolism of several amino acids.

Acetyl-CoA carbons are always oxidized to CO_2 and energy and never contribute carbon skeletons to gluconeogenesis. Therefore, fatty acid carbons cannot be used for glucose synthesis even though the fatty acids can be used to energize this pathway.

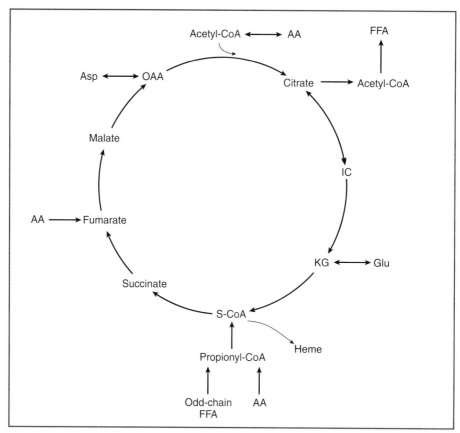

Figure 7-7. Intersection of the citric acid cycle with other metabolic pathways. See text for expansion of abbreviations.

Electron Transport Chain and Oxidative Phosphorylation

The ETC has three intermediates that interface with other pathways of metabolism: NADH, $FADH_2$, and ADP.

NADH Interfaces

NADH input to the ETC is primarily derived in the mitochondrial matrix from the CAC, the PDC, and β-oxidation. A second source of NADH is the cytoplasm, but it has to be supplied indirectly by a shuttle mechanism because the mitochondrial inner membrane is impermeable to NADH. The shuttle that transports NADH into the mitochondrion is termed the malate-aspartate shuttle (Fig. 7-8), since it relies on specific transporters for malate and aspartate in the mitochondrial inner membrane.

- OAA in the cytosol is reduced to malate, regenerating NAD^+ from NADH.
- Malate is transported to the mitochondrial matrix and oxidized back to OAA, producing NADH in the mitochondrial matrix.
- OAA is then transaminated to aspartate, which is transported to the cytoplasm by exchange with glutamate.
- The shuttle cycle is completed by transamination of aspartate back to OAA, which can then be reduced again by cytoplasmic NADH.
- All reactions in the malate-aspartate shuttle are reversible and can reverse to increase cytoplasmic NADH under abnormal conditions that increase the matrix concentration of NADH (e.g., hypoxia).

HISTOLOGY

Mitochondrial Composition
The mitochondrial inner membrane is structurally and functionally more complex than the outer membrane. It is composed of about 80% protein and is highly selective in its permeability. The ETC is located entirely within foldings of the inner membrane called cristae, structures that are more prominent in metabolically active cells. While NADH-Q reductase is specified by the mitochondrial DNA, the remainder of the enzymatic composition of the inner membrane is specified by the nuclear DNA.

Flavine Adenine Dinucleotide Interface

$FADH_2$ input to the ETC is primarily derived from the citric acid cycle and β-oxidation. However, another source of $FADH_2$ is from the cytoplasm, and it is supplied by a second shuttle mechanism that is designed to transport electrons from cytoplasmically generated NADH. This is termed the glycerol phosphate shuttle (see Fig. 7-8), since it relies on both a cytoplasmic and a mitochondrial form of glycerol phosphate dehydrogenase (GPDH).

- NADH is used by the cytoplasmic form of GPDH to reduce dihydroxyacetone phosphate (DHAP) to glycerol 3-phosphate.
- Glycerol 3-phosphate then diffuses into the intermembrane space.

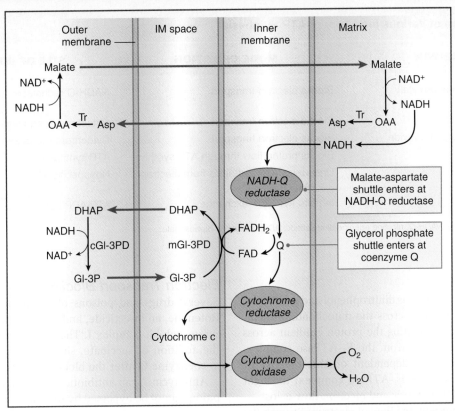

Figure 7-8. Shuttle mechanisms for cytoplasmic nicotine adenine dinucleotide (*NADH*). The malate-aspartate shuttle *(top)* produces NADH in the matrix for entry into the electron transport chain at NADH-Q reductase. The glycerol phosphate shuttle *(bottom)* produces flavine adenine dinucleotide (*FADH₂*) in the mitochondrial inner membrane so that it enters the electron transport chain at complex II by reducing coenzyme Q. *Gl-3P*, glycerol 3-phosphate; *cGl-3PD*, cytoplasmic glycerol-3-phosphate dehydrogenase; *mGl-3PD*, mitochondrial glycerol-3-phosphate dehydrogenase; *IM*, intermembrane; *Tr*, transaminase; DHAP, dihydroxyacetone phosphate.

- The mitochondrial GPDH localized in the inner mitochondrial membrane oxidizes the glycerol 3-phosphate to DHAP with a transfer of electrons to $FADH_2$. This $FADH_2$ is localized within the membrane and donates its electrons directly to coenzyme Q through complex II.

Adenosine Diphosphate/Adenosine Triphosphate Translocation

ADP has access to the F_1-ATPase only from the matrix side of the inner membrane. Therefore, the cytoplasmic ADP has to be transported into the matrix by ATP-ADP translocase. This membrane transporter operates by facilitated exchange diffusion (antiport). It is specific for ADP and ATP; thus the exchange of ATP and ADP is tightly coupled.

●●● RELATED DISEASES

Citric Acid Cycle

The crucial and central role of the CAC in metabolism is underscored by the fact that there are few identified enzyme deficiencies in this complex pathway. Thus a deficiency in any of the CAC enzymes will either be incompatible with life or will produce a mitochondrial myopathy that impairs energy metabolism.

The importance of the CAC in metabolism is underscored by a potent environmental poison, fluoroacetate.

It is considered to be a suicide substrate, since it is activated to fluoroacetyl-CoA, which then undergoes condensation with OAA to produce fluorocitrate, a potent inhibitor of aconitase. This inhibition blocks any conversion of citrate to isocitrate, thus preventing any CAC activity. Fluoroacetate is formed in some plants after uptake of fluoride from water, air, or soil. This has resulted in the poisoning of field workers and livestock. Fluoroacetate also enters aquatic ecosystems by way of atmospheric degradation of hydrofluorocarbons to fluoroacetate. Originally used in purified form as a rodenticide, this compound has been banned because of its extreme toxicity.

Electron Transport Chain and Oxidative Phosphorylation

Abnormalities associated with the ETC and oxidative phosphorylation are caused by inherited enzyme deficiencies, drugs, or poisons (Table 7-1).

Inherited Defects

Leber Hereditary Optic Neuropathy

A mutation in mitochondrial DNA reduces the activity of complex I (NADH-Q reductase). It is characterized by a loss of central vision and eventual blindness due to degeneration of the optic nerve.

TABLE 7-1. Action of Various Inhibitors of ATP Synthesis

INHIBITOR	MODE OF ACTION	SITE OF INHIBITION
Rotenone, amobarbital (Amytal) (barbiturate)	Blocks electron transport	NADH-Q reductase
Antimycin A (antibiotic)	Blocks electron transport	Cytochrome reductase
Cyanide, azide, carbon monoxide	Blocks electron transport	Cytochrome oxidase
Oligomycin	Blocks proton flow through ATP synthase	ATP synthase
Dinitrophenol	Uncouples ATP synthesis from electron transport	Nonspecific site
Atractyloside	Inhibits ATP-ADP exchange	ATP-ADP translocase

ATP, adenosine triphosphate; *NADH-Q*, nicotine adenine dinucleotide; *ADP*, adenosine diphosphate.

Uncouplers

Lipophilic organic acids, such as dinitrophenol and pentachlorophenol, can carry protons across the mitochondrial membrane effectively, short-circuiting the proton gradient across the membrane at sites away from the F_1-ATPase complex. Since respiratory control is dependent on the integrity of the proton flow through the F_1-ATPase complex, the tight coupling between ATP synthesis and electron flow is lost.

Uncouplers allow unregulated flow of electrons through the ETC to O_2. Because the flow of protons through the F_1-ATPase synthase complex is reduced, the P/O ratio is reduced. The energy that would have been captured in the ATP high-energy bond is lost as heat, resulting in hyperthermia.

PHARMACOLOGY

Cyanide Antidotes

The inhibitory action of cyanide on electron transport is due to its tight binding to the copper ions in cytochrome oxidase. Since this poison blocks at the last step in the ETC, there is no effective antidote that will bypass the block. The only effective antidotes aim to remove the cyanide with nitrates (inducing methemoglobin formation to bind the cyanide) or thiosulfate (which hastens the conversion of cyanide to the less toxic thiosulfate). In general, treatment involves the use of both compounds.

PHARMACOLOGY

Pentachlorophenol Poisoning

Pentachlorophenol is a volatile lipophilic wood preservative that is readily absorbed through the lungs. Since it uncouples oxidative phosphorylation from the ETC, the transfer of electrons to O_2 proceeds unregulated, greatly increasing the O_2 demand of the tissues. Any of the energy from the proton gradient that would have been captured in ATP is released as heat, creating a potentially fatal hyperthermia. There is no specific antidote for pentachlorophenol poisoning.

Electron Transport Blockers

Several drugs and poisons block the ETC at various sites. Rotenone, an insecticide, and amobarbital (Amytal), a barbiturate, inhibit complex I. The inhibition can be bypassed by the addition of succinate, since its electrons enter the ETC at coenzyme Q after the block (Fig. 7-9).

Antimycin A, an antibiotic, inhibits complex III. This inhibition cannot be bypassed by succinate, since it is downstream

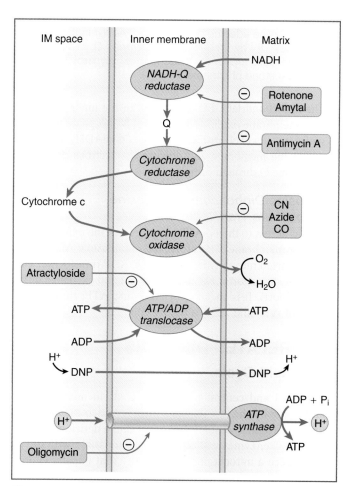

Figure 7-9. Inhibitors of adenosine triphosphate synthesis. *IM*, intermembrane. See text for expansion of other abbreviations.

from coenzyme Q, but the inhibition can be bypassed by ascorbate, which can reduce cytochrome c directly.

All carriers upstream of the block become highly reduced, and all carriers downstream from the block become oxidized. Owing to the tight coupling of respiratory control, ETC blockers reduce the synthesis of ATP.

Adenosine Triphosphate/Adenosine Diphosphate Translocase Inhibition

Inhibition of the ATP/ADP translocase by atractyloside, a plant toxin, depletes the supply of ADP in the matrix as it is converted to ATP. As ATP synthesis slows owing to the lack of ADP, respiratory control also slows the flow of electrons through the ETC. Addition of an uncoupler such as deoxyribonucleoprotein will allow electron transport and O_2 consumption to resume.

Adenosine Triphosphate Synthase Complex Inhibition

Proton flow through the F_1-ATPase complex is blocked by the antibiotic oligomycin. This blocks ATP synthesis and the flow of electrons through the ETC. As in the case of atractyloside inhibition, addition of deoxyribonucleoprotein uncouples respiratory control and allows electron transport and O_2 consumption to resume.

Self-assessment questions can be accessed at www. StudentConsult.com.

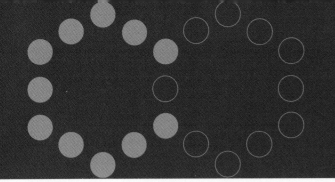

Gluconeogenesis and Glycogen Metabolism

8

●●● PATHWAY REACTION STEPS

Gluconeogenesis—Oxaloacetate to Glucose

Gluconeogenesis is an anabolic pathway that synthesizes glucose from nonglucose precursors (lactate, amino acids, and glycerol). Since the nonglucose precursors must be mobilized and transported to the liver, this source of glucose does not have the rapid response found with glycogen mobilization (covered later in more detail).

The gluconeogenic pathway is not a simple reversal of glycolysis (Fig. 8-1). There are three steps in glycolysis that are energetically irreversible: hexokinase, phosphofructokinase (PFK), and pyruvate kinase. The gluconeogenic pathway is thus a mixture of six enzymes that are needed to bypass these three irreversible steps, plus the remainder of the glycolytic steps, which are reversible.

Bypass for Pyruvate Kinase (Phosphoenolpyruvate → Pyruvate)
Pyruvate carboxylase
Carboxylation of pyruvate produces oxaloacetate (OAA). This is an energy-requiring reaction that uses adenosine triphosphate (ATP).

Malate dehydrogenase (mitochondrial)
Reduction of OAA produces malate, which can be transported out of the mitochondrion. This step simultaneously transports carbon skeletons and reduces equivalents to the cytoplasm for gluconeogenesis.

Malate dehydrogenase (cytoplasmic)
Oxidation of malate in the cytoplasm regenerates OAA and nicotine adenine dinucleotide. The latter is needed at reaction step 8 (glyceraldehyde-3-phosphate dehydrogenase; see later discussion).

Phosphoenolpyruvate carboxykinase
Decarboxylation of OAA to produce phosphoenolpyruvate is accompanied by phosphorylation using guanosine triphosphate (GTP) instead of ATP.

KEY POINTS ABOUT GLUCONEOGENESIS

- Gluconeogenesis is not a simple reversal of glycolysis; three irreversible glycolytic steps must be bypassed.

- The gluconeogenic pathway begins in the mitochondrion and ends in the cytoplasm; it consumes 6 ATP per glucose.

- Gluconeogenesis is regulated at the pyruvate carboxylase step, where acetyl-CoA from fatty acid oxidation serves as an allosteric activator; glycolysis is reciprocally regulated to avoid futile cycles.

- The carbon skeletons come from amino acids, lactate, and glycerol, and never from acetyl-CoA.

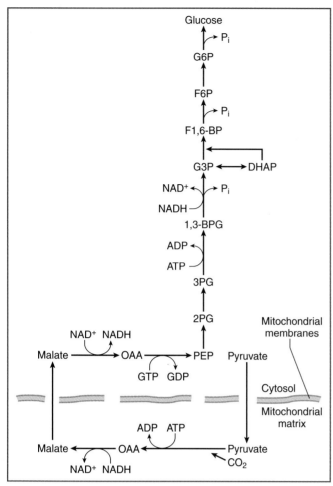

Figure 8-1. The gluconeogenic pathway. P_i, inorganic phosphate; *F6P,* fructose 6-phosphate; *NADH,* nicotine adenine dinucleotide; *PEP,* phosphoenolpyruvate; *GDP,* guanosine diphosphate; *BPG,* bisphosphoglycerate; *PG,* phosphoglycerate. See text for expansion of other abbreviations.

Bypass for Phosphofructokinase (*F1,6-BP → F6P*)
Fructose 1,6-bisphosphatase

Dephosphorylation of fructose 1,6-bisphosphonate (F1,6-BP) produces fructose 6-phosphate and inorganic phosphate.

Bypass for Hexokinase (*G6P → Glucose*)
Glucose-6-phosphatase

Dephosphorylation of glucose 6-phosphate (G6P) produces free glucose that can be released into the bloodstream.

Glycogen Metabolism—Glucose 6-Phosphate to and from Glycogen

Glycogen serves the unique purpose of providing a rapid source of glucose. The liver stores glycogen to provide rapid replenishment of blood glucose during fasting. Muscle and other tissues store glycogen as a source of intracellular glucose to be oxidized for energy. As noted above, gluconeogenesis provides a delayed source of glucose. The requirement for mobilization of free fatty acids and amino acids delays any significant supply of glucose from gluconeogenesis for several hours.

Glycogen synthesis (glycogenesis) involves the creation of an activated precursor and then the linking of the precursor into a linear growing polymer. Branching is achieved by removing and rejoining short sections from the end of the linear polymers. Glycogenolysis is likewise relatively simple. Only one enzyme is needed to release most of the glucose from glycogen; a second enzyme is needed to remove the branching sugar (Fig. 8-2).

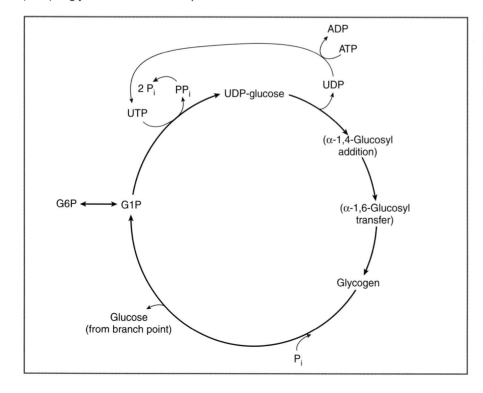

Figure 8-2. Glycogen synthesis and glycogenolysis pathways. *PP_i,* inactivated phosphorylase; *UTP,* uridine triphosphate; *P_i,* inorganic phosphate. See text for expansion of other abbreviations.

Three Reactions Create the Glucose Donor Uridine Diphosphate Glucose
Phosphoglucomutase
G6P is converted to glucose 1-phosphate (G1P) in a reversible reaction.

Uridine diphosphate glucose pyrophosphorylase
G1P is esterified with uridine triphosphate to produce uridine diphosphate (UDP)-glucose and pyrophosphate.

Pyrophosphatase
This irreversible reaction produces inorganic phosphate and provides the driving force for glycogen synthesis.

Two Reactions Use Uridine Diphosphate Glucose to Build Glycogen
Glycogen synthase
Glucose units from UDP-glucose are always transferred in an α-1,4 linkage to the C4 terminus of an existing amylose chain. Since the UDP is released from carbon 1, the ring structure of the newly added glucose residue is held closed in the ring form (nonreducing).

Branching enzyme
As the linear polymer grows, seven terminal residues are removed from an 11-residue amylose chain; it is reattached in an α-1,6 linkage to form a branch point. Branches are always at least four residues from the previous branch point.

One Reaction Depolymerizes Glycogen to Produce Glucose 1-Phosphate
Glycogen phosphorylase
The glycosidic α-1,4 bond is cleaved with inorganic phosphate to produce G1P monomers. Phosphorylase requires pyridoxal 5′-phosphate as a cofactor.

One Enzyme Catalyzes Two Reactions to Debranch Glycogen
Debranching enzyme contains two functional domains, a glucosyltransferase and a glucosidase, that remove the branches in glycogen.

Oligo 1,4 → 1,4 glucan transferase (glucosyltransferase)
Phosphorylase stops four glycosyl residues from branch points, producing a structure called a limit dextrin. Each branch point has two four-glycosyl residue branches. Glucosyltransferase moves three glycosyl residues from one branch to the end of the other branch.

α-1,6–Glucosidase (amylo-1,6–glucosidase)
The remaining glycosyl residue is released as free glucose. Thus about 80% of glucose is released from glycogen in the activated form: G1P.

One Reaction Converts Glucose 1-Phosphate Back to Glucose 6-Phosphate
Phosphoglucomutase
G1P is freely interconverted with G6P in a reversible equilibrium.

KEY POINTS ABOUT GLYCOGEN METABOLISM

- Glycogen synthesis and degradation flow through G1P, which is in equilibrium with G6P.
- The D form of glycogen synthase can react quickly to sudden changes in blood glucose; it is allosterically activated by G6P.
- The highly branched structure of glycogen allows for rapid release of glucose, since phosphorylase acts on the end terminal residues.
- In addition to its role as a precursor for glycogen synthesis, UDP-glucose helps detoxify waste products and drugs.
- Two high-energy bonds are consumed for each glucose stored in glycogen.
- cAMP-directed phosphorylation has reciprocal regulatory effects on glycogen synthase (inhibition) and phosphorylase (activation).

●●● REGULATED REACTIONS
Regulation of Gluconeogenesis

Since gluconeogenesis and glycolysis have opposite directions, their response to regulatory signals must be opposite or they would work against each other in futile cycles (i.e., energy would be used to synthesize a product, which is then immediately hydrolyzed by a reaction that effectively reverses the biosynthetic reaction. Reciprocal regulation refers to coordinated regulation of opposing pathways by the same metabolic signal (Fig. 8-3).

The gluconeogenesis pathway is primarily regulated at the pyruvate carboxylase reaction. This enzyme controls the entry of pyruvate into gluconeogenesis, and it requires acetyl–Coenzyme A (CoA) as a positive allosteric effector. Thus when fatty acids are mobilized to provide the energy for glucose synthesis, the acetyl-CoA produced during β-oxidation serves as a chemical signal to increase this first step in gluconeogenesis (Fig. 8-4). Overexpression of pyruvate carboxylase in mice produces diabetes.

Regulation also occurs at the fructose 1,6-bisphosphatase reaction. To prevent futile cycling with the PFK reaction during the fasting state, glucagon action causes fructose 2,6-bisphosphate (F2,6-BP) concentrations to decrease. This simultaneously removes both the inhibition of fructose 1,6-bisphosphatase and the stimulation of PFK by F2,6-BP.

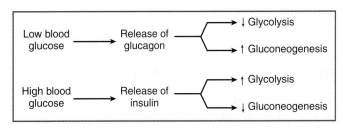

Figure 8-3. Reciprocal regulation of glycolysis and gluconeogenesis.

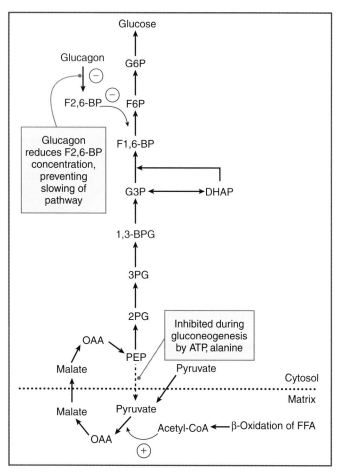

Figure 8-4. Regulation of pyruvate carboxylase and fructose 1,6-bisphosphatase *(F1,6-BP)* during gluconeogenesis. *F6P*, fructose 6-phosphate; *BPG*, bisphosphoglycerate; *PG*, phosphoglycerate; *PEP*, phosphoenolpyruvate; *FFA*, free fatty acid. See text for expansion of other abbreviations.

The flow of carbon skeletons for glucose synthesis into the gluconeogenic pathway is favored by an increased supply of amino acids from skeletal muscle to provide increased amounts of OAA. The inhibition of pyruvate dehydrogenase also prevents a flow of pyruvate carbons into the citric acid cycle, which is already supplied with acetyl-CoA from mobilized free fatty acids.

PHYSIOLOGY

Insulin/Glucagon Ratio

The insulin/glucagon ratio regulates gluconeogenesis and glycogenolysis to maintain blood sugar. High ratios reduce glucose formation, and low ratios increase glucose formation.

Regulation of Glycogen Metabolism

Glycogen synthesis is regulated with respect to both number and size of the glycogen particles (molecules) and the rate of polymerization.

All new glycogen molecules begin with a primer glycoprotein, glycogenin. When glycogen synthase acting at the nonreducing ends becomes separated from the glycogenin primer, synthesis stops. This requirement for glycogenin contact limits the size of the glycogen molecule and prevents indefinite growth. The total number of glycogen particles is determined, therefore, by the number of glycogenin primers.

The rate of polymerization is determined by phosphorylation of glycogen synthase (Fig. 8-5). The phosphorylated form, the D (dependent) form, is a less active form, but is not inactive—it has basal activity and can be stimulated by G6P. Eventually glycogen synthase is dephosphorylated to the I (independent) form that is fully active, even at low G6P concentration.

Glycogenolysis is regulated by controlling glycogen phosphorylase activity.

Phosphorylation of glycogen phosphorylase, under the influence of glucagon, activates it to remove glucosyl residues from the nonreducing ends of the glycogen particle. Dephosphorylation converts the enzyme to an inactive form.

Glycogen synthesis and glycogenolysis are controlled reciprocally. The cyclic adenosine monophosphate (cAMP) signal causes glucose to be mobilized from glycogen by its reciprocal regulation of glycogen synthase and phosphorylase.

Either glucagon (liver) or epinephrine (liver and muscle) stimulates an increase in the cellular cAMP levels (see Chapter 5).

cAMP activates protein kinase A to phosphorylate both the synthase and phosphorylase, but with opposite effects. The synthase is inactivated, whereas the phosphorylase is activated.

As insulin levels rise and glucagon and epinephrine levels decrease, the intracellular cAMP levels also drop. This leads to the activation of protein phosphatase 1 that dephosphorylates both enzymes, activating the synthase and inactivating the phosphorylase (see Fig. 8-5).

●●● UNIQUE CHARACTERISTICS

Energy Cost of Gluconeogenesis

Gluconeogenesis requires a total of six high-energy bonds to synthesize glucose from pyruvate: four from ATP (pyruvate carboxylase and 3-phosphoglycerate-dehydrogenase) and two from GTP (phosphoenolpyruvate carboxykinase).

Carbon Skeletons for Glucose

Although acetyl-CoA from fatty acid oxidation provides the energy for gluconeogenesis, it does not supply the carbon skeletons for net synthesis of glucose. Acetyl-CoA is metabolized in the citric acid cycle. Both carbons from acetyl-CoA are released as CO_2 during the cycle, leaving no residual carbon for gluconeogenesis. The carbon skeletons come only from molecules that can be converted to *OAA* (pyruvate, amino acids) or dihydroxyacetone phosphate (glycerol).

Location of Glucose 6–Phosphatase

G6Pase is found only in gluconeogenic tissues that release free glucose into the bloodstream: the liver, kidney, and small intestinal epithelium. G6Pase is absent in skeletal muscle, preventing any G6P produced from muscle glycogen mobilization from being released into the bloodstream.

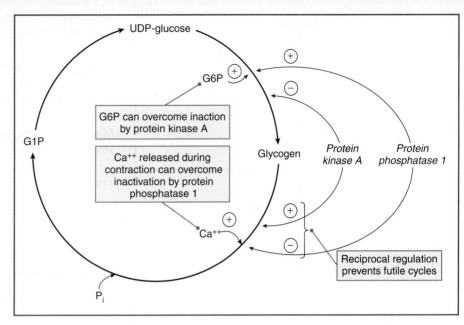

Figure 8-5. Regulation of glycogen metabolism. Inactivated glycogen synthase can be allosterically stimulated by glucose 6-phosphate (*G6P*), and inactivated phosphorylase (*PP$_i$*), (dephospho-form) can be stimulated by calcium ions (*Ca^{++}*). *P$_i$*, inorganic phosphate. See text for expansion of other abbreviations.

Function of Branched Glycogen Structure

Branching of the glycogen molecule serves several functions: it increases its solubility compared with a linear molecule, and it also increases the rate of both synthesis and breakdown. The nonreducing ends are the site of action for both processes. Note that branching occurs by a transfer reaction, not by polymerization.

Energy Cost of Storing Glucose as Glycogen

Each glucose added to the glycogen molecule expends two high-energy phosphate bonds from uridine diphosphate.

Allosteric Control of Glycogen Synthase Covalent Regulation

The D form of glycogen synthase in both liver and muscle responds quickly to change in glucose availability. It is allosterically activated by G6P (see Fig. 8-5). This allows immediate reactivation when glucose concentrations rise quickly after a meal, even before release of insulin from the pancreas.

The inactive (dephospho-) form of phosphorylase in muscle can be temporarily activated by Ca^{++} ions that directly stimulate phosphorylase kinase b, the enzyme that activates the

phosphorylase enzyme (Fig. 8-6). The release of Ca^{++} from the sarcoplasmic reticulum is triggered by the nerve impulse that contracts the muscle fiber, and the activation of phosphorylase provides glucose via glycogenolysis (see Fig. 8-5).

Glycogen Reducing End Versus Nonreducing Ends

Because of the polymerization of each new glucose monomer at the carbon 1 position, all sugar residues in the glycogen molecule are in the form of cyclic acetals, making them non-reducing ends. The only end that could be called the reducing end is the glucose residue attached to glycogenin. That is because if it were hydrolyzed from the glycogenin, it would be able to open at carbon 1 and undergo a redox color reaction with Fehling reagent (see Chapter 2).

●●● INTERFACE WITH OTHER PATHWAYS

Gluconeogenesis

The gluconeogenic pathway has several interfaces with other pathways (Fig. 8-7). For other glucogenic amino acids, see Chapter 12.

Figure 8-6. Cascade activation of glycogen phosphorylase. Each step in the cascade produces an amplification since the product of the reaction is also a catalyst. *PP$_i$*, inactivated phosphorylase; *P$_i$*, inorganic phosphate. See text for expansion of other abbreviations.

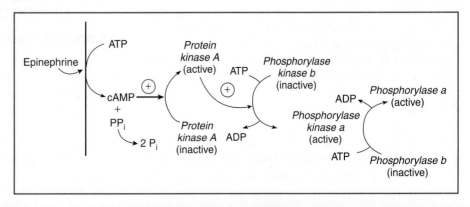

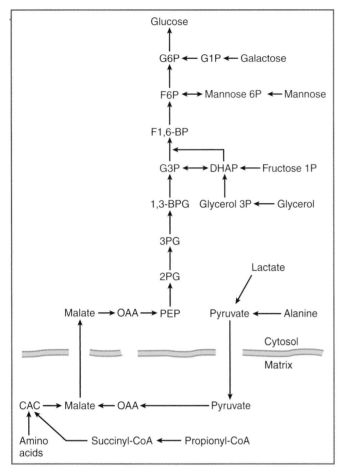

Figure 8-7. Interface of gluconeogenesis with other metabolic pathways. *F6P*, fructose 6-phosphate; *BPG*, bisphospho glycerate; *PG*, phosphoglycerate; *PEP*, phosphoenol pyruvate.

Lactate

The conversion of lactate to pyruvate provides about 30% of the glucose for gluconeogenesis in liver. Lactate is cycled from skeletal muscle and red blood cells to liver for conversion to glucose in a process known as the Cori cycle.

Alanine

Alanine is the primary amino acid that supplies carbon atoms for glucose by transamination to pyruvate. Alanine also serves a major role in transporting amino acid nitrogen from tissues to the liver for disposal in the urea cycle (see Chapter 12).

Propionyl-Coenzyme A

Propionyl-CoA is a product of odd- and branched-chain fatty acid oxidation and is also produced by the catabolism of several amino acids. Its conversion to succinyl-CoA, a citric acid cycle intermediate, allows production of malate that is transported to the cytosol and converted to OAA.

Glycerol

Free glycerol is released from triglycerides in fasting or starvation conditions due to the mobilization of fatty acids. It is phosphorylated by glycerol kinase, found only in the liver, to form glycerol 3-phosphate. Glycerol 3-phosphate

dehydrogenase then converts it to dihydroxyacetone phosphate (DHAP) for gluconeogenesis.

Dihydroxyacetone Phosphate

Fructose 1-phosphate is converted during fructose catabolism to glyceraldehyde and DHAP.

Mannose 6-Phosphate

Fructose 6-phosphate is interconverted with mannose 6-phosphate (converted to guanosine diphosphate mannose, a precursor for mannose and fucose residues in glycoproteins).

Galactose

G1P is the end product of galactose metabolism.

Glycogen Metabolism

The pathways of glycogen metabolism interface with glycolysis, gluconeogenesis, and the uronic acid pathway.

Glucose 1-Phosphate

The reversible interconversion between G1P and G6P can route glucose released during glycogenolysis to gluconeogenesis or glycolysis.

In muscle, G6P cannot be dephosphorylated, since it lacks the G6P enzyme. Thus, it is routed entirely through the glycolytic pathway to produce energy for muscle contraction.

In the liver, G6P is converted to glucose by G6Pase and released into the blood.

G1P is also produced during galactose metabolism, providing a route either for storage in glycogen or for conversion to G6P (see Chapter 9).

Uridine Diphosphate Glucose

UDP-glucuronic acid is formed from UDP-glucose by oxidation of its glucose moiety. UDP-glucuronate reacts with metabolic waste products and drugs; this results in a water-soluble conjugate called a glucuronide. Glucuronides are formed in liver and excreted in bile (e.g., bilirubin, morphine, and steroid hormones are excreted as glucuronides).

Glucuronic acid is a source of L-ascorbic acid in most mammals, except in primates (including humans) and guinea pigs.

●●● RELATED DISEASES OF GLUCONEOGENESIS AND GLYCOGEN METABOLISM

Idiopathic Neonatal Hypoglycemia

Newborns have a critical need for gluconeogenesis. The supply of glucose from the placenta is interrupted, but no glucose is immediately available from the diet. Since the brain must have a sustained source of glucose from blood, the genes for the gluconeogenic enzymes are simultaneously activated at birth. Occasionally this activation does not occur, and the newborn must be fed a glucose solution or it will experience hypoglycemia.

Glycogen Storage Diseases

Genetic deficiencies of the enzymes involved in glycogen metabolism result in abnormalities in the amount and/or structure of glycogen in tissues and in other metabolic abnormalities related to the use of glycogen, such as hypoglycemia or muscle weakness. The most serious of these diseases, von Gierke disease, results from deficiency of G6Pase that is needed to release glucose into the bloodstream. This prevents glucose from either glycogenolysis or gluconeogenesis from being released by the liver. The hypoglycemia that is produced causes an excess of free fatty acids to be released, leading to ketosis (Table 8-1).

PATHOLOGY

Glucose 6-Phosphatase Deficiency

G6P deficiency (von Gierke disease) leads to a glycogen storage disease accompanied by lactic acidosis. Patients also have ketoacidosis, hyperlipidemia (tendon xanthomas), prolonged prothrombin time (due to platelet abnormalities), and hyperuricemia (gout).

MICROBIOLOGY & IMMUNOLOGY

Amylopectinosis

A defective branching enzyme produces abnormal glycogen (amylopectinosis), leading to an autoimmune attack on the liver, which produces cirrhosis.

HISTOLOGY

Lysosomal Glycogen Digestion

A deficiency of α-1,4-glucosidase (generalized glycogenosis, or Pompe disease) prevents lysosomal digestion of glycogen. Although glycogen is synthesized and degraded enzymatically, it is continuously digested in the lysosomes as part of its normal cellular turnover.

Self-assessment questions can be accessed at www. StudentConsult.com.

TABLE 8-1. Glycogen Storage Diseases

ENZYME DEFICIENCY	BIOCHEMICAL FEATURES	CLINICAL FEATURES	GLYCOGEN STRUCTURE
G6Pase deficiency (von Gierke disease)	Inability to release free glucose into bloodstream; buildup of G6P stimulates significant resynthesis (and accumulation) of glycogen by G6P-dependent form of glycogen synthase; also prevents blood glucose regulation from gluconeogenic pathway.	Hepatomegaly, severe fasting hypoglycemia, ketosis, hyperlipidemia, hyperuricemia, lactic acidosis	Normal
Lysosomal α-1,4-glucosidase deficiency (Pompe disease)	Results in accumulation of lysosomal glycogen deposits; emphasizes importance of lysosomal digestion in normal turnover of glycogen	Hypotonia, cardiomegaly, death by age 2 years	Normal
Debranching enzyme deficiency (Cori disease)	Only terminal glycogen branches used for blood sugar regulation; gluconeogenesis makes up the difference	Mild hypoglycemia, hepatomegaly that diminishes with age	Many short-branched chains (limit dextrins)
Branching enzyme deficiency (Andersen disease)	Very long amylopectin chains cause liver to become cirrhotic	Cardiac or liver failure, lethal within 2 years	Abnormal, many long chains with few branches
Muscle glycogen phosphorylase deficiency (McArdle syndrome)	Glycolytic pathway deprived of ready supply of G6P from glycogen	Muscle cramps, absent normal anaerobic production of lactate during exercise, abnormal amount of glycogen in muscle	Normal
Liver glycogen phosphorylase deficiency (Her disease)	Causes glycogen storage	Hepatomegaly, mild hypoglycemia	Normal

G6Pase, glucose 6-phosphatase.

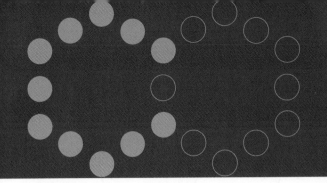

Minor Carbohydrate Pathways: Ribose, Fructose, and Galactose

9

●●● PENTOSE PHOSPHATE PATHWAY

Although the pentose phosphate pathway does not generate adenosine triphosphate (ATP), it does capture useful energy in the form of nicotinamide adenine dinucleotide (NADH), which is a coenzyme for many biosynthetic reactions in intermediary metabolism. NADH phosphate (NADPH) must be generated directly from $NADP^+$, since there is no mechanism for interconversion with NADH. In addition, it is a de novo source of ribose to be used in the synthesis of nucleotides. This pathway occurs entirely in the cytosol. (Note: The pathways in this chapter are not grouped together because they lack the functional relationship of those discussed in preceding chapters.)

Pathway Reaction Steps—Glucose 6-Phosphate to NADPH and Ribose

Oxidative Branch

Three reactions produce ribulose 5-phosphate (Rbl5P) and NADPH (Fig. 9-1):

- *Glucose 6-phosphate dehydrogenase (G6PD)*: Glucose 6-phosphate (G6P) is oxidized to 6-phosphogluconolactone with reduction of $NADP^+$ to NADPH.
- *Lactonase*: The lactone ring is then oxidized to form 6-phosphogluconic acid.
- *6-Phosphogluconate dehydrogenase*: 6-Phosphogluconate is oxidatively decarboxylated to yield Rbl5P, CO_2, and another NADPH.

Nonoxidative Branch

Either production of ribose or a sequence of reactions interconverting 3-, 4-, 5-, 6-, and 7-carbon sugars produces glyceraldehyde 3-phosphate (G3P) and fructose 6-phosphate (F6P):

- *Phosphopentose isomerase*: Rbl5P is isomerized to ribose 5-phosphate (R5P), an end product.
- *Phosphopentose epimerase*: Rbl5P is epimerized to form xylulose 5-phosphate (Xy5P).
- *Transketolase (contains thiamine pyrophosphate)*: A 2-carbon exchange between Xy5P (5C) and R5P (5C) produces G3P (3C) and sedoheptulose 7-phosphate (7C).
- *Transaldolase*: A 3-carbon exchange between G3P (3C) and sedoheptulose 7-phosphate (7C) produces erythrose 4-phosphate (4C) and F6P (6C).
- *Transketolase*: A 2-carbon exchange between Xy5P (5C) and erythrose 4-phosphate (4C) produces G3P (3C) and F6P (6C).

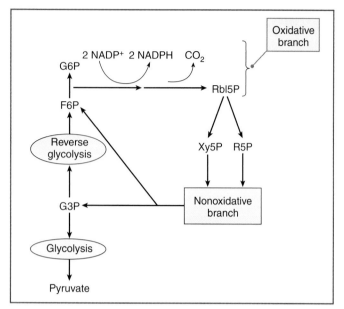

Figure 9-1. The pentose phosphate pathway. See text for expansion of abbreviations.

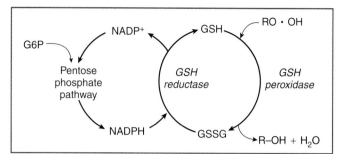

Figure 9-2. Role of nicotinamide adenine dinucleotide phosphate (*NADPH*) in the regeneration of reduced glutathione (*GSH*). See text for expansion of abbreviations.

Regulated Reactions—Glucose 6-Phosphate Dehydrogenase

The only regulation of the pentose phosphate pathway occurs at the first enzyme, G6PD. The reaction is regulated by the supply of $NADP^+$. The $NADP^+$ concentrations are normally very low in liver cells ($NADP^+$/NADPH ratio of 1:70), so any increase in this coenzyme allows the reaction to proceed spontaneously.

Unique Characteristics—Production of NADPH or Ribose or Both

The pentose phosphate pathway, also called the hexose monophosphate shunt, is a shunt from glycolysis designed to produce either NADPH or ribose or both. The direction of flow of the metabolites depends on the need for the end products.

Production of NADPH Only

The tissues with the greatest pentose phosphate pathway activity reveal its function in producing NADPH for reductive biosynthesis (see Fig. 9-1):

- Lactating mammary: fatty acid biosynthesis
- Gonads and adrenal cortex: steroid hormone synthesis
- Liver: fatty acid and cholesterol biosynthesis
- Red blood cells: reduction of glutathione (GSH) (Fig. 9-2)

When NADPH only (and no ribose) is being consumed, the products of the nonoxidative branch are recycled either through reversed glycolysis to G6P or through glycolysis to pyruvate. No energy is required to convert G3P and F6P to G6P.

Production of Ribose Only

In a tissue that is synthesizing ribonucleic acid (RNA) or DNA actively (e.g., during cell division or in response to hormones, ribose will be pulled into pathways for the synthesis of

ribonucleotides (see Chapter 14). To accommodate this, fructose 6-phosphate and G3P enter the nonoxidative branch directly (i.e., they bypass G6PD) and their carbons flow through it in the reverse direction. The Xy5P produced is converted to R5P through its equilibrium with Rbl5P. NADPH is not needed for RNA synthesis, but it is needed when the RNA ribose is converted to DNA deoxyribose (Fig. 9-3).

Production of Both NADPH and Ribose

In a tissue that is undergoing active DNA synthesis, ribose is pulled into pathways for the synthesis of deoxyribonucleotides. Thioredoxin, a cofactor in reduction of ribonucleotides to deoxyribonucleotides, requires NADPH for its regeneration (see Chapter 14). Both NADPH and R5P are produced when G6P is routed through the oxidative branch with all carbons flowing directly to R5P, bypassing the nonoxidative branch entirely (Fig. 9-4).

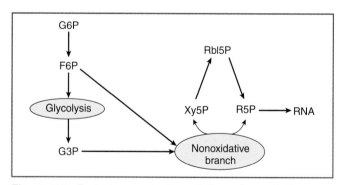

Figure 9-3. Exclusive production of ribose through the nonoxidative branch. See text for expansion of abbreviations.

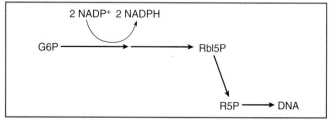

Figure 9-4. Balanced production of nicotinamide adenine dinucleotide phosphate (*NADPH*) and ribose. See text for expansion of abbreviations.

Interface with Other Pathways—Glycolysis

The reversible formation of glycolytic intermediates allows flow of carbon in either direction between glycolysis and the nonoxidative branch of the pathway.

Related Diseases

G6PDH Deficiency (Primaquine Sensitivity)

GSH serves a protective function in red blood cells by serving as a cofactor for GSH peroxidase (see Fig. 9-2). This reaction, which neutralizes hydroperoxides, oxidizes the thiol groups in GSH, causing it to become a disulfide. NADPH is required for generation of the reduced form of GSH to inhibit peroxide formation. Some drugs, such as the antimalarial quinone, primaquine, induce peroxide formation. In patients with a deficiency in the G6PD enzyme, a damaging sequence results.

1. First, primaquine raises the concentration of peroxides in the red blood cell.
2. GSH peroxidase acts to neutralize the peroxides, creating oxidized GSH.
3. Oxidized GSH, which normally is reduced back to the active thiol form by GSH reductase, remains in the oxidized form because of the lack of NADPH.
4. Reduced GSH is depleted, allowing the peroxide radicals to attack cellular components (e.g., unsaturated fatty acids in membrane lipids, cellular proteins).
5. The weakened cell membranes break, and the red blood cells lyse—a condition called hemolysis.

MICROBIOLOGY

Infection-Induced Hemolysis

Oxidant stress on red blood cells can come from internal and external sources (drugs, toxins). During an infection, the activated neutrophils and macrophages create superoxide and peroxide radicals to kill the infectious agents. Exposure to these active O_2 species will also lead to hemolysis in a G6PD-deficient red blood cell.

PHARMACOLOGY

Dapsone Side Effects

Dapsone, a drug used to treat *Mycobacterium leprae* infection in leprosy patients and *Pneumocystis jiroveci* infections in AIDS patients, can induce hemolytic anemia in those patients through the production of peroxides and the subsequent oxidation damage. In patients who have G6PD deficiency, the incidence of hemolytic anemia is approximately doubled owing to the depletion of GSH.

HISTOLOGY

Heinz Bodies

Patients with G6PD deficiency have Heinz bodies in their red blood cells. Heinz bodies are clumps of denatured hemoglobin resulting from exposure to high oxidant levels that oxidize sulfhydryl groups on adjacent molecules, joining them with a covalent disulfide bond. The oxidation process may cause enough damage to the erythrocyte plasma membrane to result in hemolysis.

KEY POINTS ABOUT THE PENTOSE PHOSPHATE PATHWAY

- The source of NADPH and ribose is the pentose phosphate pathway; NADPH is used in reductive biosynthesis, and ribose is used in nucleotide synthesis.
- The pentose phosphate pathway has two branches: the oxidative branch, which produces NADPH, and ribose, and the nonoxidative branch, which uses reversible transfer reactions to produce F6P and G3P; each branch can operate independently or together.
- The cellular concentration of NADP$^+$ determines the rate of glucose entry into the pentose phosphate pathway; two NADPH are produced for each glucose that enters the oxidative branch.
- Transketolase is a thiamine-requiring enzyme in the nonoxidative pathway.
- Primaquine sensitivity results from a G6PD deficiency; its primary symptom is hemolytic anemia resulting from the inability to maintain reduced GSH.

●●● GALACTOSE METABOLISM

Galactose is supplied in the diet from dairy products that contain the disaccharide lactose. Digestion of lactose produces glucose and galactose, both of which are transported through the hepatic portal vein directly to the liver. Galactose is metabolized by conversion initially to glucose 1-phosphate (G1P), which can then be converted either to G6P or to glycogen.

Pathway Reaction Steps—Galactose to Glucose 1-Phosphate

Conversion of Galactose to Glucose 1-Phosphate

Galactokinase

Galactose is phosphorylated with ATP to produce galactose 1-phosphate (Gal1P) (Fig. 9-5).

Galactose 1-phosphate uridyl-transferase

Gal1P is exchanged with uridine diphosphate (UDP)-glucose to produce UDP-galactose and G1P.

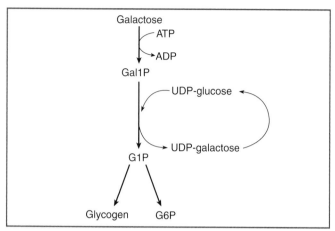

Figure 9-5. The galactose pathway. See text for expansion of abbreviations.

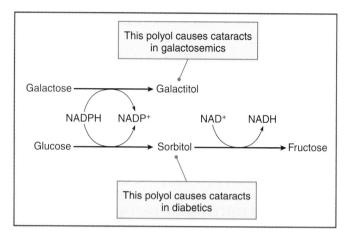

Figure 9-6. Conversion of galactose to galactitol and glucose to sorbitol by the polyol pathway. See text for expansion of abbreviations.

Uridine diphosphate-galactose 4-epimerase

UDP-galactose is converted to UDP-glucose, which can then undergo the transferase reaction again.

Regulated Reactions—No Regulation

There is no known regulated step in the conversion of galactose to glucose intermediates. The fate of glucose from dietary galactose, toward either glycolysis or glycogenesis, is determined by pathways regulating glucose metabolism in the liver.

Unique Characteristics—Uridine Diphosphate-Glucose Intermediate

Although the galactose pathway forms UDP-glucose, there is no net synthesis of this intermediate, since it is recycled. The net output of this pathway is in the conversion of a mole of Gal1P to G1P.

Interface with Other Pathways—Polyol Pathway

Free galactose can be reduced by aldose reductase in the polyol pathway to galactitol (Fig. 9-6). The polyol pathway is widely distributed in the body including in the lens, where it contributes to the formation of cataracts (see Related Diseases below) in both galactosemia and diabetes.

Related Diseases

Deficiencies in galactose pathway enzymes produce a disease called galactosemia, since they lead to an elevation in blood galactose concentration.

Classic galactosemia results from a deficiency in Gal1P uridyl-transferase. It is characterized by an accumulation of both galactose and Gal1P in blood and tissues. Gal1P is cytotoxic and produces liver and neural damage. Galactose is also converted to galactitol by aldose reductase. Accumulation of galactitol in the lens causes osmotic and oxidative stress,

leading to cataracts as a result of denaturation and precipitation of lens crystallin (see Fig. 9-6).

A secondary form of galactosemia results from a deficiency in galactokinase. Since the toxic Gal1P does not increase, there is no liver or neural damage, but the patients nevertheless develop cataracts owing to the elevated blood galactose.

Although unrelated to galactosemia, diabetic patients with chronically poor glycemic control may also develop cataracts. In this case, the increased blood glucose leads to an increased activity of the polyol pathway with the production of sorbitol.

●●● FRUCTOSE METABOLISM

Fructose is supplied in the diet from fruits, sucrose (table sugar), and honey (which contains sucrose). Digestion of sucrose produces glucose and fructose, both of which are transported through the hepatic portal vein directly to the liver. The fructose is then metabolized in a modified pathway similar to the first half of glycolysis to produce intermediates that then enter the last half of glycolysis.

Pathway Reaction Steps—Fructose to Dihydroxyacetone Phosphate and Glyceraldehyde

Glyceraldehyde 3-Phosphate Production (Fig. 9-7)
Fructokinase

Fructose is phosphorylated with ATP to produce fructose 1-phosphate (F1P).

Fructose 1-phosphate aldolase (aldolase B)
Aldol cleavage of F1P produces dihydroxyacetone phosphate and glyceraldehyde.

Triose kinase
Glyceraldehyde is phosphorylated from ATP to produce G3P.

Fructose Synthesis

Fructose is produced from glucose through the polyol pathway in the seminal vesicles; it serves as the primary energy source for spermatozoa (see Fig. 9-6).

Regulated Reactions—No Regulation

Fructose metabolism is notable for having no regulation. Thus it bypasses the normal phosphofructokinase regulation of glycolysis and can accelerate fat synthesis.

Unique Characteristics—Aldolase B Specificity

Fructokinase, like glucokinase, is found primarily in the liver. Unlike hexokinase and glucokinase, it phosphorylates the sugar at the C-1 position. Aldolase B, which is specific to the liver, works on both F1,6-BP and F1P. In extrahepatic tissues such as muscle or adipose tissue, fructose is phosphorylated to F6P by hexokinase (see Fig. 9-7).

Interface with Other Pathways—Amino Sugars in Glycoproteins and Glycolipids

F6P is a precursor for amino sugars in glycoproteins and glycolipids.

Related Diseases

Hereditary Fructose Intolerance

A deficiency in aldolase B produces hereditary fructose intolerance. The increase in F1P results in liver and kidney damage comparable to that seen with increased Gal1P in galactosemia.

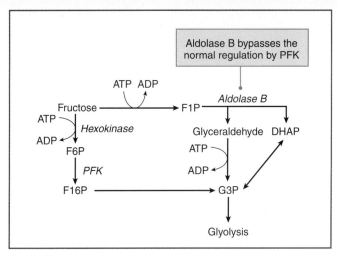

Figure 9-7. The fructose pathway. *DHAP*, dihydroxyacetone phosphate; *PFK*, phosphofructokinase. See text for expansion of other abbreviations.

Essential Fructosuria

A deficiency of fructokinase produces a benign condition marked only by an increase in fructose in the blood and urine.

KEY POINTS ABOUT GALACTOSE AND FRUCTOSE METABOLISM

- Classic galactosemia is characterized by liver and neural damage and the development of cataracts.
- Classic fructose intolerance is due to a deficiency in the liver aldolase, aldolase B, and is characterized by liver and kidney damage.

Self-assessment questions can be accessed at www. StudentConsult.com.

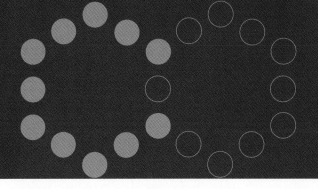

Fatty Acid and Triglyceride Metabolism

10

HISTOLOGY

Red Blood Cell Metabolism

Red blood cells have no mitochondria and therefore cannot use FFAs for energy. They are totally reliant on anaerobic glycolysis for their energy source.

●●● FATTY ACID METABOLISM

Fatty acid chains are polymerized in the cytoplasm and oxidized in the mitochondrial matrix. This prevents competing side reactions between pathway intermediates and allows separate regulation of both pathways. However, since the precursor for fat synthesis, acetyl-coenzyme A (CoA), arises in the matrix, it must first be transported to the cytoplasm for incorporation into a fatty acid. Likewise, free fatty acids (FFAs) mobilized for oxidation must be transported into the mitochondrion to undergo oxidation. Each of the fatty acid metabolic pathways must therefore be preceded by a transport process. (Note: The synthetic and oxidative pathways are treated separately to facilitate comparisons.)

Pathway Reaction Steps in Fatty Acid Synthesis—Acetyl-Coenzyme A to Palmitate

Acetyl-Coenzyme A Shuttle
Four reactions shuttle acetyl-CoA from mitochondrial matrix to cytoplasm (Fig. 10-1).

Citrate synthase
Acetyl-CoA (e.g., from glucose following a meal) is condensed with oxaloacetate to form citrate. Citrate is then transported through the mitochondrial membrane to the cytoplasm.

Citrate cleavage enzyme (citrate lyase)
Acetyl-CoA and oxaloacetate are regenerated from citrate in the cytoplasm in a reaction that requires adenosine triphosphate (ATP) and CoA.

Malate dehydrogenase
Oxaloacetate is reduced with nicotine adenine dinucleotide (NADH) to produce malate. Malate can be transported directly back into the mitochondrion, or it can undergo oxidative decarboxylation with malic enzyme.

Malic enzyme
Oxidative decarboxylation of malate produces pyruvate, CO_2, and nicotinamide adenine dinucleotide phosphate (NADPH). The pyruvate is transported back into the mitochondrion and converted back to oxaloacetate with pyruvate carboxylase.

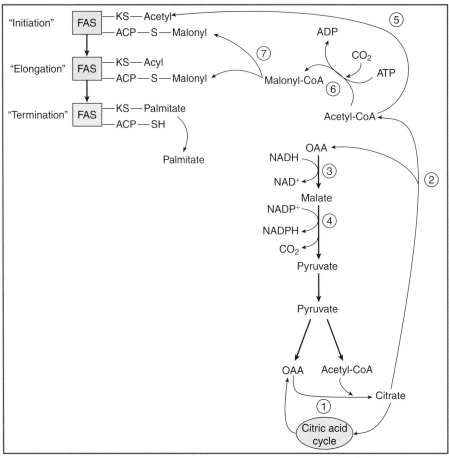

Figure 10-1. Metabolic steps in the synthesis of fatty acids. Ketoacyl site contains an acetyl group during initiation, an acyl group during elongation, and palmitate before release as free palmitate. *Step 1*, citrate synthase; *Step 2*, citrate cleavage enzyme (citrate lyase); *Step 3*, malate dehydrogenase; *Step 4*, malic enzyme; *Step 5*, acetyl-coenzyme A (*CoA*)–acyl carrier protein (*ACP*) transacylase; *Step 6*, acetyl-CoA carboxylase; *Step 7*, malonyl-CoA-ACP transacylase. FAS, fatty acid synthesis. KS, 3-ketoacyl synthase; *ADP* adenosine diphosphate; *ATP*, adenosin triphosphate.

PATHOLOGY

Fat Oxidation in Mitochondria

The mitochondrion contains not only the enzymes for aerobic production of energy from glucose but also the enzymes necessary for β-oxidation of fats. Because there is no alternative pathway for fats to be metabolized, any condition that impairs mitochondrial function will also impair fat oxidation. This will result in an accumulation of fat in the tissues (steatosis), generally as neutral triglyceride.

Fatty Acid Polymerization Initiation

Four reactions initiate fatty acid polymerization with condensation of acetyl and malonyl groups (Fig. 10-2) to produce an acetoacetyl group. Each enzyme function is catalyzed by individual domains of the fatty acid synthase multienzyme complex, which is a single polypeptide.

Acetyl–Coenzyme A–Acyl Carrier Protein Transacylase

The 2-carbon acetyl group is transferred from the phosphopantetheine group of acetyl-CoA to the phosphopantetheine group of acyl carrier protein (ACP). The ACP then transfers the acetyl group to the cysteine thiol group of 3-ketoacyl synthase (KS).

Acetyl-coenzyme A carboxylase

CO_2 is attached to acetyl-CoA to produce malonyl-CoA. ATP provides the energy input. Note that this same CO_2 will be removed when the malonyl group condenses with the growing acyl chain. Like all carboxylases, acetyl-CoA carboxylase requires biotin as a cofactor.

Malonyl-coenzyme A–acyl carrier protein transacylase

The malonyl group of malonyl-CoA is transferred from phosphopantetheine in the CoA to the phosphopantetheine in the active site of the ACP.

3-Ketoacyl synthase

The acetyl group (or a longer acyl group) in the KS site is condensed with malonyl-ACP, accompanied by release of the terminal CO_2 of the malonyl group and producing a 4-carbon 3-ketoacyl chain attached to the ACP. The loss of CO_2 drives the reaction to completion. (Note: All further 2-carbon additions to the acyl chain are also from malonyl-CoA.)

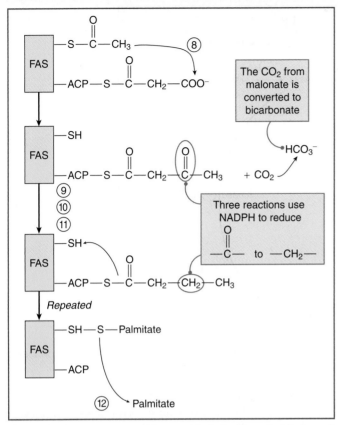

Figure 10-2. Elongation of fatty acid chain. *Step 8*, 3-ketoacyl synthase; *Step 9*, 3-ketoacyl reductase; *Step 10*, dehydratase; *Step 11*, enoyl reductase; *Step 12*, thioesterase. *NADPH*, nicotinamide adenine dinucleotide phosphate; other abbreviations as in Fig. 10-1.

β-Carbonyl Reduction
Three reactions reduce the β-carbonyl on acyl-ACP.

3-Ketoacyl reductase
The 3-ketoacyl group is reduced to a 3-hydroxyacyl group by NADPH.

Dehydratase
An unsaturated bond is created by removal of water; this is similar to the enolase reaction in glycolysis.

Enoyl reductase
The unsaturated bond is reduced with NADPH. This reduced acyl intermediate is then transferred to the free cysteine at the KS active site, and the cycle begins again.

Elongation Cycle
Repetitive condensation and reduction of malonyl-CoA units continues to produce palmitic acid.

Thioesterase
When the growing acyl chain reaches a length of 16 carbons, it is released from ACP as free palmitic acid.

Triglyceride Synthesis
Glycerol kinase
In the liver, glycerol is phosphorylated with ATP (Fig. 10-3).

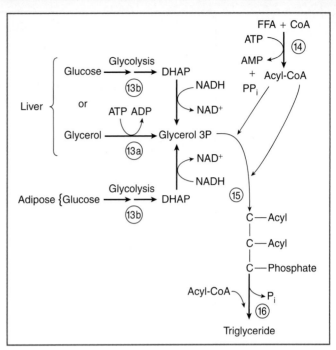

Figure 10-3. Assembly of a triglyceride. *Step 13a*, glycerol kinase; *Step 13b*, glycerol-3-phosphate dehydrogenase; *Step 14*, acetyl-coenzyme A synthase; *Step 15* and *Step 16*, acyltransferase. *FFA*, free fatty acid; *DHAP*, dihydroxyacetone phosphate; *PP_i*; inorganic pyrophosphate; *P_i*, inorganic phosphate. Other abbreviations as in Fig. 10-1.

Glycerol-3-phosphate dehydrogenase
In both liver and adipose tissue, glyceraldehyde 3-phosphate produced during glycolysis is reduced to glycerol 3-phosphate.

Acyl-coenzyme A synthase (fatty acid thiokinase)
Fatty acids are activated with CoA to acyl-CoA in an ATP-dependent reaction; adenosine monophosphate (AMP) and pyrophosphate are produced instead of adenosine diphosphate. The pyrophosphate is hydrolyzed to phosphate by pyrophosphatase, so that, in effect, two high-energy bonds are expended for production of each acyl-CoA.

Two acyl-CoA molecules are then esterified to glycerol 3-phosphate to produce a diacylphosphoglycerate.

The phosphate is then removed, and the third acyl group is added to form a triglyceride.

Regulated Reactions in Fatty Acid Synthesis—Acetyl-Coenzyme A Carboxylase

The irreversible step in fatty acid synthesis (FAS), acetyl-CoA carboxylase, is controlled by two mechanisms (Fig. 10-4).

Covalent Modification
The active dephospho- form of acetyl-CoA carboxylase is inactivated by phosphorylation catalyzed by an AMP-activated protein kinase (Note: AMP, not cyclic AMP). This ensures that under circumstances of low energy charge no acetyl-CoA will be diverted away from the citric acid cycle.
- Protein phosphatase 2A (PP2A) reactivates acetyl-CoA carboxylase.

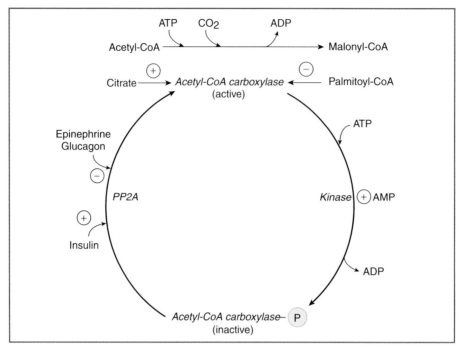

Figure 10-4. Regulation of acetyl-coenzyme A (*CoA*) carboxylase by allosteric feedback and covalent modification. *ATP*, adenosine triphosphate; *AMP*, adenosine monophosphate; *ADP*, adenosine diphosphate; *PP2A*, protein phosphatase 2A.

- Insulin reactivates acetyl-CoA carboxylase through stimulation of PP2A.
- Epinephrine and glucagon inhibit FAS by inhibiting PP2A.

Allosteric Regulation

The active dephospho- form of acetyl-CoA carboxylase is regulated by citrate and palmitoyl-CoA.

- Stimulation by citrate assures FAS when 2-carbon units are plentiful.
- Inhibition by palmitoyl-CoA coordinates palmitate synthesis with triglyceride assembly. (Note: Palmitate is the product of FAS complex.)

Unique Characteristics of Fatty Acid Synthesis

Multienzyme Complex

In humans, the enzymes for fatty acid biosynthesis exist as a single polypeptide consisting of eight catalytic domains. Thus the multiple enzymatic activities form a structurally organized complex that binds to the growing acyl chain until it is completed and released. The P domain contains the same phosphopantetheine group as in CoA. The phosphopantetheine is attached by a long, flexible arm, allowing contact with the multiple active sites in the multienzyme complex. Note that the fatty acid synthase complex is not subject to regulation, except by the availability of malonyl-CoA.

Compartmentation

FAS does not compete with fatty acid oxidation because they occur in separate compartments of the cell. Cytoplasmic synthesis ensures that NADPH will be available and that the product, palmitate, will not undergo β-oxidation.

Adipose Tissue Versus Liver

Adipose tissue does not contain glycerol kinase, an enzyme found in liver. Thus the glycerol backbone for triglyceride assembly in adipose tissue must come from dihydroxyacetone phosphate in the glycolytic pathway. In other words, uptake of glucose is essential for adipose synthesis of triglycerides.

Interface with Other Pathways

Elongation of Palmitate

When longer fatty acids are needed (e.g., in the synthesis of myelin in the brain), palmitate is elongated by enzymes in the endoplasmic reticulum. The palmitate elongation reactions also use malonyl-CoA as the 2-carbon donor and NADPH as the redox coenzyme. These extensions are carried out by enzymes in the endoplasmic reticulum, not by the fatty acid synthase complex.

Desaturation of Fatty Acids

Unsaturated fatty acids are a component of the phospholipids in cell membranes and help maintain membrane fluidity. Phospholipids contain a variety of unsaturated fatty acids, but not all of these can be synthesized in the body.

- Fatty acid desaturase, an enzyme in the endoplasmic reticulum, introduces double bonds between carbons 9 and 10 in palmitate and in stearate, producing palmitoleic acid (16:1:Δ9) and oleic acid (18:1:Δ9), respectively.
- Fatty acid desaturase requires O_2 and either NAD^+ or NADPH.

Humans lack the enzymes necessary to introduce double bonds beyond carbon 9. Thus linoleic acid (18:2:Δ9,Δ12) and linolenic acid (18:2:Δ9,Δ12,Δ15) cannot be synthesized. These are essential fatty acids. Linoleic acid can serve as a precursor for arachidonate, sparing it as an essential fatty acid.

Arachidonate is an important component of membrane lipids and, together with linoleic and linolenic acid, serves as a precursor for the synthesis of prostaglandins, thromboxanes, leukotrienes, and lipoxins.

KEY POINTS ABOUT FATTY ACID METABOLISM

■ Fatty acid chains are polymerized in the cytoplasm and oxidized in the mitochondrial matrix.

■ The precursor for fat synthesis, acetyl-CoA, arises in the matrix and must first be transported to the cytoplasm for incorporation into a fatty acid.

■ FFAs that have been mobilized for oxidation must be transported into the mitochondrion to undergo oxidation.

■ FAS in eukaryotes occurs on a multifunctional enzyme complex contained within a single polypeptide.

■ Humans lack the enzymes necessary to introduce double bonds beyond carbon 9, thus making linoleic acid (18:2:Δ9,Δ12) and linolenic acid (18:2:Δ9,Δ12,Δ15) essential fatty acids in the diet.

■ Malonyl-CoA synthesis from acetyl-CoA by acetyl-CoA carboxylase is regulated by both covalent modification and by allosteric feedback.

●●● FATTY ACID MOBILIZATION AND OXIDATION

Pathway Reaction Steps in Fatty Acid Oxidation—Palmitate to Acetyl-Coenzyme A and Ketone Bodies

Fatty Acid Transport into Mitochondria

Fatty acids are transported across the mitochondrial membrane by the carnitine cycle (Fig. 10-5). Fatty acids are first activated to an acyl-CoA in the cytoplasm.

Carnitine acyltransferase I
The acyl group is transferred to carnitine by the cytoplasmic form of the enzyme. The acylcarnitine then diffuses across the outer mitochondrial membrane.

Carnitine-acylcarnitine translocase
This membrane transporter (antiporter) exchanges cytoplasmic acylcarnitine for mitochondrial carnitine.

Carnitine acyltransferase II
The mitochondrial form of this enzyme then transfers the acyl group back to CoA. Medium-chain (6 to 12 carbons) and short-chain fatty acids (acetate propionate and butyrate) enter the mitochondrion directly and therefore bypass the carnitine cycle. They are activated in the mitochondrial matrix by acyl-CoA synthetases.

β-Oxidation of an Acyl-Coenzyme A
Acyl-coenzyme A dehydrogenase
1. Oxidation at the β-carbon of the fatty acid occurs with reduction of flavin adenine dinucleotide (FAD) (creates a trans double bond) at the Δ2 position to produce Δ2-trans-enoyl-CoA (Fig. 10-6). The electrons from FADH$_2$ are subsequently transferred to ubiquinone in the electron transport chain. A separate acyl-CoA dehydrogenase exists for long-, medium-, and short-chain fatty acids. This reaction is analogous to the succinate dehydrogenase reaction in the citric acid cycle.

Enoyl-Coenzyme A Reductase
The Δ2-trans-enoyl double bond is then hydrated to create a 3-hydroxyl group. This reaction is analogous to that of fumarase.

3-Hydroxyacyl–coenzyme A dehydrogenase
The 3-hydroxyl group is then oxidized with reduction of NAD$^+$ to NADH to produce a β-keto group. This reaction is analogous to that of malate dehydrogenase.

β-Ketothiolase
Acetyl-CoA is cleaved at the β-keto group and CoA is attached to the shortened acyl chain to reenter the β-oxidation cycle. The acetyl-CoA is in the matrix and available as a substrate for the citric acid cycle for further oxidation.

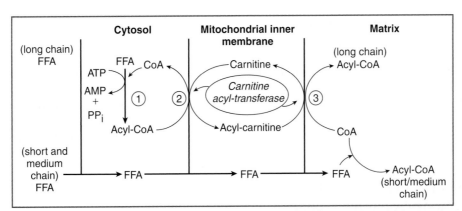

Figure 10-5. Transport of acetyl-coenzyme A (*CoA*) by the carnitine cycle. *Step 1*, carnitine acyltransferase I; *Step 2*, carnitine acyl–carnitine translocase; *Step 3*, carnitine acyltransferase II. *FFA*, free fatty acid; *ATP*, adenosine triphosphate; *AMP*, adenosine monophosphate; *PP$_i$*, inorganic pyrophosphate.

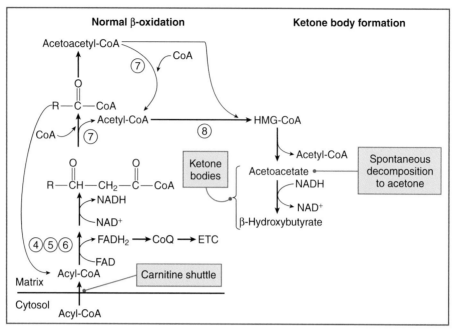

Figure 10-6. β-Oxidation of fatty acids. Acyl-coenzyme A (*CoA*) in the matrix is oxidized by a reversal of the steps involved in fatty acid synthesis, but with different enzymes and with nicotinamide adenine dinucleotide (*NAD*) as a cofactor. *Step 4*, acyl-CoA dehydrogenase; *Step 5*, enoyl-CoA reductase; *Step 6*, 3-hydroxyacyl-CoA dehydrogenase; *Step 7*, β-ketothiolase. *FMG*, β-hydroxy-β-methylglutaryl; *ETC*, electron transport chain; *NADH*, reduced *NAD*; *FAD*, in adenine nucleotide; *FADH₂*, reduced form of FAD.

Formation and Degradation of Ketone Bodies
HMG-CoA synthase
A third molecule of acetyl-CoA is condensed with acetoacetyl-CoA to form β-hydroxy-β-methylglutaryl-CoA (HMG-CoA).

HMG-CoA lysase
HMG-CoA is hydrolyzed to produce acetyl-CoA and acetoacetate, a ketone body.

β-Hydroxybutyrate dehydrogenase
Acetoacetate is further reduced to form β-hydroxybutyrate.

Acetone formation
Acetoacetate spontaneously degrades in a nonenzymatic reaction to produce acetone. When acetone accumulates in the blood, it imparts a fruity odor to the breath.

Succinyl-coenzyme A: acetoacetate-coenzyme A transferase
In peripheral tissues, acetoacetate is converted to acetyl-CoA by reaction with succinyl-CoA. Since acetoacetate is metabolized in the mitochondrial matrix, the succinate produced is metabolized as a citric acid cycle intermediate.

$$2 \text{ succinyl-CoA} + \text{acetoacetate}$$
$$\rightarrow 2 \text{ acetyl-CoA} + 2 \text{ succinate}$$

Regulated Reactions in Fatty Acid Oxidation—Hormone-Sensitive Lipase

The only site for regulation of fatty acid oxidation is mobilization that occurs at the level of hormone-sensitive lipase in

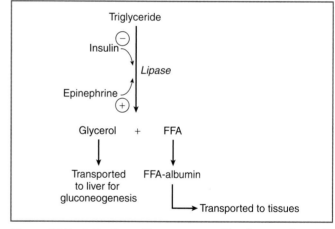

Figure 10-7. Activation of hormone-sensitive lipases. Specialized lipases remove free fatty acids (*FFA*) from the respective glycerides.

adipose tissue (Fig. 10-7). This is the underlying reason for the runaway fat mobilization that leads to ketosis in conditions such as starvation and untreated type 1 diabetes. Under fasting conditions, with minimal insulin in the blood, glucagon promotes formation of the phosphorylated, active form of hormone-sensitive lipase. When epinephrine is present, it further shifts the equilibrium to active hormone-sensitive lipase, increasing the hydrolysis of triglycerides to produce FFAs and glycerol. The glycerol is carried to the liver, where it enters gluconeogenesis, while FFAs are carried on serum albumin to the tissues where they are catabolized for energy. The liver uses some of the energy from fat mobilization to support gluconeogenesis.

The oxidation of newly synthesized FFAs is prevented by malonyl-CoA, which is present in high amounts during FAS. Carnitine acyltransferase is inhibited by malonyl-CoA, preventing transport and β-oxidation of the newly synthesized fatty acids.

Unique Characteristics of Fatty Acid Oxidation

Energy Gained from Fatty Acid Oxidation

The caloric value of neutral fat is approximately 9 kcal/g; this compares with the caloric value of carbohydrate and protein of approximately 4 kcal/g. More than half of the oxidative energy requirement of the liver, kidneys, heart, and resting skeletal muscle is provided by fatty acid oxidation. The NADH, FADH$_2$, and acetyl-CoA produced from β-oxidation create a net 129 moles of ATP for each palmitate oxidized.

Compartmentation of Ketone Body Formation and Use

The liver cannot metabolize the ketone bodies that it produces because it lacks the enzyme succinyl-CoA:acetoacetate-CoA transferase that is needed to convert acetoacetate to acetyl-CoA. This enzyme is found only in the peripheral tissues, where the energy from ketone bodies is used. Thus when acetyl-CoA produced from excessive fatty acid oxidation saturates the capacity of the citric acid cycle in the liver, it is shunted into the formation of ketone bodies that flow unidirectionally from the liver to the peripheral tissues.

Interface with Other Pathways

β-Oxidation of Dietary Unsaturated Fatty Acids

Unsaturated bonds in unsaturated fatty acids may be out of position and not recognized by β-oxidation enzymes. Any double bonds that are out of position are corrected by an isomerase, which shifts their position and configuration to produce the normal Δ2-trans-enoyl-CoA intermediate that is recognized by enoyl-CoA reductase in normal β-oxidation (see Fig. 10-6, step 5).

β-Oxidation of Odd-Chain Fatty Acids

Odd-numbered fatty acids yield propionyl-CoA (3 carbons) as the last intermediate in β-oxidation (Fig. 10-8). (Note: Propionyl-CoA is also formed from catabolism of methionine, valine, and isoleucine.) Propionyl-CoA cannot be catabolized further, so it is converted to succinyl-CoA by the following short pathway.

Propionyl-coenzyme A carboxylase
Propionyl-CoA is first converted to methylmalonyl-CoA.

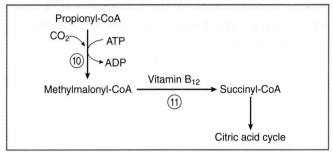

Figure 10-8. Conversion of propionyl-coenzyme A (*CoA*) to succinyl-CoA. *Step 10*, propionyl-CoA carboxylase; *Step 11*, methylmalonyl-CoA mutase. *ATP*, adenosine triphosphate; *ADP*, adenosine diphosphate.

Methylmalonyl-coenzyme A mutase
Methylmalonyl-CoA is then converted to succinyl-CoA by a vitamin B$_{12}$–dependent reaction. Succinyl-CoA enters the citric acid cycle.

Peroxisomal Oxidation of Fatty Acids

Very long chain fatty acids (20 to 26 carbons) can be degraded in peroxisomes. The process is similar to β-oxidation for fatty acids except that no NADH or FADH$_2$ is produced; instead H$_2$O$_2$ is produced and then degraded by catalase. Final products of this process are octanoyl-CoA and acetyl-CoA, which are then metabolized normally in mitochondria.

ω-Oxidation of Fatty Acids

Oxidation at the terminal carbon (ω-carbon) can be carried out by enzymes in the endoplasmic reticulum, creating a dicarboxylic acid. This process requires cytochrome p450, NADPH, and molecular O$_2$. Normal β-oxidation can then occur at both ends of the fatty acid.

α-Oxidation of Fatty Acids

Very long (>20 carbons) fatty acids and branched-chain fatty acids (e.g., phytanic acid in the diet) are metabolized by α-oxidation, which releases a terminal carboxyl as CO$_2$ one at a time. This occurs mainly in brain and nervous tissue. (Note: Few fatty acids are metabolized one carbon at a time. For example, branched-chain phytanic acids release one CO$_2$, followed by equal amounts of acetyl- and propionyl-CoA.)

PATHOLOGY

Adrenoleukodystrophy

The neurologic disorder adrenoleukodystrophy is due to defective peroxisomal oxidation of very long chain fatty acids. This syndrome demonstrates a marked reduction in plasmalogens (see Chapter 11), adrenocortical insufficiency, and abnormalities in the white matter of the cerebrum.

KEY POINTS ABOUT FATTY ACID MOBILIZATION AND OXIDATION

- To be oxidized, fatty acids are transported across the mitochondrial membrane by the carnitine cycle.

- β-Oxidation oxidizes the β-carbon of an acyl-CoA to form a carbonyl group, followed by release of acetyl-CoA.

- The only point for regulation of fatty acid oxidation is at the level of hormone-sensitive lipase in adipose tissue.

- Odd-numbered fatty acids yield propionyl-CoA (3 carbons) as the last intermediate in β-oxidation after which it is converted to succinyl-CoA.

●●● RELATED DISEASES OF FATTY ACID METABOLISM

Medium-Chain Acyl-Coenzyme A Dehydrogenase Deficiency

Long-chain fatty acids are oxidized until reaching a chain length of about 16 carbons. Because of the inability to use fatty acids to support gluconeogenesis, this deficiency produces a nonketotic hypoglycemia. It is normally dangerous only in cases of extreme or frequent fasting.

Jamaican Vomiting Sickness

The unripe fruit of the Jamaican ackee tree contains a toxin, hypoglycin, that inhibits both the medium- and short-chain acyl-CoA dehydrogenases. This inhibits β-oxidation and leads to nonketotic hypoglycemia.

Zellweger Syndrome

Associated with the absence of peroxisomes in the liver and kidneys, Zellweger syndrome results in accumulation of very long chain fatty acids, especially in the brain.

Carnitine Deficiency

Carnitine deficiency produces muscle aches and weakness following exercise, elevated blood FFAs, and low fasting ketone production. Nonketotic hypoglycemia results because gluconeogenesis cannot be supported by fat oxidation.

Refsum Disease

Also referred to as deficient α-oxidation, Refsum disease results in accumulation of phytanic acid in the brain, producing neurologic symptoms. Phytanic acid is a branched-chain fatty acid found in plants and in dairy products.

Self-assessment questions can be accessed at www. StudentConsult.com.

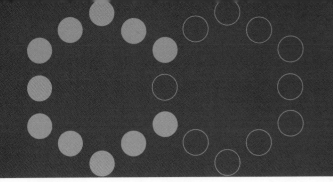

Metabolism of Steroids and Other Lipids   11

CONTENTS

●●● STEROID METABOLISM

Cholesterol is the most ubiquitous and abundant steroid found in human tissue. It serves as a nucleus for the synthesis of all steroid hormones and bile acids. The major location for the synthesis of cholesterol is the liver, although it is synthesized in significant amounts in intestinal mucosa, adrenal cortex, the testes, and the ovaries. Cholesterol is composed of a fused ring system—cyclopentanoperhydrophenanthrene (CPPP) with a hydroxyl group on carbon 3 and an aliphatic chain on carbon 17 (Fig. 11-1). All 27 carbon atoms of cholesterol originate from acetyl-coenzyme A (CoA).

The major categories of steroids are based on the side chain attached to the C_{17} position of the CPPP nucleus:

- Estrogens; C_{18} (i.e., 18-carbon) steroids
- Androgens; C_{19} steroids
- Progesterone and adrenal cortical steroids; C_{21} steroids
- Bile acids; C_{24} steroids
- Cholesterol and cholecalciferol (not shown in Fig. 11-1); C_{27} steroids

Cholesterol Synthesis

Cholesterol is synthesized in four phases, all of which are in the cytoplasm. First, the precursor mevalonate is synthesized, followed by its conversion to an isoprenoid (5 Carbons) intermediate. Then the isoprenoid intermediate is polymerized into a 30-carbon steroid carbon skeleton, squalene. The final phase consists of cyclizing and refining the 30-carbon squalene to produce the 27-carbon cholesterol. Nicotinamide adenine dinucleotide phosphate (NADPH) is a coenzyme for many of the reductive biosynthesis steps in this pathway.

Six-Carbon Mevalonate

Three reactions synthesize 6-carbon mevalonate by condensation of 3 molecules of acetyl-CoA (Fig. 11-2).

Thiolase

Two molecules of acetyl-CoA condense to form acetoacetyl-CoA.

β-Hydroxy-β-methylglutaryl (HMG)-CoA synthase. A third molecule of acetyl-CoA condenses with acetoacetyl-CoA to form β-hydroxy-β-methylglutaryl-CoA (HMG-CoA). This cytoplasmic form of HMG-CoA synthase is not involved in ketone formation (Fig. 11-3).

β-Hydroxy-β-methylglutaryl (HMG)-CoA reductase. HMG-CoA is reduced with NADPH to form mevalonic acid.

PHARMACOLOGY

Statin Side Effects

Statin drugs control cholesterol synthesis by inhibition of HMG-CoA reductase. Since this inhibition also lowers the production of isoprenoid precursors of other biomolecules, such as coenzyme Q and lipid anchors for membrane proteins, in rare cases (0.15% of patients), statin drugs can induce myopathies related to deficiencies in these cell components.

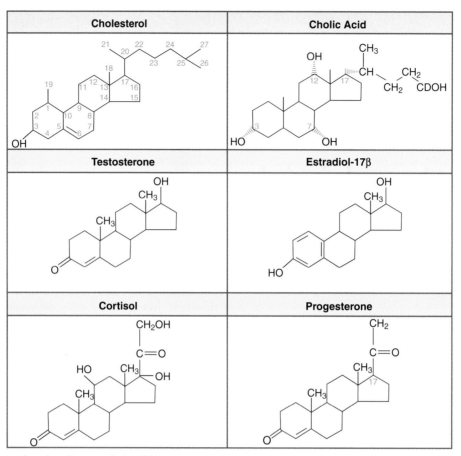

Figure 11-1. Structure of major classes of steroids.

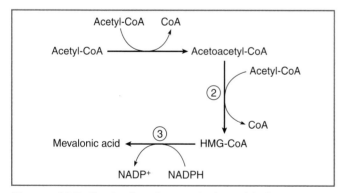

Figure 11-2. Synthesis of mevalonic acid from acetyl-coenzyme A (*CoA*). *HMG*, β-hydroxy-β-methylglutaryl; *NADP*, nicotinamide adenine dinucleotide phosphate.

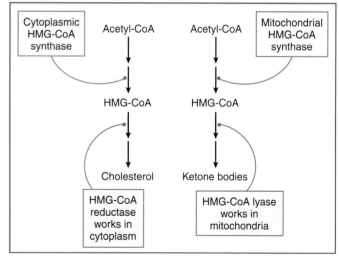

Figure 11-3. Comparison of cytoplasmic and mitochondrial β-hydroxy-β-methylglutaryl-coenzyme A (*HMG-CoA*) synthase.

Isoprenoid (5 Carbons)

Four reactions synthesize activated isoprenoid (5-carbon) units from mevalonate (Fig. 11-4). (Note: Enzyme names are generalized.)

Kinase. Mevalonic acid is phosphorylated to mevalonic acid 5-phosphate.

Kinase. Mevalonic acid 5-phosphate is then phosphorylated to mevalonic acid 5-pyrophosphate.

Decarboxylase. Mevalonic acid 5-pyrophosphate is decarboxylated to yield dimethylallyl pyrophosphate.

Isomerase. Dimethylallyl pyrophosphate is isomerized to form isopentenyl pyrophosphate.

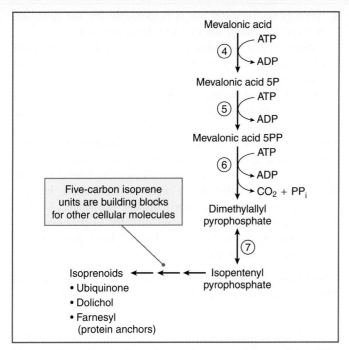

Figure 11-4. Conversion of mevalonate to isoprenoids. *ATP*, adenosine triphosphate; *ADP*, adenosine diphosphate; *PP$_i$*, inorganic pyrophosphate.

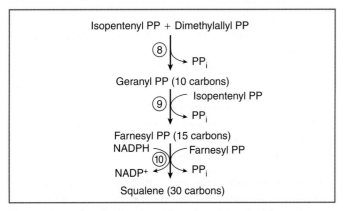

Figure 11-5. Synthesis of squalene from isoprenoid precursors. *PP*, pyrophosphate; *PP$_i$*, inorganic PP; *NADP*, nicotinamide adenine diphosphatase; *NADPH*, reduced NADP.

Squalene

The squalene molecule (30 carbons) is synthesized from six 5-carbon isopentenyl pyrophosphates (three reactions) (Fig. 11-5).

Transferase

Isopentenyl pyrophosphate and dimethylallyl pyrophosphate condense to form geranyl pyrophosphate (10-carbon intermediate).

Isopentenyl pyrophosphate condenses with geranyl pyrophosphate to yield farnesyl pyrophosphate (15-carbon intermediate).

Two molecules of farnesyl pyrophosphate combine to form squalene (30 carbons).

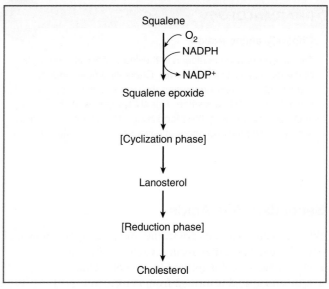

Figure 11-6. Synthesis of cholesterol from squalene. *NADP*, nicotinamide adenine dinucleotic phosphate; *NADPH*, reduced NADP.

Squalene Conversion to Cholesterol

Squalene conversion to cholesterol requires one step and two phases (Fig. 11-6).

Squalene monooxygenase. Squalene epoxide is formed from squalene; reaction requires O_2 and NADPH.

Cyclization phase. Concerted intramolecular cyclization of squalene epoxide produces lanosterol.

Reduction phase. Lanosterol is converted to cholesterol (27 carbons); NADPH is involved in the reduction and removal of three methyl groups as CO_2.

Bile Acids

Approximately 70% to 80% of liver cholesterol is converted to bile acids. These 24-carbon steroids have 5-carbon side chains on C_{17} that terminate in a carboxyl group.

Bile acids facilitate digestion and absorption of fats and fat-soluble vitamins (A, D, E, and K).

Bile acids prevent gallstones by solubilizing the insoluble components of bile (i.e., phospholipids and cholesterol).

Primary Bile Acids

Bile acids synthesized from cholesterol in liver are the primary bile acids. Chenodeoxycholic acid and cholic acid are the major bile acids.

Conjugation of bile acids with either taurine or glycine occurs in liver before secretion into bile. They are found in bile as water-soluble sodium or potassium salts (bile salts). The hydroxyl groups are all oriented toward the same side of the plane of the CPPP nucleus, providing a hydrophilic side that associates with water and a hydrophobic side that associates with the lipid being emulsified.

PHARMACOLOGY

Cholestyramine Action

The enterohepatic circulation in the ileum recycles about 95% of the bile salts back to the liver. Cholestyramine binds bile salts tightly, thereby preventing their recirculation and redirecting them to excretion. This shifts the flow of cholesterol in the body away from the blood lipoproteins for new bile acid synthesis and has the effect of lowering serum cholesterol.

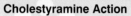

Secondary Bile Acids

When primary bile salts are further metabolized by intestinal bacterial enzymes, they form secondary bile acids:

- Deoxycholic acid is formed from cholic acid.
- Lithocholic acid is formed from deoxycholic acid.

KEY POINTS ABOUT PRIMARY AND SECONDARY BILE ACIDS

- Steroids all have the same CPPP nucleus and most function as hormones.

- HMG-CoA is synthesized in either cytosol or mitochondria. In cytosol, HMG-CoA is converted to mevalonic acid. In mitochondria, HMG-CoA is intermediate in the synthesis of ketone bodies.

- Most cholesterol synthesized in the liver is converted to bile acids, which recirculate through the enterohepatic circulation.

Steroid Hormones

There are five major classes of steroid hormones:

- *Progestagens*: Progesterone prepares the uterine lining for implantation of the ovum and also contributes to the maintenance of pregnancy.
- *Glucocorticoids*: Cortisol, a stress hormone, promotes glycogenolysis and gluconeogenesis and alters fat metabolism and storage.
- *Mineralocorticoids*: Aldosterone acts at kidney distal tubules to promote sodium reabsorption and potassium and proton excretion.

- *Androgens*: Testosterone is responsible for the development of secondary sex characteristics in males.
- *Estrogens*: 17β-Estradiol is responsible for the development of secondary sex characteristics in females and menstrual cycle regulation.

Several steroid hormones serve as precursors for the synthesis of the remaining hormones synthesized in the adrenal cortex. The first step in the synthesis of the adrenocortical hormone classes is the formation of pregnenolone from cholesterol (Fig. 11-7). This reaction is catalyzed by the enzyme desmolase (a cytochrome P450 mixed-function oxidase; see later discussion) and is stimulated by the pituitary hormone adrenocorticotropic hormone (ACTH). Pregnenolone is then converted directly to progesterone. The remaining steroids are all derived from progesterone as a precursor molecule.

Synthesis of progesterone. Progesterone is synthesized from pregnenolone by 3β-hydroxysteroid dehydrogenase (Fig. 11-8).

Synthesis of glucocorticoids. Progesterone is converted to either 17α-hydroxyprogesterone by 17α-hydroxylase or to 11-deoxycorticosterone by 21α-hydroxylase.

- 17α-Hydroxyprogesterone is then converted to 11-deoxycortisol by 21α-hydroxylase.
- 11-Deoxycortisol is then converted by 11β-hydroxylase to cortisol.
- 11-Deoxycorticosterone is converted to corticosterone by 11β-hydroxylase.

Synthesis of mineralocorticoids. Corticosterone is converted to aldosterone by 18-hydroxylase. This reaction is stimulated by angiotensin II, a hormone produced in the angiotensin by angiotensin-converting enzyme.

Synthesis of androgens and estrogens. 17α-Hydroxyprogesterone is converted to androstenedione, which is then converted to testosterone.

- Testosterone can be converted to estradiol by the action of aromatase. The major estrogen in premenopausal women is 17β-estradiol.
- Testosterone can also be converted to dihydrotestosterone by 5α-reductase. Dihydrotestosterone is a more potent androgen than testosterone.

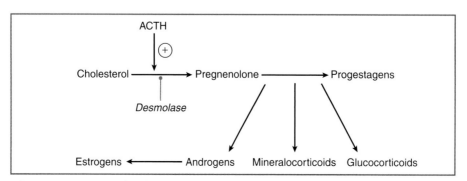

Figure 11-7. Pregnenolone as a precursor for the adrenal cortical steroids. *ACTH*, adreno corticotropic hormor.

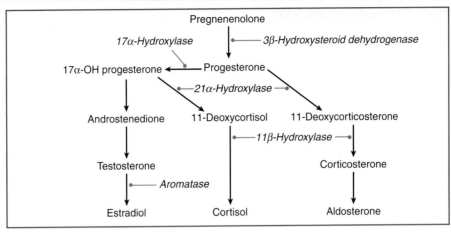

Figure 11-8. Synthesis of the adrenocortical steroids.

Cytochrome P450 mixed-function oxidases. Most reactions in steroid synthetic pathways are hydroxylations catalyzed by cytochrome P450 mixed-function oxidases (see Chapter 20).

HISTOLOGY

Steroid Hormone Production

Different classes of steroid hormones are synthesized in each layer of the adrenal cortex. Mineralocorticoids (mostly aldosterone) are synthesized in the zona glomerulosa (outer layer), glucocorticoids (such as cortisone) are synthesized in the zona fasciculata (middle layer), and the reproductive steroids (weak androgens) are synthesized in the zona reticularis (inner layer).

HISTOLOGY

Thecal Cell Function

Thecal cells of graafian follicles convert testosterone to 17β-estradiol and androstenedione to estrone (and estrone to 17β-estradiol).

PHARMACOLOGY

5α-Reductase Inhibitors

Dihydrotestosterone is the active androgen in the prostate. For patients with benign prostatic hyperplasia, its effects can be reversed with a 5α-reductase inhibitor, such as finasteride or the plant sterol β-sitosterol.

Adrenogenital Syndrome

A deficiency in several of the enzymes involved in the synthesis of the adrenal steroid hormones leads to adrenogenital syndrome, also known as congenital adrenal hyperplasia, caused by increased secretion of ACTH. All known deficiencies have in common a reduction in the synthesis of cortisol, which is the major feedback regulator of ACTH secretion detected by the pituitary. Deficiency of cortisol results in the characteristic increase in the release of ACTH. In general, any deficiency produces an increase in hormones before the block and a deficiency of hormones distal to the block.

- *3β-Hydroxysteroid deficiency.* Patients have female genitalia (no androgens or estrogens) and marked salt excretion in urine (no mineralocorticoids).
- *17α-Hydroxylase deficiency.* Patients have hypertension (increased mineralocorticoids) and female genitalia (no androgens or estrogens).
- *21α-Hydroxylase deficiency (most common, several variants known).* Overproduction of androgens leads to masculinization of female external genitalia and early virilization of males. Deficient mineralocorticoids lead to loss of sodium and volume depletion.
- *11β-Hydroxylase deficiency.* Patients have marked hypertension, masculinization, and virilization.

KEY POINTS ABOUT STEROID HORMONES

- Pregnenolone is the first major derivative of cholesterol for the synthesis of the steroid hormones; progesterone, which is derived from pregnenolone, is the precursor for all other steroid hormones.

- Female hormones are derived from male hormones, which are derived from female hormones.

●●● PHOSPHOGLYCERIDE METABOLISM

Phosphoglycerides are polar lipids. They differ from triglycerides in that one of the ester bonds on the glycerol moiety is esterified to phosphate instead of an acyl group. As described in Chapter 10, phosphatidic acid is an intermediate in the synthetic pathway for triglycerides. However, it also serves as a precursor to numerous other phosphoglycerides that serve various structural functions in cell membranes and blood lipids.

Synthesis of Simple Phosphoglycerides

Cytidine Diphosphate Diglyceride-Glyceride Precursor

The phosphatidyl alcohols can be synthesized from the precursor cytidine diphosphate diglyceride (CDP-diglyceride), the activated form of phosphatidic acid (Fig. 11-9). Phosphatidic acid reacts with cytidine triphosphate to produce CDP-diglyceride and pyrophosphate:

- CDP-diglyceride reacts with choline to form phosphatidylcholine.
- CDP-diglyceride reacts with ethanolamine to form phosphatidylethanolamine.
- CDP-diglyceride reacts with serine to produce phosphatidylserine.
- CDP-diglyceride reacts with inositol to form phosphatidylinositol.

Phosphatidylcholine from Phosphatidylserine

Phosphatidylserine is first decarboxylated in a reaction that requires pyridoxal phosphate (vitamin B$_6$) to form phosphatidylethanolamine. Phosphatidylcholine can then be formed from phosphatidylethanolamine with the addition of three methyl groups from S-adenosyl methionine to the primary amino group of ethanolamine (Fig. 11-10).

Cytidine Diphosphate Diglyceride-Alcohol Precursors

Choline from the diet or choline and ethanolamine salvaged from turnover of phospholipids can be activated with kinases to CDP-choline and CDP-ethanolamine. In this pathway,

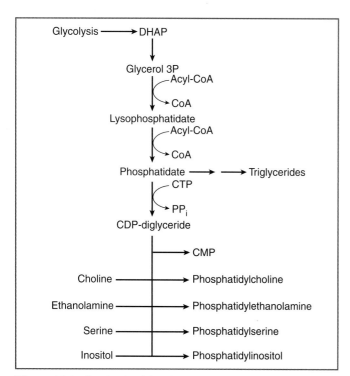

Figure 11-9. Synthesis of the phosphatidyl alcohols from cytidine diphosphate (CDP)-diglyceride. DHAP, dihydroxyacetone phosphate; CoA, coenzyme A; CTP, cytidine triphosphate; PP$_i$, inorganic pyrophosphate; CMP, cytidine monophosphate.

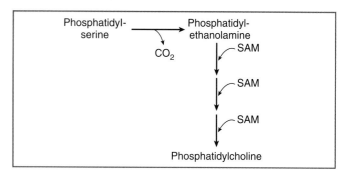

Figure 11-10. Synthesis of phosphatidylcholine from phosphatidylserine. SAM, S-adenosyl methionine.

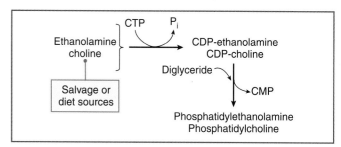

Figure 11-11. Salvage of choline and ethanolamine with cytidine diphosphate (CDP) conjugation. CTP, cytidine triphosphate; CMP, cytidine monophosphate; inorganic phosphate

CDP-choline adds choline to diglyceride with release of free cytidine monophosphate (Fig. 11-11).

Complex Phospholipids

Glycerol Ethers

If the acyl group on the glycerol carbon 1 is replaced with an unsaturated acyl group joined with an ether linkage instead of an ester linkage, the product is a plasminogen. The most common plasminogens, phosphatidylethanolamine and phosphatidylcholine, are found in large concentrations in nerves and the heart, respectively, where they are thought to provide protection against oxidative stress.

If the ether at carbon 1 is joined to a saturated acyl group and an acetyl group is esterified to carbon 2, the product is platelet-activating factor. Platelet activating factor causes platelet aggregation at concentrations of 10 to 11 mol/L (Fig. 11-12).

Cardiolipin

Two molecules of phosphatidic acid joined by ester linkages to glycerol create a symmetric molecule called cardiolipin. This phospholipid, originally described in heart mitochondria, is present at high concentrations in the inner mitochondrial membrane.

Phospholipases

Phospholipase enzymes are found in pancreatic secretions and in tissues. They play a role in toxins and venoms in digesting membranes to allow the spread of infection. In addition to

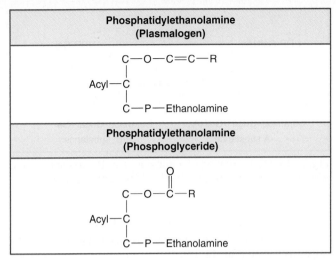

Figure 11-12. Comparison of plasmalogen and phosphoglyceride structures.

Phosphatidylethanolamine
(Plasmalogen)

$$C-O-C=C-R$$
$$Acyl-C$$
$$C-P-Ethanolamine$$

Phosphatidylethanolamine
(Phosphoglyceride)

$$C-O-\overset{\overset{\textstyle O}{\|}}{C}-R$$
$$Acyl-C$$
$$C-P-Ethanolamine$$

Figure 11-13. Action of phospholipases.

their digestive function in recycling precursors, they have roles in signal transduction.

- Phospholipase A_1 and A_2 remove acyl groups to form lysophospholipids (Fig. 11-13). This is the first step in the remodeling of phospholipids, where different acyl groups can be esterified at C_1 and C_2 to produce a variety of phospholipids.
- Phospholipase A_2 releases arachidonic acid, a precursor for prostaglandin synthesis. Arachidonate and other polyunsaturated fatty acids are found primarily at the C_2 position of glycerol in phospholipids.
- Phospholipase C liberates two potent intracellular signals, diacylglycerol and inositol triphosphate, from phosphatidylinositol 4,5-bisphosphate (see Chapter 5).
- Phospholipase D generates phosphatidic acid from various phospholipids.

●●● RESPIRATORY DISTRESS SYNDROME

Approximately 100,000 infants in the United States are afflicted with respiratory distress syndrome (hyaline membrane disease) annually. Respiratory distress syndrome is caused by the lack of surfactant production in the lungs of premature infants. A major component of lung surfactant is dipalmitoyl lecithin (a general term for phosphatidylcholine). The surface tension in the lung alveoli increases when the concentration of surfactant decreases. This causes portions of the lungs to collapse, severely reducing O_2 and CO_2 exchange.

KEY POINTS ABOUT RESPIRATORY DISTRESS SYNDROME

- Both triglycerides and phosphoglycerides have phosphatidic acid as a common precursor.
- Phospholipids are the major component of cellular membranes.

●●● SPHINGOLIPID METABOLISM

Sphingolipids are named for the sphingosine backbone that is the counterpart of glycerol in phospholipids (Fig. 11-14). The sphingolipids serve a structural and recognition role in membranes and are synthesized in the cells where they are needed.

Ceramide Synthesis

The sphingolipids are derived from a common precursor, ceramide (Fig. 11-15). Sphingosine is produced by condensation and modification of palmitoyl-CoA and serine. The sphingosine is converted into ceramide by the addition of an acyl group to the amino group at carbon 1 of the sphingosine backbone. The acyl group is bound in a nonsaponifiable, amide form.

Ceramide is then converted to sphingomyelin, cerebrosides, gangliosides, and sulfatides.

- Sphingomyelin is produced by reaction of phosphatidylcholine with ceramide. Sphingomyelin is a sphingophospholipid and is an important component of nerve cell myelin.

Phosphatidic Acid	Ceramide
$C_1-O-Acyl$	Attachment site for sugars and phosphorylcholine
$C_2-O-Acyl$	$HO-C_1$
$C_3-Ⓟ$	$_2C-N-Acyl$
	$HO-C_3$
	C_4
	C_5
	$Acyl\ (C_{6-18})$

Figure 11-14. Structure of a ceramide compared with phosphatidic acid.

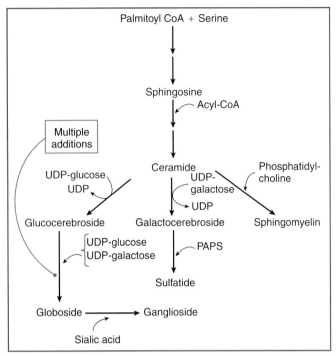

Figure 11-15. Overview of pathways for sphingolipid synthesis. *CoA*, coenzyme A, *UDP*, uridine diphosphate; *PAPS*, 3′-phosphoadenosine-5′-phosphosulfate.

- Cerebrosides are formed by addition of neutral or amino sugars to ceramide. Glucocerebroside is produced by reaction of uridine diphosphate (UDP)-glucose with ceramide. Further addition of either galactose or glucose from the UDP precursors produces a globoside.
- Gangliosides are produced by the addition of one or more sialic acid groups (also called N-acetylneuraminic acid) to a cerebroside.
- Sulfatides are produced by the addition of sulfate from the precursor 3′-phosphoadenosine-5′-phosphosulfate (Fig. 11-16) to galactocerebroside. (This glycosphingolipid is produced similarly to glucocerebroside except UDP-galactose is the precursor.)

ABO Blood Groups

The ABO antigens that determine the compatibility of red blood cells (RBCs) during transfusion are glycosphingolipids. A ceramide termed H substance, a component of the RBC

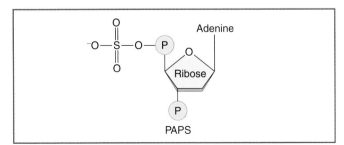

Figure 11-16. Structure of 3′-phosphoadenosine-5′-phosphosulfate (*PAPS*).

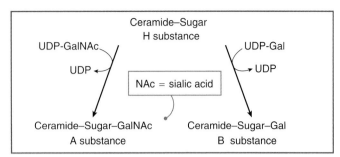

Figure 11-17. Formation of A substance or B substance of the ABO blood group antigens. *UDP*, uridine diphosphate.

membrane, is acted on by either Gal sialic acid (NAc) transferase or Gal transferase to modify the terminal sugar of the oligosaccharide (Fig. 11-17).
- Type O individuals lack either of these transferases and have only the core H substance on their RBCs.
- Type A individuals have the GalNAc transferase and have A substance on their RBCs.
- Type B individuals have the Gal transferase and have B substance on their RBCs.
- Type AB individuals have both the GalNAc and Gal transferases, and both A and B substances are on their RBCs.

Sphingolipidoses (Lipid Storage Diseases)

Sphingolipids are normally digested in lysosomes. The sugars are removed from the terminal ends of the oligosaccharide by lysosomal exoglycosidases, and a deficiency of any of these enzymes blocks the removal of any of the remaining sugars. Several genetic diseases referred to as sphingolipidoses result from deficiencies in these lysosomal enzymes (Fig. 11-18 and Table 11-1).

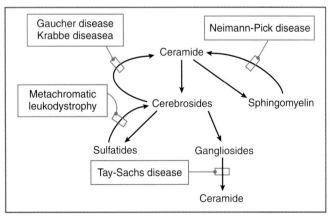

Figure 11-18. Enzyme deficiencies in the lysosomal digestion of sphingolipids.

TABLE 11-1. Common Sphingolipidoses

DEFICIENT ENZYME	NAME OF DISEASE	SYMPTOMS
Sphingomyelinase	Niemann-Pick disease	Mental retardation, liver and spleen enlargement
Hexosaminidase A	Tay-Sachs disease	Mental retardation, muscular weakness, blindness
Arylsulfatase A	Metachromatic leukodystrophy	Mental retardation, progressive paralysis
β-Galactosidase	Krabbe disease	Mental and motor deterioration, myelin deficiency, blindness and deafness
β-Glucosidase	Gaucher disease	Hepatosplenomegaly, osteoporosis of long bones

●●● EICOSANOIDS

The eicosanoids are paracrine (local diffusion to another type of cell) and autocrine (local diffusion to same cell) messenger molecules derived from 20-carbon polyunsaturated fatty acids. They have half-lives of 10 seconds to 5 minutes and act primarily within their tissue of origin. Three major classes are derived from arachidonic acid: prostaglandins, thromboxanes, and leukotrienes (Fig. 11-19).

Prostaglandins

The prostaglandin intermediate, prostaglandin H_2 (PGH_2), is produced by cyclooxygenase as a precursor for other prostaglandins and for the thromboxanes (Fig. 11-20). PGH_2 contains a cyclopentane ring formed by action of cyclooxygenase. Cyclooxygenase action is inhibited by aspirin and indomethacin, producing antiinflammatory effects and reducing menstrual cramps.

The prostaglandins influence a wide variety of biologic effects: inflammation, smooth muscle contraction, sodium and water retention, platelet aggregation, and gastric secretion.

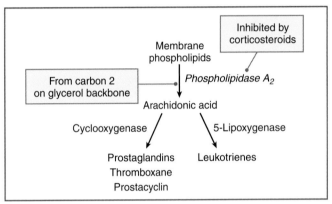

Figure 11-19. Overview of eicosanoid pathways.

Thromboxanes

Thromboxanes are formed by the action of thromboxane synthetase on PGH_2. Thromboxane A_2 is produced in platelets and causes arteriole contraction and platelet aggregation. Since the PGH_2 precursor is produced by cyclooxygenase

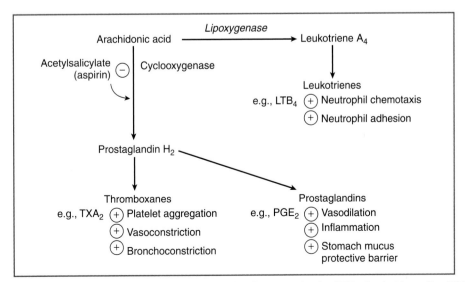

Figure 11-20. Examples of prostaglandin thromboxane and leukotriene synthesis. *LTB₄*, leukotriene B_4; *TXA₂*, thromboxane A_2; *PGE₂*, prostaglandin A_2.

action, thromboxane synthesis is also inhibited by aspirin and indomethacin; this leads to prolonged clotting time.

Leukotrienes

Leukotriene (LT) A_4 is formed by the action of lipoxygenase on arachidonic acid (see Fig. 11-20). LTB_4 stimulates neutrophil chemotaxis and adhesion. LTC_4, LTD_4, and LTE_4 are referred to as the "slow-reacting substances of anaphylaxis"; they mediate allergic reactions, chemotaxis of white blood cells, and inflammation. Lipoxygenase is not inhibited by aspirin or indomethacin.

KEY POINTS ABOUT SPHINGOLIPIDS AND EICOSANOIDS

- Ceramide forms the core structure of the sphingolipids.
- The eicosanoids are short lived, locally produced, and locally acting signal molecules that are derived from arachidonic acid.

Self-assessment questions can be accessed at www. StudentConsult.com.

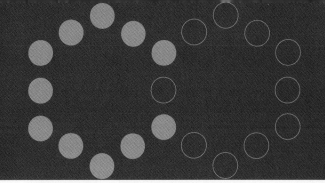

Amino Acid and Heme Metabolism

12

●●● PRODUCTION OF AMMONIUM IONS AND THE UREA CYCLE

The structure of amino acids reveals that they are simply carbohydrates with a nitrogen attached (Fig. 12-1). Thus, when amino acids are not needed for synthesis of other nitrogen-containing molecules they can be converted to carbohydrates. When the nitrogen is removed from the amino acid, the residual carbohydrate is converted either into pyruvate or into a citric acid cycle intermediate for energy production or gluconeogenesis. Ammonia is toxic, so the pathway for disposal of amino acid nitrogen is designed to convert the nitrogen to the nontoxic neutral compound urea, which is excreted in urine.

Flow of Nitrogen from Amino Acids to Urea

Amino acid nitrogen is transferred to the urea cycle in three steps: transamination, formation of ammonia, and formation of urea (Fig. 12-2).

Transamination Reactions

Amino acid nitrogen begins its path to its final incorporation into urea when amino acids undergo transamination with α-ketoglutarate to produce glutamate. These reactions are catalyzed by aminotransferases (transaminases) that transfer the α-amino group from the amino acid to α-ketoglutarate, producing glutamate. There are about 12 transaminases that catalyze the disposal of nitrogen through formation of glutamate. Two clinically important transaminases serve as markers for liver damage when they appear in high concentrations in the blood:

- Aspartate aminotransferase: Catalyzes reversible transamination of nitrogen between aspartate and glutamate (Fig. 12-3).
- Alanine aminotransferase: Catalyzes reversible transamination of nitrogen between alanine and pyruvate.

Pyridoxal phosphate, the active form of vitamin B_6 (pyridoxine), is required by transaminases as a coenzyme.

Pyruvate	Alanine
CH₃ | C=O | COOH	CH₃ | C—NH₂ | COOH
α-Ketoglutarate	**Glutamate**
COOH | C=O | CH₂ | CH₂ | COOH	COOH | C—NH₂ | CH₂ | CH₂ | COOH
Oxaloacetate	**Aspartate**
COOH | C=O | CH₂ | COOH	COOH | C—NH₂ | CH₂ | COOH

Figure 12-1. Comparison of common carbohydrate–amino acid pairs.

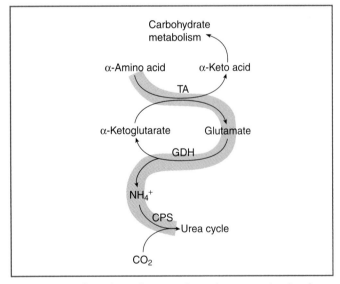

Figure 12-2. Overview of ammonia and urea production from amino acid N₂. *CPS*, carbamoyl phosphate synthetase; *GDH*, glutamate dehydrogenase; *TA*, transaminase.

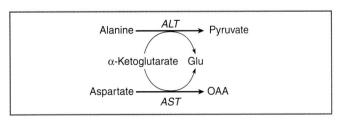

Figure 12-3. Aspartate aminotransferase (*AST*) and alanine amino-transferase (*ALT*). *OAA*, oxaloacetate.

NEUROSCIENCE

Amino Acid Neurotransmitters

γ-Aminobutyrate (GABA) is synthesized by decarboxylation of glutamate. GABA is an inhibitory neurotransmitter in the central nervous system, as are the monocarboxylic amino acids glycine, β-alanine, and taurine. This is in contrast to the dicarboxylic amino acids glutamate and aspartate, which are excitatory.

Formation of Ammonia

Oxidative deamination of glutamate to α-ketoglutarate in the mitochondrial matrix produces free ammonia (Fig. 12-4). This reaction is catalyzed by glutamate dehydrogenase, producing either nicotinamide adenine dinucleotide or nicotinamide adenine dinucleotide phosphate (NADPH). The reaction is reversible, so it can also incorporate free ammonia into α-ketoglutarate when needed to form glutamate. The ammonia that is liberated in the mitochondrial matrix serves as a precursor for the urea cycle.

Formation of Urea

The urea cycle begins in the mitochondrial matrix and ends with the formation of urea in the cytoplasm (Fig. 12-5).

1. Carbamoyl phosphate synthetase I (CPS I): Ammonium ions are joined with carbon dioxide and adenosine triphosphate to produce carbamoyl phosphate (see Fig. 12-5).
2. Ornithine transcarbamoylase: Carbamoyl phosphate and ornithine are condensed to form citrulline. Both ornithine and citrulline have specific membrane transport carriers in the mitochondrial membrane.
3. Argininosuccinic acid synthetase: In the cytoplasm, citrulline and aspartic acid condense to form argininosuccinate.
4. Argininosuccinase: Argininosuccinate is cleaved to form fumarate and arginine.
5. Arginase: Arginine is cleaved to release urea and regenerate ornithine.

Anaplerotic Replacement of Aspartate

An active urea cycle quickly depletes cytoplasmic aspartate by formation of argininosuccinate. An anaplerotic mechanism prevents this by the conversion of fumarate to oxaloacetate (OAA) (see Fig. 12-5), which can be converted to aspartate. This is a separate set of enzymes from the forms that are located in the mitochondrion.

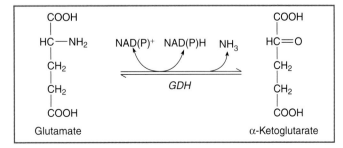

Figure 12-4. Glutamate dehydrogenase (*GDH*) reaction.

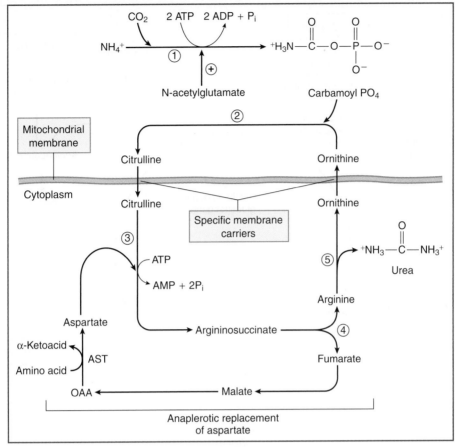

Figure 12-5. The urea cycle. See text for numbered enzymes. *ATP*, adenosine triphosphate; *ADP*, adenosine diphosphate; *Pᵢ*, inorganic phosphate; *AMP*, adenosine monophosphate; *AST*, aspartate aminotransferase; *OAA*, oxaloacetate.

Urea Cycle Regulation

Short Term

Immediately after a high protein meal, excess amino acids are catabolized, with the production of large amounts of ammonia. This is accomplished by the CPS I enzyme, which is allosterically activated by N-acetylglutamate. This positive effector is synthesized from acetyl-coenzyme A (CoA) and glutamate; the reaction is stimulated by arginine. All of these intermediates are elevated in liver after a high protein meal. (Note: The cytoplasmic CPS II enzyme associated with pyrimidine synthesis is not regulated by N-acetylglutamate.)

Long Term

Increased levels of ammonia activate the genes for urea cycle enzymes. Such a sustained increase in ammonia occurs during starvation when muscle proteins are broken down for energy.

KEY POINTS ABOUT PRODUCTION OF AMMONIUM IONS AND THE UREA CYCLE

- Amino acid nitrogen is transferred to the urea cycle in three steps: (1) transamination, (2) formation of ammonia, and (3) formation of carbamoyl phosphate.
- The carbon skeleton of aspartate is found in OAA, and the carbon skeleton of glutamic acid is found in α-ketoglutarate.

- The mitochondrial form of CPS requires a positive allosteric effector, N-acetylglutamate, for activity. The cytosolic form of CPS, which is part of the pyrimidine synthetic pathway, does not require acetylglutamate and uses glutamine as the nitrogen donor for carbamoyl phosphate synthesis.

●●● AMINO ACID DEGRADATION

Transamination of amino acid nitrogen also produces carbon skeletons of amino acids as α-keto acids. These carbon skeletons enter intermediary metabolism at various points depending on whether they are converted to pyruvate, acetyl-CoA, acetoacetyl-CoA, or citric acid cycle intermediates (Fig. 12-6). They provide substrates for gluconeogenesis or ketone body production. Ketogenic amino acids are converted to either acetyl-CoA or acetoacetyl-CoA, whereas glucogenic amino acids are converted to pyruvate or to citric acid cycle intermediates.

Alanine, Cysteine, Glycine, Serine, and Threonine Conversion to Pyruvate

Alanine yields pyruvate directly by transamination, whereas cysteine and serine must have their side chains removed first (see Fig. 12-6). Glycine interconverts with serine,

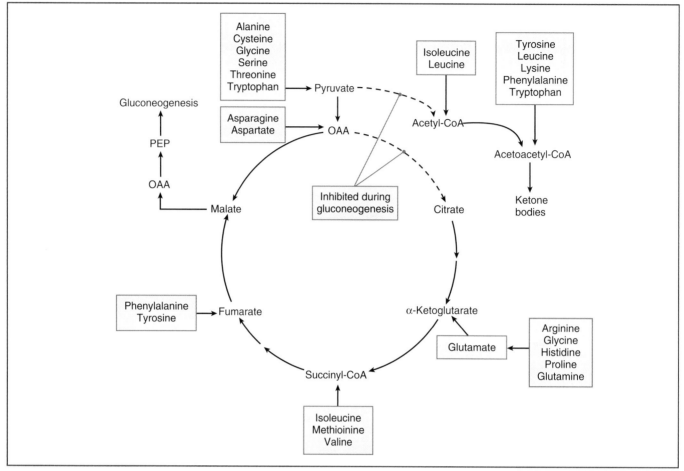

Figure 12-6. Metabolic intermediates formed from amino acid degradation. *CoA*, coenzyme A; *PEP*, peptida; *OAA*, oxaloacetate.

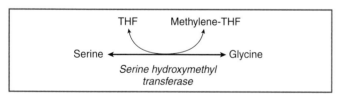

Figure 12-7. Interconversion of serine and glycine. *THF*, tetrahydrofolate.

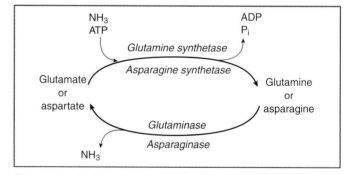

Figure 12-8. Interconversion of glutamate/glutamine and aspartate/asparagine. *ATP*, adenosine triphosphate *ADP*, adenosine diphosphate; *P₁*, inorganic phosphate.

providing a degradative route to pyruvate (Fig. 12-7). The enzyme that interconverts glycine and serine, serine hydroxymethyl transferase, requires methylene tetrahydrofolate as a cofactor. Threonine is first converted to aminoacetone and is then deaminated to pyruvate.

Conversion of Aspartate and Asparagine to Oxaloacetate

Asparaginase removes the amide nitrogen on the asparagine side chain to produce aspartate (Fig. 12-8; see also Fig. 12-6); aspartate is converted to OAA by transamination with aspartate aminotransferase.

Branched-Chain Amino Acid Degradation to Succinyl-Coenzyme A and Acetoacetyl-Coenzyme A

Transamination of leucine, isoleucine, and valine (branched-chain amino acids) yields branched-chain α-keto acids. This is followed by oxidative decarboxylation of these α-keto acids by branched-chain α-ketoacid dehydrogenase multienzyme complexes, which are similar to those that catalyze pyruvate and α-ketoglutarate oxidation. Valine and isoleucine are converted to succinyl-CoA, and leucine is converted to acetoacetyl-CoA (see Fig. 12-6).

PHARMACOLOGY

Histamine

Histidine decarboxylase produces histamine directly from histidine. Histamine is a potent vasodilator and is released by mast cells during the allergic response. This autacoid relaxes smooth muscles in the blood vessels and contracts smooth muscle in bronchi and gut. Many allergy medications block the binding of histamine to its H_1 receptor, preventing vasodilation and capillary permeability.

Conversion of Glutamine, Proline, Arginine, and Histidine to α-Ketoglutarate

Glutamine is converted to glutamate by glutaminase (see Fig. 12-8), and the side chains of proline, arginine, and histidine are also modified to produce glutamate (5-carbon). Glutamate is then converted to α-ketoglutarate by glutamate dehydrogenase (see Fig. 12-6).

The conversion of histidine to glutamate provides a test for folate deficiency (Fig. 12-9). N-formiminoglutamate (FIGLU) is the intermediate in the catabolism of histidine that produces glutamate. This reaction requires tetrahydrofolate, and FIGLU will increase in the urine in a patient who is deficient in folate when given an oral histidine load. Histidase, an enzyme in this pathway, is deficient in histidinemia.

Conversion of Methionine to Succinyl-Coenzyme A

Methionine is converted to homocysteine in the activated methyl cycle (Fig. 12-10). Cystathionine synthase converts homocysteine to cystathionine, which is then converted to propionyl-CoA. The propionyl-CoA is then converted to succinyl-CoA via methylmalonyl-CoA (see Fig. 12-6).

S-adenosyl methionine (SAM) is formed in the activated methyl cycle by transfer of the adenosyl group from adenosine triphosphate to the sulfur of methionine (see Fig. 12-10). The methyl group attached to the methionine sulfur transfers readily to the nitrogen, oxygen, or carbon of an acceptor.

$$\text{SAM} + \text{acceptor} \rightarrow \text{S-adenosyl homocysteine} + \text{methylated acceptor}$$

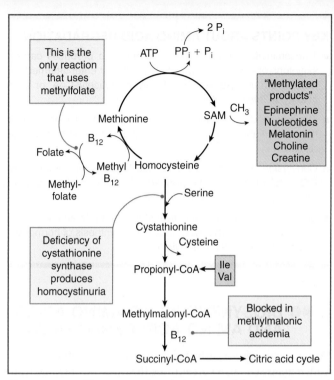

Figure 12-10. The activated methyl cycle and the degradation of methionine. P_i, inorganic phosphate; PP_i, inorganic pyrophosphate; *ATP*, adenosine triphosphate; *SAM*, S-adenosyl methionine; *CoA*, coenzyme A; *Ile*, isoleucine; *Val*, valine.

S-adenosyl homocysteine is the major donor of methyl groups in the synthesis of phospholipids, nucleotides, epinephrine, carnitine, melatonin, and creatine.

Conversion of Phenylalanine and Tyrosine to Fumarate and Acetoacetyl-Coenzyme A

Phenylalanine and tyrosine are degraded to homogentisate and ultimately to fumarate and acetoacetate (see Figs. 12-6 and 12-11).

Degradation of Tryptophan and Lysine

Both tryptophan and lysine are degraded to acetoacetyl-CoA. However, tryptophan is present in negligible amounts in proteins and its contribution to energy metabolism is of minor importance; more important is its role as precursor for niacin, serotonin, and melatonin (see later discussion; see Fig. 12-6).

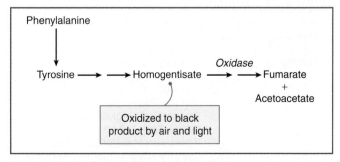

Figure 12-11. Conversion of phenylalanine and tyrosine to fumarate and acetoacetate.

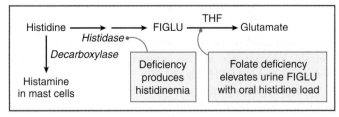

Figure 12-9. Formation of N-formiminoglutamate (*FIGLU*) in histidine metabolism.

KEY POINTS ABOUT AMINO ACID DEGRADATION

- Transamination of amino acid nitrogen also produces carbon skeletons of amino acids as α-keto acids that enter intermediary metabolism as pyruvate, acetyl-CoA, acetoacetyl-CoA, or citric acid cycle intermediates.

- The branched-chain amino acids are degraded in a pathway that has remarkable similarities to pyruvate and α-ketoglutarate oxidation.

- Conversion of histidine to glutamate involves the formation of FIGLU, an intermediate that appears in the urine of folate-deficient patients when given a histidine load.

- SAM is formed during the activated methyl cycle and serves as the major donor of methyl groups in the synthesis of hormones, nucleotides, and membrane lipids.

●●● BIOSYNTHESIS OF AMINO ACIDS AND AMINO ACID DERIVATIVES

Amino acids whose carbon skeletons can be synthesized are called nonessential, whereas those that must be obtained from the diet are termed essential (Table 12-1). Cysteine and tyrosine synthesis depend on adequate dietary methionine and phenylalanine.

Synthesis of Glutamate, Alanine, and Aspartate

Glutamate dehydrogenase incorporates free ammonium ions into α-ketoglutarate to produce glutamate by reversing oxidative deamination (see Fig. 12-4). Glutamate then serves as a source of nitrogen by transamination with pyruvate to make alanine, and OAA to make aspartate.

TABLE 12-1. Essential and Nonessential Amino Acids

ESSENTIAL AMINO ACIDS	NONESSENTIAL AMINO ACIDS AND THEIR SOURCE
Histidine (His)	Alanine (Ala) ← pyruvate
Isoleucine (Ile)	Arginine (Arg) ← urea cycle
Leucine (Leu)	Asparagine (Asn) ← oxaloacetate (OAA)
Lysine (Lys)	Aspartic acid (Asx) ← oxaloacetate (OAA)
Methionine (Met)	Glutamic acid ← α-ketoglutarate (α-KG)
Phenylalanine (Phe)	
Threonine (Thr)	Glutamine (Glx) ← α-ketoglutarate (α-KG)
Tryptophan (Trp)	
Valine (Val)	Glycine (Gly) ← pyruvate
	Proline (Pro) ← glutamate
	Serine (Ser) ← 3-phosphoglycerate
	If precursor is supplied in diet:
	Cysteine (Cys) ← methionine in diet
	Tyrosine (Tyr) ← phenylalanine in diet

Synthesis of Glutamine

Glutamine synthetase produces glutamine from glutamate in an energy-requiring reaction (see Fig. 12-8).

Synthesis of Serine and Glycine

Serine is synthesized through the conversion of 3-phosphoglycerate to 3-phosphopyruvate, which is then transaminated to form 3-phosphoserine. Serine is formed by removal of the phosphate ester. Glycine is formed from serine in a folate-requiring reaction (see Fig. 12-7).

HISTOLOGY

Erythropoiesis

Heme synthesis is coordinated with globin synthesis during erythropoiesis and as such does not occur in the mature erythrocyte. Erythropoiesis is the development of mature red blood cells from erythropoietic stem cells. The first cell that is morphologically recognizable in the red blood cell pathway is the proerythroblast. In the basophilic erythroblast, the nucleus becomes somewhat smaller, exhibiting a coarser appearance, and the cytoplasm becomes more basophilic owing to the presence of ribosomes. As the cell begins to produce hemoglobin, the cytoplasm attracts both basic and eosin stains and is called a polychromatophilic erythroblast. As maturation continues, the orthochromatophilic erythroblast extrudes its nucleus and the cell enters the circulation as a reticulocyte. As reticulocytes lose their polyribosomes, they become mature red blood cells.

Synthesis of Cysteine

Homocysteine derived from dietary methionine is combined with serine to produce cystathionine. Cystathionine is then cleaved to produce cysteine, an ammonium ion, and α-ketobutyrate. The α-ketobutyrate is decarboxylated to form propionyl-CoA.

Synthesis of Catecholamines and Melanin from Phenylalanine and Tyrosine

Phenylalanine is converted to tyrosine by phenylalanine hydroxylase. Phenylalanine hydroxylase is a mixed-function oxidase that uses the cofactor tetrahydrobiopterin to split molecular O_2, adding one atom to the phenylalanine ring and converting the other to water. Tetrahydrobiopterin contains the pteridine ring structure found in folic acid, but it is synthesized by the body and is therefore not a vitamin. Tetrahydrobiopterin is regenerated by dihydrobiopterin reductase and NADPH (Fig. 12-12).

Tyrosine hydroxylation yields 3,4-dihydroxyphenylalanine (DOPA). The DOPA pathway is active in neural tissue and adrenal medulla. DOPA is decarboxylated to produce 3,4-dihydroxyphenylethylamine (dopamine), which is then

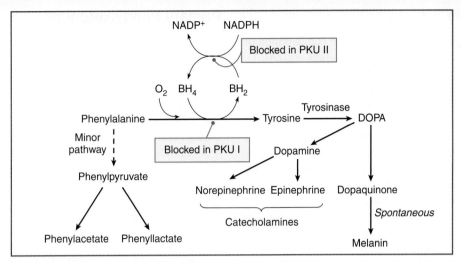

Figure 12-12. Synthesis of catecholamines, 3,4-dihydroxyphenylalanine (*DOPA*), and melanin from phenylalanine and tyrosine. *BH$_2$*, dihydrobiopterin; *BH$_4$*, tetrahydrobiopterin; *NADP*, nicotinamide adenine dinucleotide phosphate; *NADPH*, reduced NADP; *PKU*, phenylketonuria.

further hydroxylated to produce norepinephrine. Methylation of DOPA using SAM as the methyl donor produces epinephrine. In melanocytes, DOPA is oxidized to dopaquinone, which then polymerizes into the skin pigment melanin.

Synthesis of Serotonin and Melatonin

Tryptophan hydroxylase converts tryptophan to 5-hydroxytryptophan, which is then converted to serotonin (5-hydroxytryptamine). Serotonin synthesis occurs in the hypothalamus and brainstem, pineal gland, and chromaffin cells of the gut. Melatonin is produced from serotonin in the pineal gland during the dark phase of the light/dark cycle and is involved in regulating the sleep/wake cycle (Fig. 12-13).

Synthesis of Creatine Phosphate

Creatine phosphate is a high-energy storage compound in muscle that is derived from arginine, glycine, and SAM. Creatine spontaneously cyclizes to produce creatinine at a constant rate. The rate of creatinine excretion in urine is useful in evaluating renal function.

Synthesis of the Polyamines from Ornithine and Decarboxylated S-Adenosyl Methionine

Ornithine decarboxylase appears in increased concentrations as cells enter the replicative cycle. It initiates a pathway for synthesis of several polyamines that play a role in DNA

synthesis. Decarboxylation of ornithine produces putrescine, the first polyamine in the pathway. Putrescine then reacts with decarboxylated SAM to produce spermidine. Lastly, spermidine reacts with decarboxylated SAM to produce spermine.

●●● HEME METABOLISM

Heme is a cyclic planar molecule (a wheel) with an iron atom at the center hub (Fig. 12-14) and an asymmetric arrangement of side chains around the rim. Four pyrrole rings connected by methenyl bridges (a tetrapyrrole ring) compose the rim of the wheel. The iron is chelated in place by coordination-bonding with the pyrrole nitrogens of the porphyrin.

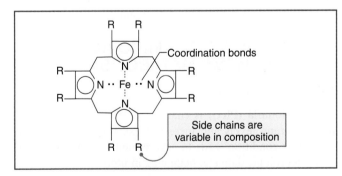

Figure 12-14. Structure of heme.

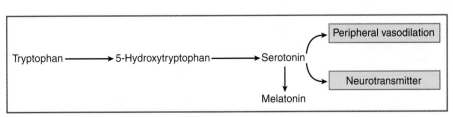

Figure 12-13. Conversion of tryptophan to serotonin and melatonin.

Heme Synthesis

The rate-limiting step in heme synthesis is the condensation of succinyl-CoA and glycine to form δ-aminolevulinic acid (ALA). This reaction is catalyzed by mitochondrial enzyme ALA synthetase. The translation of messenger RNA for ALA synthetase is inhibited by heme, thereby providing a feedback inhibition by heme for its own synthesis (Fig. 12-15).

ALA dehydratase catalyzes condensation of two molecules of ALA to form porphobilinogen in the cytoplasm. ALA dehydratase is inhibited by lead, resulting in accumulation of ALA, leading to its excretion in urine; this is diagnostic for lead poisoning.

Reactions that cyclize the porphobilinogen and modify porphyrin ring to produce coproporphyrinogen III are catalyzed in the cytoplasm. Coproporphyrinogen III is transported back into the mitochondrion to be modified to produce protoporphyrin IX. As a last step, a ferrous atom is added to protoporphyrin IX by ferrochelatase.

Heme Degradation

In the spleen, heme oxygenase opens the heme tetrapyrrole ring to produce biliverdin (verd = green) and one molecule of carbon monoxide (heme oxygenase is similar in function to cytochrome P 450 monooxygenases; the reaction requires NADPH and molecular O_2. Next, biliverdin reductase produces bilirubin in an NADPH-requiring reaction. Bilirubin, a hydrophobic molecule, is bound by albumin and transported to the liver, where it is conjugated with two molecules of glucuronic acid; this produces the water-soluble bilirubin diglucuronide (Fig. 12-16), which is excreted in bile.

Bilirubin Metabolism in the Gut

The gut floras hydrolyze bilirubin diglucuronide and reduce free bilirubin to the colorless urobilinogen. Urobilinogen is further processed to produce stercobilin, which gives feces its characteristic brown color. Some urobilinogen is reabsorbed from the gut and removed from the circulation in urine as urobilin; this is responsible for the amber color of urine.

⬤⬤⬤ DISEASES OF AMINO ACID AND HEME METABOLISM

Phenylketonuria

Phenylketonuria (PKU) is characterized by elevated blood phenylalanine levels and increased excretion of phenylalanine. This condition leads to severe mental retardation and other neurologic damage, beginning in utero.

Primary Phenylketonuria

The deficient enzyme in the primary form of the disease, PKU I, is phenylalanine hydroxylase (see Fig. 12-12). A buildup of phenylalanine causes increased flow through a minor pathway, called a shunt pathway. The shunt pathway produces neurotoxic metabolites—phenylpyruvate, phenylacetic acid, and phenyllactic acid—that normally are produced during phenylalanine metabolism but in nontoxic amounts.

A phenylalanine-restricted diet until age 6 years generally prevents neurologic damage; the brain becomes resistant to shunt pathway metabolites after this age

Secondary Phenylketonuria

A secondary form, PKU II, is due to a deficiency in dihydrobiopterin reductase (see Fig. 12-12). Phenylalanine blood levels respond to a phenylalanine-restricted diet, as expected, but the course of neurologic damage remains unchanged, since other neurotransmitters required for brain development also require tetrahydrobiopterin as a cofactor in their synthesis.

Alcaptonuria

Alcaptonuria, described by Garrod in 1902, was the first described inborn error of metabolism. It is a benign disease in which homogentisate accumulates (Fig. 12-11). Homogentisate in the urine oxidizes to a black substance, giving the urine a dark color.

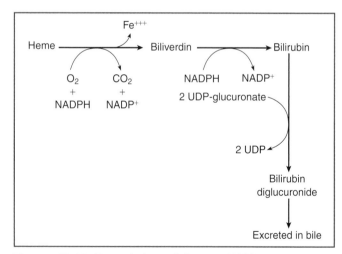

Figure 12-16. Degradation of heme. *NADP*, nicotinamide adenine dinucleotide phosphate; *NADPH* reduced NADP; *UDP*, uridine diphosphate.

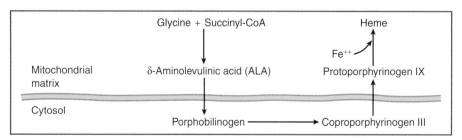

Figure 12-15. Biosynthesis of heme.

Methylmalonic Acidemia

Methylmalonic acidemia is caused by a deficiency in methylmalonyl-CoA mutase, which functions in the conversion of methionine, isoleucine, and valine to succinyl-CoA (see Fig. 12-6). The pathway involves the formation of propionyl-CoA and its conversion to methylmalonyl-CoA before the formation of succinyl-CoA. Affected newborns are characterized by recurrent vomiting, hepatomegaly, and developmental retardation owing to accumulation of methylmalonic acid. One form of this disease results from defective synthesis of 5'-deoxyadenosylcobalamin, the active form of cobalamin for the mutase reaction. Symptoms can be alleviated by administration of large doses of vitamin B_{12}. As for PKU, a diet restricted in the relevant amino acids (Met, Ile, Val) is prescribed.

Maple Syrup Urine Disease

Maple syrup urine disease is also known as branched-chain ketonuria. It is caused by a deficiency in the branched-chain α-keto acid dehydrogenase enzyme. This is a single enzyme that acts on all three branched-chain keto acids that are produced from transamination of Val, Leu, and Ile. As these keto acids accumulate, they give the urine the odor of maple syrup. Affected infants are difficult to feed and may vomit; severe mental defects develop, and the disease can be fatal. Therapy includes dietary restriction of the branched-chain amino acids.

Urea Cycle Disorders—Ammonia Disposal

All defects in the urea cycle result in interference with ammonia excretion and produce ammonia toxicity (hyperammonemia). This toxicity is most severe when the defect is in CPS or ornithine transcarbamoylase (see Fig. 12-5). Citrullinemia and argininosuccinic aciduria are treated with arginine. This creates high concentrations of ornithine that can react with carbamoyl phosphate to increase citrulline production, leading to lower free ammonia levels and resulting in the excretion of citrulline and argininosuccinate in place of urea. Treatment with sodium benzoate (Fig. 12-17) and phenylacetate also helps because these compounds are excreted in urine as adducts with glycine (hippuric acid is benzoylglycine) and glutamine, respectively, causing the amino acid metabolic pathways to consume nitrogen to replace glycine and glutamine.

Porphyrias

Porphyrias are diseases resulting from deficiencies in the heme biosynthetic pathway enzymes. They are usually dominant and are often accompanied by photosensitivity, which is

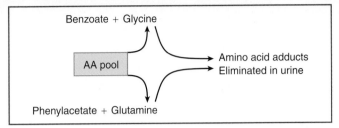

Figure 12-17. Treatment of hyperammonemia by adduct formation between benzoate and glycine and between phenylacetate and glutamate.

due to damage from oxygen radicals produced by irradiated porphyrin intermediates.

Acute intermittent porphyria is due to the buildup of porphobilinogen (not affected by light) and ALA produced buy a deficiency in uroporphyrinogen I synthase. This causes abdominal pain, constipation, and mental derangement. The symptoms occur as acute attacks and there is no photosensitivity involved. Porphyria cutanea tarda does demonstrate photosensitivity and is caused by a buildup of porphyrins (light causes production of oxidants) due to a deficiency of uroporphyrinogen decarboxylase. There are no neurologic or abdominal symptoms as in acute intermittent porphyria and the symptoms do not occur as acute attacks. Symptoms appear as a result of alcohol abuse or liver damage.

KEY POINTS ABOUT HEME METABOLISM

- Phenylalanine hydroxylation to tyrosine requires a cofactor—biopterin—that has structural similarities to folate.

- Both forms of methylmalonic acidemia result in defective conversion of methylmalonyl-CoA to succinyl-CoA by methylmalonyl-CoA mutase; one form is due to a defective enzyme and the other form to vitamin B_{12} deficiency.

- Heme is synthesized from glycine and succinyl-CoA; the cytoplasmic step catalyzed by ALA dehydrase is sensitive to lead poisoning.

- Degradation of heme produces biliverdin and bilirubin; bilirubin is eventually conjugated (direct bilirubin).

- Symptoms of all urea cycle disorders are vomiting, lethargy, irritability, and mental retardation. Treatment of all urea cycle disorders includes a low-protein diet taken in frequent, small meals to avoid rapid increases in ammonia production.

Self-assessment questions can be accessed at www. StudentConsult.com.

Integration of Carbohydrate, Fat, and Amino Acid Metabolism

13

●●● HORMONAL INFLUENCES ON METABOLISM

All metabolic pathways are coordinated by hormone signaling. The metabolic activity within various tissues is regulated to store energy when ingested fuel is plentiful and to draw on energy stores to maintain blood glucose during fasting or starvation. The actions of hormones regulate critical points in pathways to avoid competing reactions—a process called reciprocal regulation (Table 13-1). Thus if a hormone triggers a wave of phosphorylation within the cell, the effect will be to activate enzymes in one pathway and to inactivate enzymes in a competing pathway. Each hormone that affects carbohydrate and amino acid metabolism has consistent effects on its target tissues through its signaling mechanism. It is important to keep in mind that hormone action is always in concert with the underlying allosteric properties of individual enzymes.

Insulin—A Hormone for Feasting

The metabolic actions of insulin are most pronounced in liver, muscle, and adipose tissue (Fig. 13-1). The overall effect of insulin is to promote fuel storage. This involves synthesis of glycogen in liver and muscle as well as synthesis of triglycerides primarily in liver and also in adipose tissue. Simultaneous insulin activation of energy-storing enzymes (e.g., glycogen synthase) and inactivation of energy-mobilizing enzymes (e.g., glycogen phosphorylase) is the result of dephosphorylation of these enzymes. Insulin also promotes increased enzyme synthesis (e.g., glucokinase and phosphofructokinase) through effects on gene transcription. Insulin additionally increases glucose uptake by muscle and adipose tissue by promoting translocation of vesicles containing glucose transporter (GLUT4) receptors to the cell surface. Insulin also increases K^+ uptake because its signaling pathways up-regulate the Na^+/K^+-adenosine triphosphatase membrane transporter.

Insulin is a hormone that is released in response to ingestion of carbohydrates. It is synthesized by pancreatic β-cells as an inactive precursor—proinsulin. Proteolytic cleavage of proinsulin yields C peptide (C = connecting) and active insulin, composed of disulfide-linked A and B chains. The release of both insulin and C peptide is influenced primarily by the blood glucose concentration, although it is also influenced by some amino acids (e.g., arginine), gastrointestinal peptides (gastric inhibitory peptide and glucagon-like peptide-1), and neural stimulation.

The insulin receptor is a tetramer whose cytosolic domain has tyrosine kinase activity that is activated when insulin binds to the extracellular domain (see Fig. 5-10). Insulin binding triggers autophosphorylation of the cytosolic domain, followed by phosphorylation of a cytosolic signaling protein,

TABLE 13-1. Allosteric and Hormonal Regulation of Metabolic Pathways

CHARACTERISTIC	UNTREATED TYPE 1 DIABETES	STARVATION
1. Gluconeogenesis	Increased	Decreased
2. Glycogenolysis	Increased	Glycogen absent
3. Blood glucose	Above normal range	Below normal range
4. Muscle protein	Degraded for gluconeogenesis	Conserved
5. Ketone body synthesis	Pathologic ketoacidosis	Ketosis, but not ketoacidosis
6. Brain fuels	Glucose only	Glucose and ketones

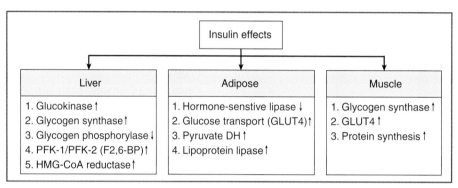

Figure 13-1. Metabolic effects of insulin in liver, adipose, and muscle tissue. *PFK*, phosphofructokinase; *F2,6-BP*, fructose-2, 6-biphosphatose; *HMG-CoA*, β-hydroxy-β-methylglutaryl coenzyme A; *DH*, dehydrogenase.

the insulin receptor substrate. This initiates signaling pathways that produce the intracellular responses to insulin. Increased adipose tissue leads to down-regulation of insulin receptor synthesis, whereas weight loss leads to up-regulation of receptor synthesis.

PHYSIOLOGY

Biphasic Insulin Secretion

Insulin is released in two phases. The first, a rapid release phase, represents preformed proinsulin, which is rapidly depleted. The second phase represents new synthesis of insulin, showing that glucose also stimulates messenger ribonucleic acid (mRNA) transcription.

Glucagon—A Hormone for Fasting

The metabolic actions of glucagon are most pronounced in the liver (Fig. 13-2). The overall effect of glucagon is to promote glycogenolysis and gluconeogenesis in the liver to prevent fasting hypoglycemia. Secretion of glucagon from pancreatic-α-cells is stimulated by below normal concentrations (<70 mg/L) of circulating glucose. Glucagon receptors are coupled to stimulatory G-proteins, which send a wave of phosphorylation through the cell by stimulating adenylate cyclase to increase intracellular cyclic adenosine monophosphate. Phosphorylation by protein kinase A simultaneously stimulates some enzymes and inhibits others. For example, phosphorylation stimulates glycogen phosphorylase to mobilize glycogen, whereas it inhibits enzymes such as glycogen synthase that store glycogen; phosphorylation also stimulates hormone-sensitive lipase in adipose tissues.

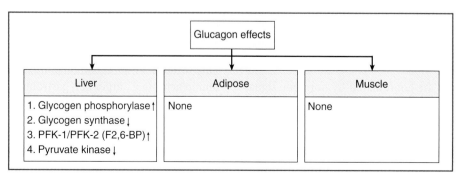

Figure 13-2. Metabolic effects of glucagon in liver, adipose, and muscle tissue. *PFK*, phosphofructokinase; *F2,6-BP*, fructose-2,6-bisphosphatase.

To provide energy for gluconeogenesis, fats must be mobilized from adipose depots.

Epinephrine—A Hormone for Fleeing or Fighting

The metabolic actions of epinephrine are most pronounced in muscle and adipose tissue, but it also acts on the liver (Fig. 13-3). Along with norepinephrine, epinephrine acts to mobilize energy for the flight-or-fight response. This includes glycogenolysis in muscle and the liver and fat mobilization in adipose tissue.

Epinephrine receptors in muscle and adipose tissue are β-adrenergic (i.e., they act through stimulatory G-proteins that, like the glucagon response, create a wave of phosphorylation through the cell by stimulating adenylate cyclase). This leads to the mobilization of glucose from glycogen for energy in muscle and the mobilization of free fatty acids (FFAs) from adipose tissue for use as an energy source both in muscle and the liver.

Epinephrine receptors in the liver are α_1-adrenergic (i.e., they act through the G_q-proteins that activate phospholipase C and stimulate a Ca^{++}-dependent protein kinase). This also leads to glycogen phosphorylase activation as seen with glucagon.

PHYSIOLOGY

Epinephrine Secretion

Secretion of epinephrine from the adrenal medulla is triggered by impulses from preganglionic sympathetic nerves in response to stress, prolonged exercise, hypoglycemia, or trauma.

Glucocorticoids—Hormones for Sustained Stress

The glucocorticoids are steroid hormones produced by the adrenal glands to help tissues respond to long-term metabolic stress (Fig. 13-4). They are synthesized in response to adrenocorticotropic hormone that is released from the pituitary; thus they have a response time of days rather than minutes as with epinephrine. Since one action of the glucocorticoids is to down-regulate insulin receptor substrate the general effect of the glucocorticoids is anti-insulin or "counter-regulatory." Rather than exert their effects through second messenger pathways, glucocorticoids act on nuclear DNA to alter the rates of enzyme synthesis.

KEY POINTS ABOUT HORMONAL INFLUENCES ON METABOLISM

- Insulin and glucagon are the key hormones in the short-term regulation of blood glucose concentration under normal physiologic conditions.
- Insulin acts to reduce blood glucose (hypoglycemic effect); glucagon acts to increase blood glucose (hyperglycemic effect).
- Insulin primarily dephosphorylates enzymes, whereas glucagon primarily phosphorylates them.

●●● THE WELL-FED STATE

The regulation of metabolism in the well-fed state (Fig. 13-5) is determined primarily by the influx of glucose from the gut. The period extending for up to 4 hours after ingestion of a normal meal is marked by a high insulin/glucagon ratio, which is caused by the absorption of dietary glucose.

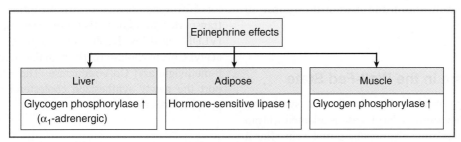

Figure 13-3. Metabolic effects of epinephrine in liver, adipose, and muscle tissue.

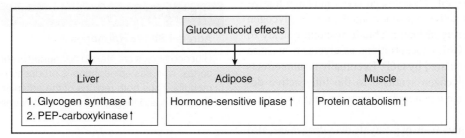

Figure 13-4. Metabolic effects of glucocorticoids in liver, adipose, and muscle tissue. *PEP*, phosphoenolpyruvate.

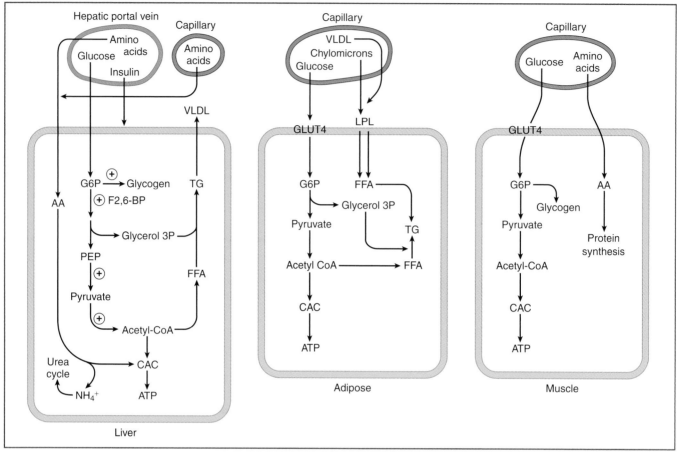

Figure 13-5. Liver, adipose, and muscle metabolism in the well-fed state. Hormones and fuels in the hepatic portal vein are delivered directly to the liver, whereas those in the capillaries are from the general circulation. *VLDL*, very-low-density lipoprotein; *AA*, amino acid; *G6P*, glucose 6-phosphate; *F2,6-BP*, fructose-2,6-bisphosphatase; *PEP*, phosphoenolpyruvate; *FFA*, free fatty acid; *CoA*, coenzyme A; *ATP*, adenosine triphosphate; *GLUT4*, glucose transporter; *TG*, triglyceride; *LPL*, lipoprotein lipase; *CAC*, citric acid cycle.

With the exception of long-chain fatty acids, all other digestible dietary components, such as amino acids and medium-chain plus short-chain fatty acids, are also transported directly to the liver. Epinephrine and glucocorticoids do not play a significant role in the hormonal response to the fed state.

Liver Metabolism in the Well-Fed State

In the well-fed state, insulin causes the liver to synthesize glycogen, fat, and cholesterol. Glucokinase is adapted to trap the large glucose influx from the hepatic portal vein after a meal. This enzyme is active only at high (10 to 20 mmol/L) glucose concentrations and is not inhibited by its product, glucose 6-phosphate (G6P) (as is hexokinase, found in other tissues). Also, the less active phosphorylated form of glycogen synthase, formed during fasting, is able to respond quickly to store the increased G6P concentrations as glycogen because it is allosterically stimulated by G6P. Eventually insulin effects the conversion of glycogen synthase to the fully active dephospho- form through a generalized increase in phosphatase activity.

The active dephospho- form of pyruvate dehydrogenase, also induced by insulin, provides abundant acetyl-coenzyme A

(CoA) for FFA synthesis and cholesterol synthesis. The increased G6P also provides the substrate needed by the oxidative branch of the pentose phosphate pathway to provide the nicotinamide adenine dinucleotide phosphate required for FFA synthesis. FFAs are esterified as triglyceride and transported to adipose tissue in very-low-density lipoprotein (VLDL) particles. Insulin also stimulates the conversion of acetyl-CoA to cholesterol through the activation of β-hydroxy-β-methylglutaryl CoA reductase. The VLDL particles transport the newly synthesized cholesterol and triglycerides to peripheral tissues.

HISTOLOGY

Adrenal Stress Hormones

Glucocorticoids are steroid hormones produced in the adrenal cortex, whereas epinephrine is produced in the adrenal medulla. Thus both regions of the adrenals participate in the short-term and long-term response to stress.

ANATOMY

Hepatic Portal Vein

The hepatic portal vein carries blood directly from the capillary bed in the gut to the capillary bed in the liver without passing through the heart. This arrangement ensures that, with the exception of long-chain fatty acids, the liver sees everything in the diet first. That includes not only nutrients but also xenobiotics (both drugs and toxins) that need detoxification. Even the release of insulin and glucagon is by way of the hepatic portal vein, thus ensuring that the liver sees newly released insulin and glucagon first.

Adipose Tissue Metabolism in the Well-Fed State

Following a meal, the high insulin/glucagon ratios stimulate pathways in adipose tissue, leading to triglyceride synthesis and storage. Increased glucose uptake by insulin-mobilized GLUT4 increases glycolysis for the production of glycerol 3-phosphate, the backbone for esterification of FFAs. Increased activity of pyruvate dehydrogenase provides acetyl-CoA for fatty acid synthesis, which can supplement the synthesis of fatty acids in the liver. Increased insulin levels also inhibit hormone-sensitive lipase, preventing fat mobilization. Up-regulation of lipoprotein lipase by insulin promotes release and uptake of fatty acids from chylomicrons and VLDL (see Lipoproteins section in Chapter 20) for incorporation into triglycerides.

Muscle Metabolism in the Well-Fed State

The high insulin/glucagon ratio promotes energy storage in muscle. Increased glucose uptake by insulin-mobilized GLUT4 coupled with activation of glycogen synthase leads to formation of glycogen. Increased amino acid incorporation into muscle protein leads to muscle growth. This muscle mass also serves as a source of carbon skeletons for hepatic gluconeogenesis during fasting. Thus protein synthesis serves, in part, as an energy storage mechanism.

Brain Metabolism in the Well-Fed State

The brain cannot use FFAs for energy, and it has no stored glycogen reserves. Aerobic glucose metabolism is its only source of energy (except in periods of extreme starvation, when it can use ketone bodies). This is evident from the overlap in symptoms for hypoxia and hypoglycemia, such as confusion, motor weakness, and visual disturbances.

●●● THE FASTING STATE

The regulation of metabolism in the fasting state (Fig. 13-6) is determined primarily by the disappearance of glucose from the blood, signaling an end to fuel absorption from the gut. Fasting begins approximately 3 hours after the last meal (post-prandial) and can extend to 4 to 5 days before entering the starvation state. The declining insulin/glucagon ratio causes metabolism to shift to increasing reliance on glycogenolysis followed by gluconeogenesis to maintain blood glucose.

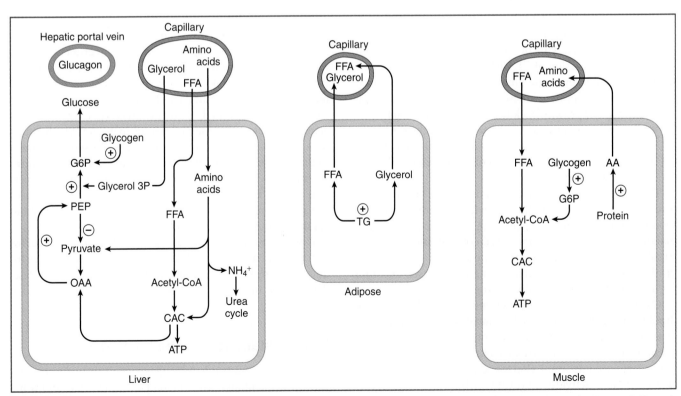

Figure 13-6. Liver, adipose, and muscle metabolism in the fasting state. Hormones and fuels in the hepatic portal vein are delivered directly to the liver, whereas those in the capillaries are from the general circulation. Abbreviations as in Figure 13-5.

Because extended fasting is physiologically stressful, epinephrine can play a role in fasting metabolism.

ANATOMY

Lymphatic Dietary Uptake

Long-chain fatty acids are esterified back to triglycerides after absorption from the gut and repackaged into chylomicron particles. They enter the lymphatic circulation and pass through the thoracic duct into the junction of the left subclavian and internal jugular veins. Other fat-soluble components of the diet such as fat-soluble vitamins are also absorbed through this route.

Liver Metabolism in the Fasting State

In the fasting state, glucagon causes the liver to mobilize glucose from glycogen (glycogenolysis) and to synthesize glucose from oxaloacetate and glycerol (gluconeogenesis). Glucagon stimulates an increase in cyclic adenosine monophosphate leading to an increase in phosphorylation by protein kinase A. The wave of phosphorylation that spreads through the liver cell activates enzymes such as glycogen phosphorylase that are involved in glycogen degradation while simultaneously inhibiting glycogen synthesis. Inhibition of glycogen synthase prevents futile resynthesis of glycogen from glucose 1-phosphate (G1P) via uridine diphosphoglucose. Glucose 6-phosphatase (G6Pase), a gluconeogenic enzyme that is present in the liver but not in muscle, then converts G6P to glucose for release into the blood.

Gluconeogenesis, a second source of glucose, is stimulated by glucagon via two mechanisms:

1. Reduction of fructose-2,6-bisphosphatase (F2,6-BP) formation. Reduced F2,6-BP synthesis simultaneously removes the stimulation of phosphofructokinase-1 while increasing the activity of F1,6-BP. This results in an increase in conversion of F1,6-BP to F6P.
2. Inactivation of pyruvate kinase. Phosphorylation of pyruvate kinase by protein kinase A reduces futile recycling of phosphoenolpyruvate back to pyruvate. Instead phosphoenolpyruvate is converted to F1,6-BP through reverse glycolysis. Pyruvate kinase is further inhibited by alanine and adenosine triphosphate (ATP), both of which are elevated during gluconeogenesis.

The increased liver uptake of amino acids (derived from protein catabolism in muscle) during fasting provides the carbon skeletons for gluconeogenesis (e.g., alanine is transaminated into pyruvate). The increased concentrations of NH_4^+ resulting from deamination of amino acids are metabolized in the liver by the urea cycle, leading to increased excretion of urea in urine and a negative nitrogen balance.

Oxidation of fatty acids derived from adipose tissue lipolysis provides the energy for gluconeogenesis. Thus fatty acid oxidation elevates ATP concentrations and the concentration of both acetyl-CoA and citrate. ATP, acetyl-CoA, and citrate are important effectors during gluconeogenesis:

- Acetyl-CoA activates pyruvate carboxylase, which converts pyruvate to oxaloacetate for use in the gluconeogenic pathway.
- Inhibition of pyruvate dehydrogenase by acetyl-CoA also increases shunting of pyruvate toward oxaloacetate.
- Citrate allosterically inhibits phosphofructokinase-1, preventing a futile cycle with F1,6-BP.
- Increased ATP concentrations inhibit glycolysis while providing energy for gluconeogenesis.

The glycerol that is derived from lipolysis in adipose tissue is taken up by the liver and phosphorylated by glycerol kinase, thus contributing additional carbon skeletons for hepatic gluconeogenesis.

Some ketogenesis occurs in the liver, especially with prolonged fasting, with ketone bodies primarily going to muscle as an alternative fuel. At this point, ketosis is mild and not clinically important.

Adipose Tissue Metabolism in the Fasting State

A low insulin/glucagon ratio and release of epinephrine promote formation of the active phosphorylated form of hormone-sensitive lipase, which splits triglycerides into glycerol and FFAs. The FFAs are transported in the circulation bound to serum albumin. Liver and muscle use released FFAs as a major energy source during fasting via β-oxidation in the mitochondria. Glycerol is converted to glycerol 3-phosphate in the liver and is used as a substrate for gluconeogenesis.

Muscle Metabolism in the Fasting State

In the absence of insulin, an inducer of protein synthesis, there is a shift toward net degradation of muscle protein. The increased supply of amino acids provides the carbon skeletons needed for hepatic gluconeogenesis. Most amino acids released from muscle protein are transported directly to the liver, where they are transaminated and converted to glucose. Alanine and glutamine are the major amino acids released from muscle, indicating extensive reshuffling of carbon and nitrogen in muscle tissue. The branched-chain amino acids (isoleucine, leucine, and valine) are converted to their α-keto acids in muscle by transamination of pyruvate, yielding alanine, which is transported to the liver. The transport of alanine to the liver followed by its conversion to glucose that returns to muscle to form more pyruvate is called the alanine cycle (Fig. 13-7). The alanine cycle results in a net transport of nitrogen from branched-chain amino acids to the liver but results in no net production of glucose.

While glycogen degradation can provide glucose as fuel for short periods of exertion, FFAs serve as a major fuel source for muscle during fasting. Because skeletal muscle lacks G6Pase, degradation of muscle glycogen cannot contribute to blood glucose.

Brain Metabolism in the Fasting State

The brain depends on hepatic glycogenolysis and gluconeogenesis to maintain normal blood glucose concentrations because it continues to use glucose as an energy source during periods of fasting.

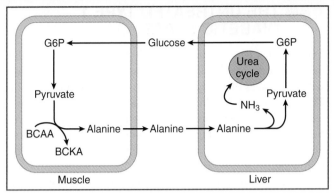

Figure 13-7. The alanine cycle as a nitrogen transport mechanism. Alanine is created in muscle to transport the nitrogen from the branched-chain amino acids (*BCAA*). These must be metabolized in muscle because the liver lacks the necessary enzymes. After transamination in muscle, the branched-chain keto acids (*BCKA*) that are produced enter the citric acid cycle to produce adenosine triphosphate. Alanine is converted to glucose in the liver, leading to its release into the blood and conversion to pyruvate in muscle. Thus no net glucose synthesis occurs. *G6P*, glucose 6-phosphate.

KEY POINTS ABOUT THE WELL-FED AND FASTING STATES

- Liver tissue responds to increased insulin by storing glycogen and synthesizing fat; it responds to increased glucagon by synthesizing glucose and burning fat.

- Adipose tissue responds to insulin by increasing uptake of fat and storing it; it responds to epinephrine by mobilizing fat.

- Muscle tissue responds to insulin by synthesizing protein and glycogen; it responds to epinephrine by mobilizing its own glycogen for energy.

- The brain uses glucose exclusively for fuel except during starvation, when it burns ketone bodies to use less blood glucose.

●●● THE STARVATION STATE

Starvation metabolism is not just extended fasting metabolism. Fasting metabolism anticipates the next meal and is able to shift quickly back to the well-fed state. Starvation metabolism, on the other hand, cannot anticipate the next meal. Thus, instead of breaking down protein to maintain blood glucose, metabolism shifts to conserve blood glucose and to spare protein from continual degradation (Fig. 13-8).

After 3 to 5 days of fasting, increasing reliance on fatty acids and ketone bodies for fuel enables the body to maintain blood glucose at 60 to 65 mg/dL (normal 70 to 100 mg/dL) and to save muscle protein for prolonged periods without food. Less NH_4^+ is produced, and therefore less urea is excreted in the urine.

Liver Metabolism in the Starvation State

Ketosis resulting from increased hepatic production of ketone bodies is the hallmark of starvation. In the absence of insulin, mobilization of FFAs from adipose tissue continues to increase. Because the only site for regulation of fat oxidation is at the level of adipose tissue, oxidation of fatty acids in the liver continues unabated. Accumulating acetyl-CoA is

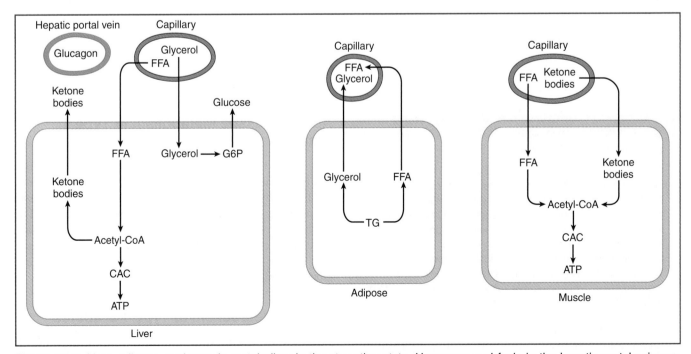

Figure 13-8. Liver, adipose, and muscle metabolism in the starvation state. Hormones and fuels in the hepatic portal vein are delivered directly to the liver, whereas those in the capillaries are from the general circulation. Abbreviations as in Figure 13-5.

shunted through ketogenesis to produce the ketone bodies acetoacetate and β-hydroxybutyrate. These substrates, which are water-soluble forms of fat, are metabolized to acetyl-CoA and used for energy production by many tissues (e.g., muscle, brain, kidney) but not by red blood cells or the liver. Acetone, a ketone formed spontaneously by decomposition of acetoacetate, gives a fruity odor to the breath.

Gluconeogenesis slows down as the supply of amino acid carbon skeletons from muscle protein catabolism decreases. However, glycerol released by lipolysis in adipose tissue supports a low level of gluconeogenesis in liver, which is the only tissue that contains glycerol kinase (glycerol → glycerol 3-phosphate →→→ glucose).

Adipose Tissue Metabolism in the Starvation State

The combined effects of the absence of insulin and elevated epinephrine concentrations due to the stress of starvation activate hormone-sensitive lipase, the only site for hormonal regulation of fatty acid oxidation. The mobilized FFAs serve not only as a source of ketone body formation in the liver but also as a fuel for most other tissues, such as muscle and heart (but not red blood cells). Glycerol released from lipase activity is the only significant adipose source of carbons for gluconeogenesis.

Muscle Metabolism in the Starvation State

Degradation of muscle protein is decreased in starvation, with most of its energy supplied by FFA and ketone bodies. As starvation persists, muscle relies increasingly on FFAs, saving glucose and ketone bodies for use by the brain.

Brain Metabolism in the Starvation State

Increasing ketone body use by the brain saves blood glucose for use by red blood cells, which rely solely on glucose for energy production. Decreasing glucose use by the brain reduces the need for hepatic gluconeogenesis from muscle and thus indirectly spares muscle protein.

PATHOLOGY

Protein-Calorie Malnutrition

Protein-calorie malnutrition is a condition involving inadequate intake of protein and/or carbohydrate. This occurs in some trauma or surgical patients that are in a highly catabolic state or in populations of underdeveloped countries. Kwashiorkor is a form of malnutrition in which the protein deficiency is greater than the carbohydrate deficiency. Although many tissues suffer from degeneration, the key characteristic of these patients is a swollen abdomen from edema (ascites) produced by a reduced serum albumin concentration. Marasmus is a form of malnutrition in which the carbohydrate deficiency is greater than the protein deficiency. Ascites is not seen in this form of starvation, although tissue degeneration such as muscle wasting still occurs. Most of the protein in a marasmus patient is spent on gluconeogenesis.

●●● THE UNTREATED TYPE 1 DIABETIC STATE

Type 1 diabetes, sometimes still referred to as insulin-dependent diabetes mellitus, is caused by β-cell destruction, which removes the body's only source of endogenous insulin. The absence of insulin also typifies the starvation state, leading to some similarities between untreated type 1 diabetes and starvation (Fig. 13-9). Four characteristic metabolic abnormalities caused by the absence of insulin are the following:

1. Hyperglycemia is caused by increased hepatic glucose production and reduced glucose uptake by insulin-sensitive GLUT4 in adipose tissue and muscle.
2. Muscle wasting results from excessive degradation of muscle protein.
3. Ketoacidosis results from excessive mobilization of fatty acids from adipose tissue.
4. Hypertriglyceridemia is caused by reduced lipoprotein lipase activity in adipose tissue and excessive fatty acid esterification in liver.

However, upon closer inspection, the metabolic response in diabetes is different from that in starvation in several ways because starvation is due to a lack of fuel, not of insulin. Thus when fuel is plentiful and insulin is lacking, the normal mechanisms for fasting and starvation respond abnormally.

Liver Metabolism in Type 1 Diabetes

The liver interprets the low insulin/glucagon ratio as a signal of low blood sugar, leading to stimulation of gluconeogenesis. Thus the hepatic output of glucose is increased despite ample or excessive glucose in the blood. Amino acids mobilized from muscle are used as the carbon skeletons, as described for fasting metabolism. Excessive amounts of acetyl-CoA produced by mobilization of FFAs are shunted away from the already saturated citric acid cycle and into production of ketone bodies. Significantly, the rate of ketone production in diabetes is much greater than in starvation, making this a life-threatening condition.

Adipose Tissue Metabolism in Type 1 Diabetes

The absence of insulin leads to uncontrolled mobilization of FFAs, which serves as the source of excess ketone body production by the liver. Lipoprotein lipase, which is increased by insulin, is decreased in its absence, leading to an elevation in chylomicrons and VLDL levels. Because glucose uptake in adipose cells is insulin dependent, the defective transport further contributes to an abnormally elevated blood glucose level.

Muscle Metabolism in Type 1 Diabetes

The lack of insulin prevents glucose uptake by muscle tissue, further contributing to abnormally high blood glucose concentrations. Protein synthesis is decreased and

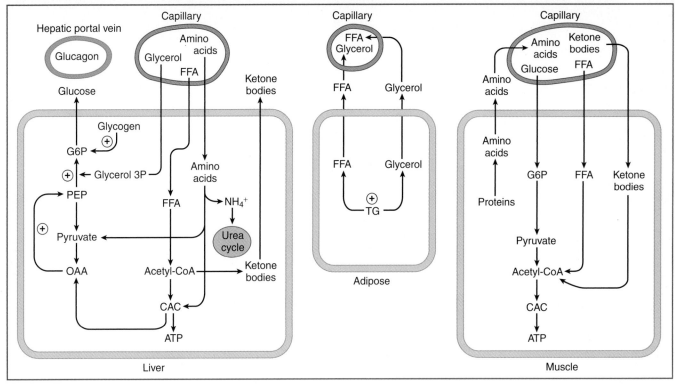

Figure 13-9. Liver, adipose, and muscle metabolism in the untreated type 1 diabetic state. Hormones and fuels in the hepatic portal vein are delivered directly to the liver, whereas those in the capillaries are from the general circulation. Abbreviations as in Figure 13-5.

degradation increased in the diabetic state, as would be seen during fasting, to mobilize carbon skeletons for use in gluconeogenesis, even though it is not needed. Muscle amino acids are also consumed in the citric acid cycle to make up for the loss of glucose, which cannot be transported into the cell.

Brain Metabolism in Type 1 Diabetes

In the untreated diabetic, blood glucose remains the sole source of fuel because it is in plentiful supply. Therefore ketones are not used by the brain as they are during starvation.

KEY POINTS ABOUT THE STARVATION STATE AND UNTREATED TYPE 1 DIABETES

- During starvation, fatty acids mobilized from adipose tissue and ketone bodies produced in the liver supply the energy needs of all tissues except red blood cells and the liver.

- Type 1 diabetes is characterized by an absence of insulin and therefore displays characteristics of both fasting and starvation.

- People with diabetes are threatened by short-term damage from ketoacidosis and electrolyte imbalances and by long-term damage from hyperglycemia and hypertriglyceridemia.

Self-assessment questions can be accessed at www. StudentConsult.com.

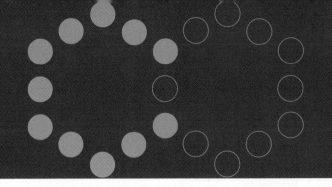

Purine, Pyrimidine, and Single-Carbon Metabolism

14

Purines and pyrimidines are cyclic nitrogen-containing molecules that form the core structure of nucleotides. Nucleotides serve numerous key roles in the cell: they serve as high-energy substrates for many anabolic reactions; they serve as precursors for DNA and ribonucleic acid (RNA) synthesis; they function in intracellular signaling (e.g., cyclic adenosine monophosphate); and they contribute to the structure of several coenzymes such as nicotinamide adenine dinucleotide, flavin adenine dinucleotide, and coenzyme A. Since both purines and pyrimidines are produced in adequate amounts from de novo synthesis, no dietary requirement exists. When available from the diet or from metabolic degradation, they can be recycled through salvage pathways.

●●● PURINE SYNTHESIS

5-Phosphoribosyl-1-Pyrophosphate Synthesis

The precursor molecule for both de novo synthesis and salvage of purines and pyrimidines is the activated form of ribose 5-phosphate, 5-phosphoribosyl-1-pyrophosphate (PRPP). It is produced by pyrophosphorylation of ribose 5-phosphate (Fig. 14-1). The reaction consumes two high-energy bonds by transferring a pyrophosphate group to the ribose sugar.

Phosphoribosylamine Synthesis

The first component of the purine ring, an amine, is added to PRPP by an amidotransferase enzyme to form 5-phosphoribosylamine (Fig. 14-2). This is also the committed and rate-limiting step in purine synthesis. Feedback regulation of this reaction by the end products of the pathway—adenosine monophosphate (AMP), guanosine monophosphate (GMP), and inosine monophosphate (IMP)—prevents their overproduction. Feed-forward regulation by high concentrations of PRPP will override AMP, GMP, and IMP inhibition.

The purine pathway involves nine reactions that incorporate the various components of the purine ring, leading to the production of IMP (Fig. 14-3). The purine ring includes contributions from the entire glycine skeleton, the amino nitrogen of aspartate, the amide nitrogen of glutamine, carbon and O_2 from CO_2, and two single-carbon additions from tetrahydrofolate. The end product of this pathway, IMP, serves as an intermediate for synthesis of both AMP and GMP.

PATHOLOGY

Gout in Von Gierke Disease

Von Gierke patients have a buildup of PRPP due to an increase in the nonoxidative branch of the pentose phosphate pathway. The buildup of glucose 6-phosphate results in excess concentrations of all glycolytic intermediates, including glyceraldehyde 3-phosphate and fructose 6-phosphate, both of which can lead to an elevation of ribose 5-phosphate. This in turn increases the concentration of PRPP, which forces overproduction of purines, leading to elevation of uric acid and gout.

Production of AMP and GMP from a Common IMP Precursor

IMP represents a "fork in the road" because it is converted to either GMP or AMP, with both pathways requiring only two steps. The output of both forks in the pathway is kept in

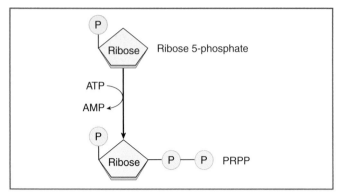

Figure 14-1. Synthesis of 5-phosphoribosyl-1-pyrophosphate *(PRPP)*. Ribose 5-phosphate from the pentose phosphate pathway is pyrophosphorylated in one step. *ATP*, adenosine triphosphate; *AMP*, adenosine monophosphate.

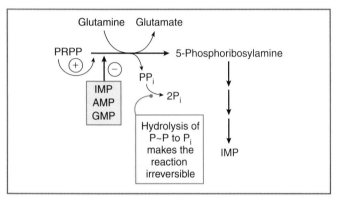

Figure 14-2. Formation of 5-phosphoribosylamine from 5-phosphoribosyl-1-pyrophosphate *(PRPP)*. Feed-forward regulation by PRPP is balanced by feedback inhibition by inosine monophosphate *(IMP)*, guanosine monophosphate *(GMP)*, and adenosine monophosphate *(AMP)*. ~ Signifies a high-energy bond. P_i, inorganic phosphate; PP_i, inorganic pyrophosphate.

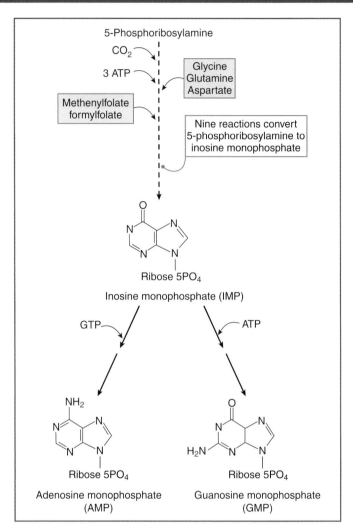

Figure 14-3. Formation of IMP from amino acids, CO_2, and single-carbon folate. *ATP*, adenosine triphosphate; *GTP*, guanosine triphosphate.

balance by cross-regulation, a process in which the end product of one pathway is required for completion of the other pathway. GMP synthesis requires adenosine triphosphate (ATP) in a step that adds the amino group from glutamine; AMP synthesis requires guanosine triphosphate in a step that adds the amino group from aspartate (Fig. 14-4). Thus the adenylate pool limits the concentration of the guanylate pool and vice versa.

The adenylate pool also helps keep the concentrations of uridine monophosphate (and thymidine monophosphate [TMP]) and cytidine monophosphate in balance with the purine nucleotides, since ATP acts as a positive allosteric effector for the pyrimidine synthetic pathway (see Pyrimidine Synthesis section). The result of the allosteric feedback regulation loops is to provide balanced replacement of nucleotides as they are consumed.

Purine Salvage

Normal turnover of both RNA and DNA molecules produces abundant amounts of preformed purine and pyrimidine bases. Salvage pathways allow these bases to be recycled and used for resynthesis of nucleotides. Purine salvage involves two

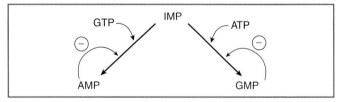

Figure 14-4. Cross-regulation of the synthesis of adenosine monophosphate *(AMP)* and guanosine monophosphate *(GMP)* from inosine monophosphate *(IMP)*. Guanosine triphosphate *(GTP)* is required for AMP synthesis, and adenosine triphosphate is required for GMP synthesis. The end products also act to slow their own synthesis.

phosphoribosyl transferase enzymes. Their function is to transfer phosphoribosyl groups from PRPP to the free bases formed from nucleic acid degradation. This produces a mononucleotide, as shown in Figure 14-5. Adenine has its own enzyme, adenine phosphoribosyl transferase, that produces adenylate from adenine. Hypoxanthine and guanine share an enzyme, hypoxanthine-guanine phosphoribosyl transferase, that produces inosinate and guanylate, respectively.

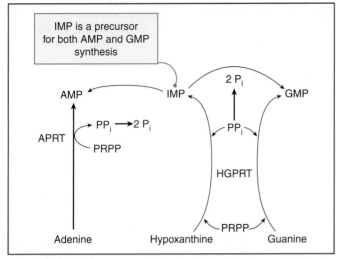

Figure 14-5. Purine salvage pathway. The free bases adenine, hypoxanthine, and guanine are converted to adenosine mono-phosphate (*AMP*), inosine monophosphate (*IMP*), and guanosine monophosphate (*GMP*), respectively. 5-Phosphoribosyl-1-pyrophosphate (*PRPP*) serves as a ribose-phosphate donor. *APRT*, adenine phosphoribosyl transferase. *P$_i$*, inorganic phosphate; *PP$_i$*, inorganic pyrophosphate; *HGPRT*, hypoxanthine-guanine phosphoribosyl transferase.

KEY POINTS ABOUT PURINES

- Purines are assembled on the ribose 5-phosphate molecule; this is in contrast with the pyrimidines, which undergo considerable assembly and refinement of the ring before attachment to the ribose molecule.

- IMP is the first purine intermediate with an intact ring.

- Increased throughput from phosphoribosylamine to IMP, as seen in gout, results in an increased conversion of IMP to uric acid rather than an overproduction of AMP and GMP, since these end products regulate their own synthesis.

●●● DEGRADATION OF PURINES TO URIC ACID

Cells can dispose of purines that are not needed for salvage. The end product for the degradation of all of the purines is uric acid, which is excreted in the urine.

Although adenine degradation can occur through multiple routes (Fig. 14-6), all these pathways ultimately converge to form inosine. Inosine, a nucleoside, is then converted to hypoxanthine, a purine base, by removal of the ribose sugar as ribose 1-phosphate. Hypoxanthine is acted on, in turn, by xanthine oxidase to form xanthine. Xanthine is also formed from the other purine, guanine, by deamination. Xanthine additionally is acted on by xanthine oxidase to form uric acid, which is then excreted in the urine. The xanthine oxidase reaction also produces hydrogen peroxide, which is converted to water and O$_2$ by the enzyme catalase.

$$2H_2O_2 \rightarrow 2H_2O + O_2$$

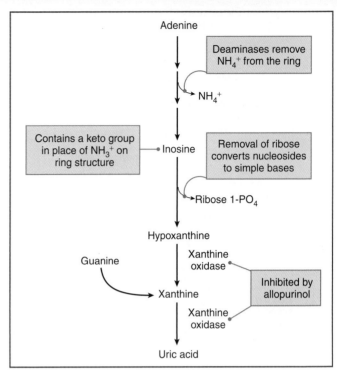

Figure 14-6. Purine degradation to uric acid. The purine intermediates are all routed to xanthine, which is then converted to uric acid.

●●● PYRIMIDINE SYNTHESIS

Formation of Carbamoyl Aspartate

Carbamoyl aspartate has all of the components of the final pyrimidine ring (Fig. 14-7). It is formed from the condensation of aspartate with carbamoyl phosphate. Once the ring has been closed, it is converted through the synthetic pathway to the end products uridine triphosphate (UTP), cytidine triphosphate (CTP), and thymidylate.

The immediate precursor to carbamoyl aspartate is carbamoyl phosphate. This precursor is formed in the cytoplasm in a reaction catalyzed by cytoplasmic carbamoyl phosphate synthetase. Similarly to the mitochondrial form that functions in the urea cycle, the cytoplasmic carbamoyl phosphate synthetase uses ATP and bicarbonate (CO$_2$) in the formation of carbamoyl phosphate. The difference in these two enzymes is the nitrogen source. Compared with the use of ammonia as a nitrogen source for the urea cycle, which serves as a disposal process for nitrogen in the form of urea (see Chapter 12), the formation of carbamoyl phosphate is a synthetic process that uses glutamine as the nitrogen source. N-acetylglutamate has no effect on the activity of the cytoplasmic form of carbamoyl phosphate synthetase, in contrast with its stimulatory effect on the mitochon-drial form.

Aspartate transcarbamoylase combines the entire structure of aspartate with carbamoyl phosphate to form carbamoyl aspartate. This reaction, like that for carbamoyl phosphate synthetase, is regulated so that purines and pyrimidines are formed in balanced concentrations in the cell.

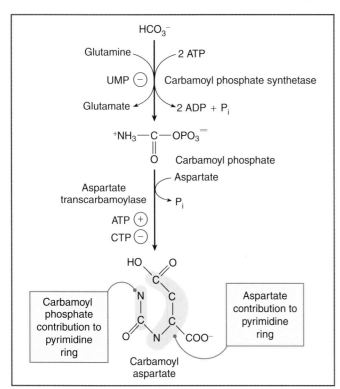

Figure 14-7. Formation of carbamoyl aspartate. Carbamoyl phosphate formed from ammonia, bicarbonate, and glutamine is converted to carbamoyl aspartate. The pyrimidine end products, uridine monophosphate (*UMP*) and cytidine triphosphate (*CIP*) feedback, inhibit the pathway. The purine adenosine triphosphate (*ATP*) stimulates pyrimidine synthesis, helping to keep a balanced amount of purines and pyrimidines. P_i, inorganic phosphate.

PATHOLOGY

Sodium Urate Crystals

In patients with gout, uric acid accumulates in the blood and tissues. Because of its low pH of 5.4, uric acid exists in the sodium urate form, which makes needle-shaped crystals when it precipitates from a solution. Normal concentrations of sodium urate do not form crystals, but either increased production or decreased excretion can elevate these concentrations. Since synovial fluid is a poorer solvent for sodium urate than is plasma and peripheral joints tend to be at a lower temperature, sodium urate is more likely to precipitate and cause irritation and arthritis in peripheral joints (e.g., toes and fingers).

PHARMACOLOGY

Treatment of Gout

Elevated urate concentrations are brought under control with either colchicine or allopurinol. Colchicine works by inhibiting inflammation through prevention of neutrophil migration and phagocytosis. The phagocytic process requires the formation of microtubules, but colchicine causes microtubules to disassemble. Allopurinol works by inhibiting xanthine oxidase.

This creates a distribution of end products between hypoxanthine, xanthine, and urate, thereby reducing urate concentrations. Elevations in hypoxanthine and xanthine, which also are excreted in the urine, do not lead to crystal formation in the tissues.

Synthesis of Pyrimidine Nucleotides from Orotate

Carbamoyl aspartate undergoes ring closure and oxidation to form orotic acid (Fig. 14-8). Uridylate is formed when PRPP is added to the orotate ring structure, followed by decarboxylation. Thus, in only a few reaction steps, the open structure of carbamoyl aspartate is converted to the pyrimidine nucleotide—uridylic acid. Continued phosphorylation by ATP converts uridylate to UTP, which can in turn be aminated with the amido group from glutamine to produce CTP.

Thymidylate Synthesis

Because DNA requires thymine, the methylated form of uracil, the pathway for pyrimidine synthesis branches at uridine diphosphate (UDP). Thus UDP not only serves as the precursor to UTP and CTP, but it is also the precursor to thymidylate. UDP is first converted to deoxyuridine diphosphate (dUDP) by ribonucleotide reductase (see Deoxyribonucleotide Synthesis section and Fig. 14-8). Dephosphorylation of dUDP produces deoxyuridine monophosphate. Thymidylate synthase then transfers a methyl group from 5,10-methylene tetrahydrofolate, forming dTMP; dTMP is commonly abbreviated as TMP because thymine is found only in DNA. Thymidylate synthase is irreversibly inactivated by the cancer drug fluorouracil.

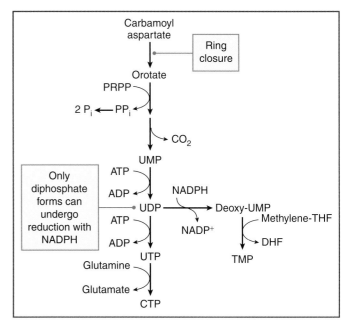

Figure 14-8. Formation of pyrimidine nucleotides from carbamoyl aspartate. See text for expansion of abbreviations.

Pyrimidine Salvage

Uracil and thymine can be salvaged by pyrimidine phosphoribosyl transferase, which uses PRPP to form the respective nucleotides.

KEY POINTS ABOUT PYRIMIDINE SYNTHESIS

- N-acetylglutamate, which stimulates the mitochondrial form of carbamoyl phosphate synthetase (urea cycle), is not an allosteric activator of the cytoplasmic form (pyrimidine synthesis).

- Cross-regulation refers to the requirement for ATP in the synthesis of GMP and the requirement for guanosine triphosphate in the synthesis of AMP; one pathway has a requirement for the end product of the coordinated pathway.

PHARMACOLOGY

Methotrexate Action

The action of thymidylate synthase leaves folate in the form of dihydrofolate, which must be regenerated to tetrahydrofolate before it can become a single-carbon donor again. The regeneration is catalyzed by the enzyme dihydrofolate reductase, an enzyme that is sensitive to the competitive inhibitor methotrexate. For this reason, methotrexate serves as an effective antineoplastic agent. Methotrexate is usually used in combination with other agents because some cancer cells can develop a resistance to it.

●●● DEOXYRIBONUCLEOTIDE SYNTHESIS

Only ribonucleotide diphosphates are recognized by ribonucleotide reductase. This enzyme uses reduced thioredoxin as a cofactor to convert ribonucleotide diphosphates to 2′-deoxyribonucleotide diphosphates (Fig. 14-9). Oxidized thioredoxin, produced by this reaction, is recycled back to its reduced form by thioredoxin reductase in a reaction that requires reduced nicotine adenine dinucleotide phosphate.

●●● NUCLEOSIDE PHOSPHATE INTERCONVERSION

Although the nucleotides are created as monophosphates, ATP can serve as a universal phosphoryl donor. Thus monophosphates are converted to diphosphates by nucleoside monophosphate kinase enzymes:

$$\text{Nucleoside monophosphate} + \text{ATP}$$
$$\rightarrow \text{nucleoside diphosphate} + \text{ADP}$$

and nucleoside diphosphates are converted to nucleoside triphosphates by nucleoside diphosphate kinase enzymes:

$$\text{Nucleoside diphosphate} + \text{ATP}$$
$$\rightarrow \text{nucleoside triphosphate} + \text{ADP}$$

PHARMACOLOGY

Nucleotide Base Analogs

Structural analogs of nucleotide bases enter intracellular pathways to exert their effects. The bases or nucleosides are generally used, since they are transported more readily into cells and then activated. Examples of some purine analogs are methylxanthines (caffeine, theobromine, theophylline), 6-thioguanine, and 6-mercaptopurine. Examples of some pyrimidine analogs are 5-fluorouracil (uracil analog), bromodeoxyuridine (thymidine analog), and the anti-HIV drugs β-D-arabinofuranosylcytosine (Ara-C) and 2′,3′-dideoxy-3′-azidothymidine (zidovudine [AZT]).

●●● DISEASES RELATED TO NUCLEOTIDE METABOLISM

Several diseases are caused by genetic deficiencies in enzymes associated with nucleotide metabolism.

Lesch-Nyhan Syndrome

Lesch-Nyhan syndrome is a lethal disease caused by a deficiency in the salvage enzyme hypoxanthine guanine phosphoribosyl transferase. Patients have symptoms of gout,

Figure 14-9. The ribonucleotide reductase reaction. Thioredoxin (reduced form) acts as a redox cofactor in the reduction of the 2′-ribose position. Nicotinamide adenine dinucleotide phosphate (*NADP*) generated by the pentose phosphate pathway is used to regenerate reduced thioredoxin. *UDP*, uridine diphosphate; *NADPH*, reduced NADP.

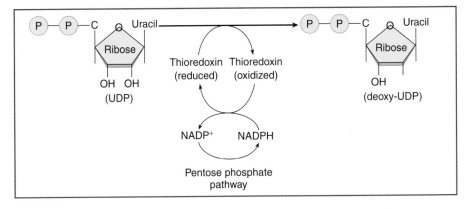

self-mutilation, and mental retardation. The uric acid elevations in their blood and urine are caused by the increased concentrations of hypoxanthine and guanine that cannot be salvaged and therefore must be excreted as uric acid.

Adenosine Deaminase Deficiency

Adenosine deaminase deficiency produces severe combined immunodeficiency disease. The absence of this enzyme causes buildup of deoxy-ATP in lymphocytes, which inhibits ribonucleotide reductase, leading to inhibition of DNA synthesis. Since lymphocytes undergo cell division during a normal immune response, the slowed synthesis of DNA leads to cell death and immune deficiency.

Gout

Patients with gout develop painful, arthritis-like inflammation and destruction of joint tissues. The tissue damage is caused by the precipitation of needle-shaped Na^+ urate crystals; because precipitation of urate is temperature dependent, the distal (coldest) joints in the feet are affected first. The increased urate concentrations are caused by either a genetically altered increase in the formation of PRPP or a decrease in the renal clearance of urate. The latter is more common.

KEY POINTS ABOUT DEOXYRIBONUCLEOTIDE SYNTHESIS, NUCLEOTIDES, AND NUCLEOSIDES

- UMP cannot be converted to TMP by thymidine kinase. It must first be converted to the deoxy- form.

- Deoxyribose is produced by reduction of ribonucleoside diphosphates.

- Tetrahydrofolate contributes single carbons to the purine ring structure and the methyl functional group on thymine.

- The amino acids that contribute carbon and nitrogen to the nucleotide structure are glycine, glutamine, and aspartate.

Self-assessment questions can be accessed at www. StudentConsult.com.

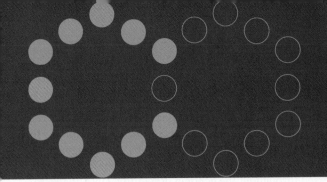

Organization, Synthesis, and Repair of DNA

15

●●● DNA ORGANIZATION

The organization of eukaryotic deoxyribonucleic acid (DNA) reflects two of its major characteristics: extreme length and a predominance of noncoding sequences. Its extreme length must be compacted to fit within the confines of the nucleus and still remain accessible for selective expression of genetic information. This is accomplished by supercoiling of DNA around histones to form nucleosomes.

Noncoding sequences account for more than 98% of the haploid genome. Some of the noncoding DNA is associated with the coding sequences in two ways:
- It divides the coding regions (exons) by acting as intervening regions, or introns.
- It serves a regulatory function.

The remainder of the noncoding DNA is present in two forms:
- Pseudogenes
- Families of repeated sequences, known as repetitive DNA

Nucleosomes

When purified DNA and histone proteins are mixed, they associate to form nucleosomes, the basic structural unit of chromatin. DNA forms a supercoil that wraps twice around an octet

of histones to form an individual nucleosome. Chromatin contains one nucleosome every 200 bases along the DNA. This is enough DNA to wrap around the octet core and still have 30 base pairs left over to form a "linker" with the next nucleosome. A fifth histone, histone H_1, is associated with the linker region.

- The histones composing the octet are named H_2A, H_2B, H_3, and H_4.
- The amino acid sequence of each histone is highly conserved (kept similar) across all species.
- The formation of nucleosomes is not dependent on the base sequence of DNA.

DNA is further compacted through coiling into a solenoid structure, a regular cylindrical arrangement of nucleosomes assembled in 30-nm fibers (Fig. 15-1). The packing of the nucleosomes within these fibers is stabilized by histone H_1. When the fibers are attached to nuclear scaffold proteins, they form chromatin fibers, which can undergo further condensation to form either heterochromatin or euchromatin (Table 15-1). The highly compacted state of heterochromatin renders it genetically inactive in contrast with euchromatin, which has a more open and extended structure.

Pseudogenes

Other than the single-copy DNA that constitutes introns, exons, and regulatory sequences, the remainder of single-copy DNA is present in the form of pseudogenes. A pseudogene contains the intact sequence for a functional polypeptide, but it cannot be expressed because it has no promoter to initiate ribonucleic acid (RNA) synthesis. Pseudogenes are produced by retroviruses (see Reverse Transcriptase section) that make a DNA copy of messenger RNA. This produces a DNA sequence that has no promoter site (see Chapter 16) or introns, but does possess a polyA tail. All these features are present in messenger RNA, but they are not characteristic of the structure of the corresponding normal gene. Thus the term "pseudogene" describes a DNA sequence in the genome that represents a mature messenger RNA (mRNA).

The reason that pseudogenes appear in the genome is that the retrovirus that creates them can insert them into the DNA helix in the same way that they insert copies of their own retroviral chromosome. These pseudogenes are permanently incorporated into the DNA, but they remain dormant and inert and have no ability to be expressed.

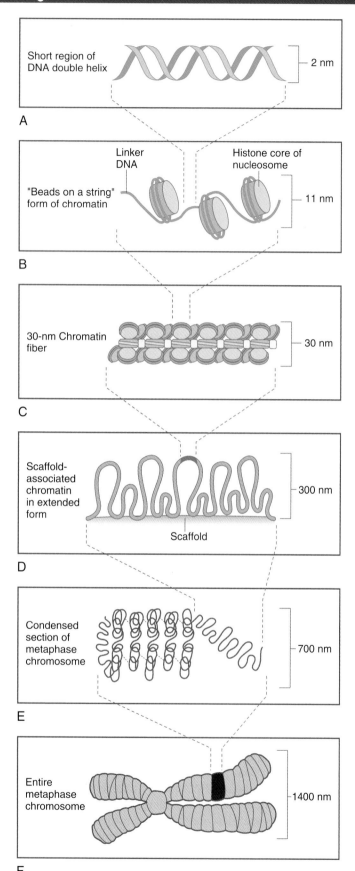

A

Short region of DNA double helix — 2 nm

B

Linker DNA
Histone core of nucleosome
"Beads on a string" form of chromatin — 11 nm

C

30-nm Chromatin fiber — 30 nm

D

Scaffold-associated chromatin in extended form — 300 nm
Scaffold

E

Condensed section of metaphase chromosome — 700 nm

F

Entire metaphase chromosome — 1400 nm

Figure 15-1. Compacting of DNA into chromatin and metaphase chromosomes by formation of nucleosomes, 30-nm fibers, and scaffold-associated fibers.

Repetitive DNA and Transposons

Repetitive DNA is composed of tandem, repeated sequences of from two to several thousand base pairs and is estimated to constitute about 30% of the genome. Many of these sequences are localized in centromeres and telomeres, but they are also dispersed throughout the genome. Repetitive DNA is also referred to as satellite DNA because it was discovered as a small satellite band during density gradient centrifugation. This centrifugation technique allows both isolation and analysis of DNA through centrifugation in cesium chloride solutions. The high forces generated in the centrifuge (greater than 200,000 g) cause the cesium chloride to form a density gradient, and the DNA migrates to a point in the centrifuge tube that exactly matches its own density. Most of the genomic DNA forms a single thick band, but the satellite that forms is denser (higher guanine-cytosine content) and much smaller. Repetitive DNA is created by randomly occurring, unequal crossover events during cell division, producing a deletion on one chromosome and a duplication on the other. The duplications create localized or grouped tandem sequences, which can continue to expand by duplicating the tandem arrangement and doubling it with each recombination event.

Transposons, like pseudogenes, are also produced by retroviruses. In contrast to pseudogenes, which represent host messenger RNA, the transposon is the retrovirus itself. The transposon differs from a functional retrovirus because it has lost its ability to make viral coat proteins and has thus become trapped inside the cell. Transposons can still leave the chromosome and reenter it at a different site and thus are called jumping genes. When they leave the chromosome, they can also take flanking sequences with them, creating deletion mutations, or insertion mutations if they are inserted into a gene. There are two major classes of transposons, which make up about 10% of the genome:

- Short interspersed nuclear elements (SINEs) are 100 to 500 base pairs in length. A well-known example is the 280 base pair Alu sequence, which has about 1 million copies dispersed throughout the genome, including locations within many introns. This major family of SINEs is readily identified, since it contains the Alu restriction enzyme recognition sequence. It is thought to be derived from the 7 S RNA that is found in signal recognition particles (see Chapter 17).
- Long interspersed nuclear elements (LINEs) are 6000 to 7000 base pairs in length. They contain the reverse transcriptase gene, indicating that they are derived from retroviruses. The L1 family of LINEs is a major family of repetitive DNA that constitutes about 5% of the genome.

PATHOLOGY

Repetitive DNA and Disease

A number of genetic diseases are associated with an increase in repetitive DNA sequences. The repeat sequence CpGpG is associated with fragile X syndrome; other examples are Huntington chorea (CAG), myotonic dystrophy (CTG), and spinobulbar muscular dystrophy (CAG). Note that the last is the same type of repeat as in Huntington chorea, indicating that the location of the repeat is significant.

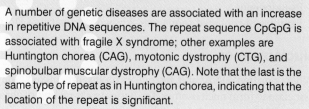

TABLE 15-1. Comparison Between Heterochromatin and Euchromatin

CHARACTERISTIC	HETEROCHROMATIN	EUCHROMATIN
Gene transcription	Inactive	Active
Degree of condensation	Condensed	Dispersed
DNase sensitivity	No	Yes
Cytosine methylation	Hypermethylated	Hypomethylated

KEY POINTS ABOUT DNA ORGANIZATION

- Eukaryotic DNA is coiled around histones to form nucleosomes, which can compact further to form higher order structures resulting in the chromatin of the nucleus. The majority of DNA is transcriptionally inactive as highly compacted, highly methylated, DNase-resistant heterochromatin.

- Approximately 2% of the eukaryotic genome codes for polypeptides (exons), with the remainder as noncoding DNA; noncoding DNA is associated with genes as regulatory sequences or as intervening (intron) sequences, with the remainder as either pseudogenes or repetitive DNA.

●●● DNA SYNTHESIS

Cellular DNA synthesis occurs in response to two types of signals. One is a signal for cell division to occur, and the other is a signal for the repair of damaged DNA. In either case, the DNA, which is highly compacted within chromatin, must be made physically available to the replication or repair enzymes. DNA replication and DNA repair occur at distinct times during the cell cycle.

Cell Cycle

The cell cycle consists of a timed sequence of events that occur during interphase and mitosis (M). Interphase is made up of the G_1 (G = gap) phase, the S (synthesis) phase, and the G_2 phase (Fig. 15-2). Both G phases contain checkpoints that govern whether the cell moves into DNA replication (G_1 checkpoint) or into mitosis (G_2 checkpoint).

- The G_1 and G_2 phases involve the synthesis of RNA and proteins but not of DNA.
- The S phase involves the replication of DNA.
- The M phase involves the separation of the chromosomes during cell division.

Progression through the cell cycle is controlled by cyclins, proteins whose concentrations rise and fall during the cell cycle. Cyclins activate cyclin-dependent protein kinases (Cdks) by binding to them. The activated cyclin-Cdk complexes then phosphorylate various target proteins whose activity is essential for progression through the cell cycle.

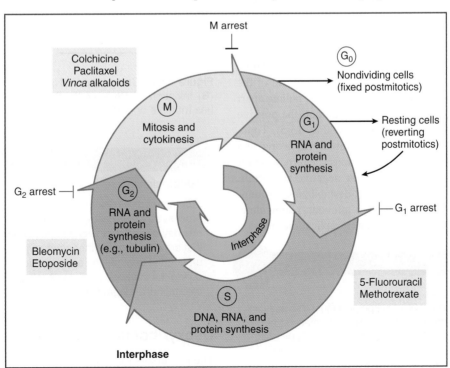

Figure 15-2. The cell cycle in eukaryotic cells. Damage to DNA or improper mitotic spindle formation will cause arrest at checkpoints. Various anticancer drugs exert their effect at different stages of the cell cycle. The G_0 phase is entered by nondividing cells, but some cells can reenter the G_1 phase and resume cell division. *M*, mitosis.

Checkpoints in the cell cycle prevent formation of abnormal daughter cells when DNA is damaged by inhibiting the activity of activated cyclin-Cdks. One well-known protein that functions at both G_1 and G_2 checkpoints is the nuclear phosphoprotein p53. It serves as a transcription factor to increase the expression of genes for growth arrest, for DNA repair, or for apoptosis (a process leading to cell death). By causing the arrest of the cell cycle, p53 allows time for DNA repair and reduces the chances for damaging mutations. Because it has this antimutagenic activity, *Tp53* is known as a tumor suppressor gene. Thus many human cancers are associated with mutations in the *Tp53* gene.

Formation of the Replication Fork

Entry into the S phase initiates the process of DNA replication. Since the two strands of the DNA helix must separate to serve as templates (semiconservative replication), the higher order packing of the chromatin must be reduced to allow access by the replication enzymes. Semiconservative replication results in one parent (original) strand and one daughter (new) strand in each new double helix.

Since the two strands of the DNA helix are antiparallel, each direction contains a template strand. Thus DNA synthesis is bidirectional starting from an origin of replication for both eukaryotic and prokaryotic DNA (Fig. 15-3). Eukaryotic DNA synthesis differs primarily by having multiple origins of replication in order to reduce the time necessary to replicate the much larger chromosome.

For the DNA helix to be accessible by polymerization enzymes, the supercoiling is relaxed by the action of DNA gyrase (topoisomerase II), an enzyme that induces negative (opposite direction to right-handed twist) supercoils in DNA. The relaxation of the supercoiled DNA allows helicase to bind and continue to unwind the helix in an energy-requiring reaction (Fig. 15-4). Helicase is not a topoisomerase because it does not break and rejoin the strands—it simply spreads the DNA strands apart. This action results in the formation of positive supercoils (same direction as right-handed twist) ahead of the replication fork. This can be illustrated by quickly pulling apart two strands from a string or rope, causing a knot (the positive supercoil) to form ahead of the separation (Fig. 15-5). Topoisomerase I relieves the strain by repeatedly breaking and rejoining one strand of the helix as it unwinds one turn, and thus is capable of relaxing either positive or negative supercoils. As helicase unwinds the helix, helix-destabilizing proteins bind to the single-stranded DNA to prevent reannealing. The point of separation is referred to as a replication fork.

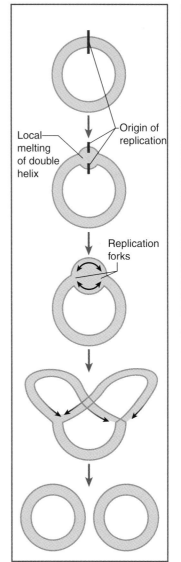 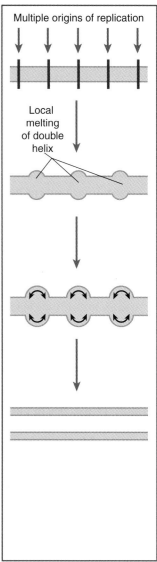

A   B

Figure 15-3. Comparison of prokaryotic (**A**) and eukaryotic (**B**) initiation of DNA synthesis. The eukaryotic chromosome has multiple origins of replication.

HISTOLOGY

Apoptosis

Programmed cell death, apoptosis, refers to an orderly, natural process by which cells commit suicide. For example, after only one day of existence, neutrophils form blebs on their surface that are digested by other phagocytic cells. Their DNA also undergoes degradation and digestion. Another event seen during the stepwise process of cellular apoptosis is mitochondrial degradation.

Deoxyribonucleotide Polymerization

The precursors for synthesis of DNA are 5′-deoxyribonucleotide triphosphates. DNA polymerase creates a phosphodiester bond by cleaving off a pyrophosphate from the precursor and attaching it to the free 3′-hydroxy group on the growing

HISTOLOGY

Mitosis (M)

After a cell has passed the G_2 checkpoint, it must also pass an M checkpoint that detects improper spindle formation to prevent mis-segregation of the chromatids to daughter cells. If the M checkpoint is passed, cells may enter mitosis and proceed through metaphase (where chromosomes line up on metaphase plate) and anaphase (where chromosomes separate as they are pulled to opposite spindle poles).

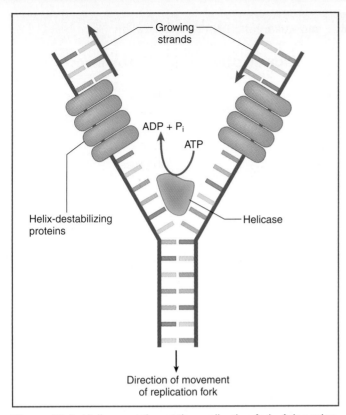

Figure 15-4. Helicase action at the replication fork. Adenosine triphosphate *ITP*) energy is used to overcome the resistance of the helix to unwinding. Helix-destabilizing proteins prevent reannealing. *ADP*, adenosine diphosphate; *P_i*, inorganic phosphate.

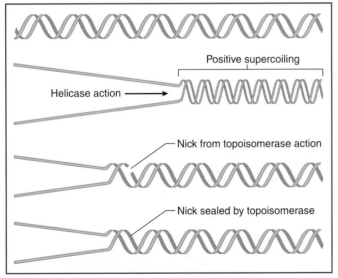

Figure 15-5. Comparison of helicase and topoisomerase action. Positive supercoiling of DNA results from strand separation. Topoisomerase breaks and reseals the strands to allow unwinding one turn at a time.

polypeptide (Fig. 15-6). This leaves a free 3′-hydroxy group on the newly added nucleotide ready to receive the next 5′-deoxyribonucleotide.

Because of the nature of the polymerase, the direction of DNA synthesis is always in the 5′ to 3′ direction; thus nucleotide

sequences are typically represented with the 5′ end on the left and the 3′ end on the right. The DNA strand that is synthesized with the 3′ end advancing in the same direction as the replication fork is called the leading strand. As might be expected, leading strand synthesis is continuous, or highly processive. In prokaryotes, this is catalyzed by DNA polymerase III (Table 15-2), which encircles the DNA helix and moves along the template strand to add the new nucleotides to the growing daughter strand.

The direction of the opposite strand creates a replication dilemma. It requires that the direction of synthesis is initiated and extended away from the direction in which the replication fork is advancing (Fig. 15-7). This strand is called the lagging strand and, because it must be continuously restarted, this process is referred to as discontinuous synthesis (compared with processive synthesis with the leading strand). Lagging strand synthesis requires sequential action of series of enzymes that initiate, elongate, and join pieces of DNA of about 1000 nucleotides called Okazaki fragments.

The synthesis of a new DNA molecule may lead to some errors, which, if not corrected, would lead to mutations in the genome. DNA polymerase needs to be attached to a helix with one complete turn, requiring from 9 to 10 nucleotides. This initial helix is provided by synthesizing an RNA primer that is subsequently removed, instead of a DNA primer that would be permanent. The removal of the primer and replacement with the corresponding DNA sequence allows for high-fidelity base pairing and a reduction in potentially damaging mutations. The primer for each new Okazaki fragment is synthesized in the 5′ to 3′ direction by primase (a DNA-dependent RNA polymerase), which is also component of the primosome along with helicase and other DNA binding proteins (Fig. 15-8). Thus each primer originates at or near the replication fork and is extended in the opposite direction. The primosome functions to keep lagging strand synthesis in synchrony with leading strand synthesis at the replication fork.

Extension of the new Okazaki fragment is accomplished by DNA polymerase III (a DNA-dependent DNA polymerase). The polymerization of deoxynucleotides continues until it reaches the 3′ hydroxyl of the primer on the prior Okazaki fragment. The primer on the prior Okazaki fragment is removed one base at a time by DNA polymerase I, which has 5′ to 3′ exonuclease activity. Each ribonucleotide is replaced with the corresponding deoxyribonucleotide, and any errors associated with the RNA primer are corrected. The last deoxyribonucleotide is joined by a different enzyme, DNA ligase, which uses one ATP to join the Okazaki fragment into the growing lagging strand.

MICROBIOLOGY

Relaxation of Supercoiling

The action of gyrase during DNA synthesis relieves the strain from positive supercoiling by inducing negative supercoils. If DNA gyrase is blocked by fluoroquinolone antibiotics, bacterial growth is inhibited. An example is ciprofloxacin, which is used to treat urinary tract and other bacterial infections.

TABLE 15-2. Comparison Between Enzymes for Prokaryotic and Eukaryotic DNA Polymerization

ENZYME ACTION	PROKARYOTIC	EUKARYOTIC
Leading strand synthesis	DNAP III	DNAP δ
Lagging strand synthesis—RNA primer formation	Primase	DNAP α
Lagging strand synthesis—elongation from primer	DNAP III	DNAP δ
Lagging strand synthesis—replacement of RNA primer with DNA	DNAP I	DNAP ε
Joining of Okazaki fragments to lagging strand	DNA ligase	DNA ligase

DNAP, DNA polymerase.

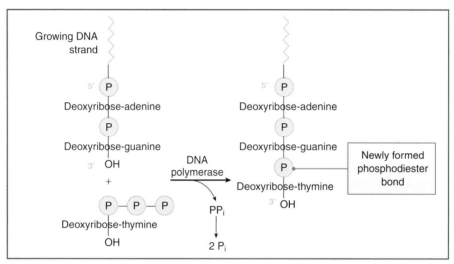

Figure 15-6. Action of DNA polymerase. The 5′ triphosphate reacts with the 3′ end of the growing DNA strand, forming a phosphodiester bond. Cleavage of the pyrophosphate to monophosphate ensures that the reaction is irreversible. P_i, inorganic phosphate; PP_i, inorganic pyrophosphate.

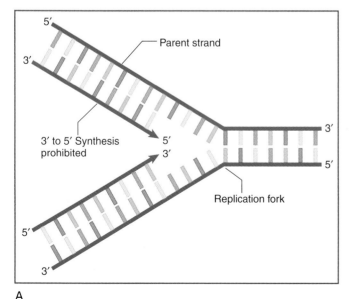

A

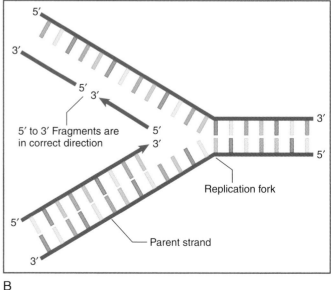

B

Figure 15-7. The replication dilemma (**A**). DNA synthesis must occur in the same direction, but the DNA strands are in opposite directions. Lagging strand synthesis (**B**) is required to piece together short 5′ to 3′ Okazaki fragments.

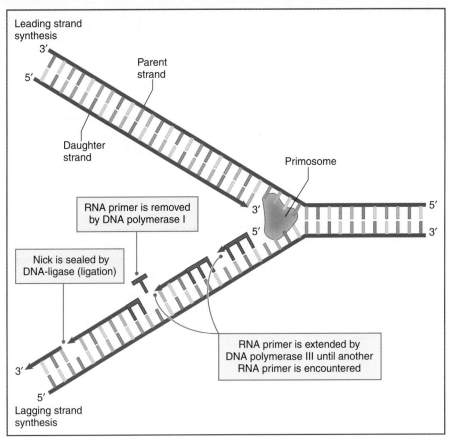

Figure 15-8. Lagging strand synthesis in prokaryotic cells. New Okazaki fragments are initiated with a primer, extended by DNA polymerases, and sealed with DNA ligase.

Proofreading

Mispairing occurs during DNA synthesis because keto-enol and amino-imino tautomeric forms occasionally cause mismatching during the base-pairing process (Fig. 15-9). These mismatches would result in a mutation if they were not detected and corrected by a process called proofreading. Both DNA polymerases I and III proofread base-pair mismatches because any base pairs other than adenosine-thymine (AT) and guanine-cytosine (GC) create an irregularity in the shape of the DNA helix. As the helix is synthesized, it passes through a channel in the DNA polymerase enzymes that requires a precise fit. Any irregularity in the helix results in the activation of a 3′ to 5′ exonuclease activity in both DNA polymerase enzymes (Fig. 15-10). In other words, the polymerase backs up (3′ to 5′ direction), removes the incorrect nucleotide, and then reinserts the correct nucleotide.

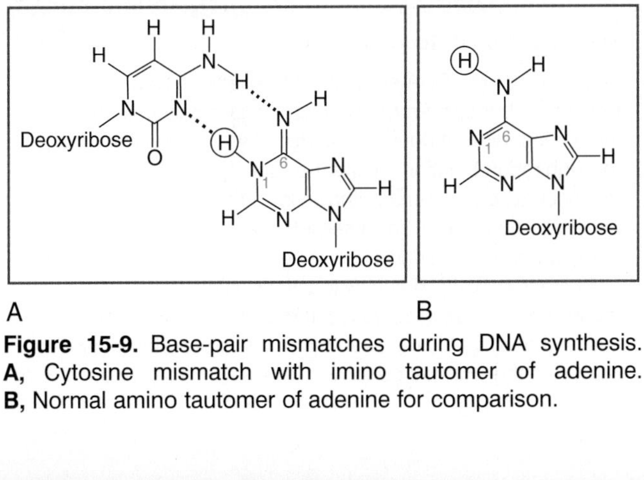

Telomerase and Telomeres

As the replication fork approaches the end of the eukaryotic chromosome, a problem arises with regard to the initiation of the last Okazaki fragment. The primosome, which contains the primase needed to initiate the last Okazaki fragment, dissociates from the DNA molecule when the strands finally separate and the replication fork no longer exists. This presents a situation in which the leading strand is synthesized completely to the end of the molecule, but the lagging strand is shortened by the length of one Okazaki fragment. After a succession of cell divisions, the length of the chromosome will become shorter until a critical sequence is lost, thus leading to the death of the cell. This is, in fact, what happens during cell senescence and programmed cell death (apoptosis).

Cells that are undergoing active proliferation possess an enzyme—telomerase—that solves the problem associated with lagging strand synthesis at the end of the chromosome. Telomerase contains an RNA sequence as a prosthetic group that it uses as a template to synthesize tandemly repeating

Figure 15-9. Base-pair mismatches during DNA synthesis. **A,** Cytosine mismatch with imino tautomer of adenine. **B,** Normal amino tautomer of adenine for comparison.

A

B

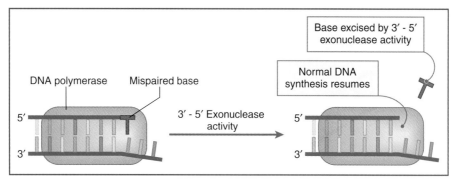

Figure 15-10. Proofreading by DNA polymerase enzymes.

six-base sequences that extend the end of the chromosome well beyond the genomic DNA sequence. This allows the replication fork and the associated primosome to remain intact long enough to initiate the synthesis of the terminal Okazaki fragments. The DNA repeats sequences at the ends of the chromosomes are thus called telomeres. As long as proliferating cells maintain the synthesis of telomeres, erosion of the terminal genomic sequence is avoided.

Reverse Transcriptase

A special type of DNA polymerase, reverse transcriptase, is found in retroviruses that have an RNA chromosome. Its name implies a reversal of the direction of information flow from the classic central dogma that states that the flow of genetic information is from DNA to RNA to protein. Reverse transcriptase (an RNA-dependent DNA polymerase) uses an RNA template to direct the synthesis of a DNA molecule. It first synthesizes a DNA-RNA hybrid using the RNA chromosome as the template. Then RNAase H, a retroviral enzyme, degrades the RNA strand, and it is replaced with DNA to form a DNA helix. The new DNA molecule can then be inserted into the host chromosome as a permanent modification of the DNA for the infected cell, or it can serve as a template to direct the synthesis of viral mRNA.

Reverse transcriptase activity results in a high mutation rate because it lacks the 3' to 5' exonuclease activity necessary for proofreading. It has the highest error rate of any DNA polymerase and makes possible the genetic adaptability of retroviruses, such as HIV.

KEY POINTS ABOUT DNA SYNTHESIS

- DNA synthesis occurs during chromosome replication and during DNA repair; replication of the genome occurs during the S phase of the cell cycle if cyclin-Cdk complexes are present to allow the cell to pass the G_1 checkpoint, and repair occurs throughout the cell cycle wherever damage is detected.

- DNA polymerization enzymes are given access to the individual strands of DNA by helicase, an enzyme that opens the helix and unwinds it; this creates a replication fork during DNA synthesis at multiple sites along the chromosome.

- DNA polymerization occurs in the 5' to 3' direction using 5'-deoxyribonucleotide triphosphates that base pair with the parent DNA template; the leading strand is synthesized continuously, whereas the lagging strand (oriented in the opposite direction) is synthesized in short Okazaki fragments that are joined together by DNA ligase.

- DNA polymerase can proofread the new strand and repair any mismatches that are detected; reverse transcriptase that uses RNA as a template for DNA synthesis lacks proofreading ability.

- Telomeres composed of repetitive DNA are synthesized at the ends of the chromosomes to allow for completion of lagging strand synthesis; telomerase is found in actively dividing cells and is absent in senescent cells.

PHARMACOLOGY

Nucleoside Reverse Transcriptase Inhibitors

Among the drugs that inhibit DNA synthesis, the 3'-deoxy drugs act to terminate the growing polynucleotide chain. Lacking a 3' hydroxyl group, they cannot form a 5' to 3' phosphodiester bond and thus become chain terminators. Each requires intracellular activation to the triphosphate precursor form. They are used primarily for treating HIV infection, and an important side effect is lactic acidosis and hepatomegaly resulting from their inhibition of mitochondrial DNA synthesis. They also inhibit nuclear DNA synthesis in proliferating cells.

MICROBIOLOGY

Transpositional Recombination

Transposons are DNA sequences that lack an origin of replication but contain the RT enzyme and enzymes that can induce insertion of double-stranded DNA into the genome through recombination. This is the same type of recombination that occurs normally in dividing cells and that leads to crossing-over in germinal cells. The inserted gene can create a complete RNA copy of itself, which is converted to a DNA copy by RT. The ability to reinsert itself at new locations within the genome has led to the term jumping genes. If the transposon lands in a critical part of the DNA, it can block the expression of and inactivate the affected gene.

●●● DNA MUTATION AND REPAIR

A change in the base sequence of DNA that escapes detection and correction by proofreading becomes "locked in" to a cell's genome as a permanent mutation at the next cell division. Errors that escape correction by proofreading or that appear after replication has been completed are corrected by repair enzymes. Some of the major categories of repair are mismatch repair, base excision repair, nucleotide excision repair, and direct repair.

Mismatch Repair

Mismatch repair enzymes detect distortions caused by mismatched bases inserted during DNA synthesis. Although the enzyme can find the site of the mutation by detecting the distortion caused by the mismatched bases, additional information must be available to indicate which strand is incorrect. This information is present in the form of adenine methylation in guanine, adenine, thymine, and cytosine (GATC) sequences and occurs just after DNA synthesis (Fig. 15-11). The repair enzymes must detect the mismatched bases and repair the unmethylated strand before methylation of the new strand takes place. The repair is initiated by a GATC endonuclease, which makes a single-strand cut in the strand bearing the incorrect base at the nearest GATC sequence. (Note: Specific sequences are always represented 5′ to 3′. Even more specificity can include the position of the phosphodiester bonds (e.g., GpApTpC). An endonuclease then digests the damaged strand past the site of damage. The gap is then filled in by the normal cellular enzymes,

and the new sequence is joined with the existing strand by DNA ligase.

Base Excision Repair

Cytosine spontaneously deaminates at a constant rate to produce uracil. If left uncorrected, future base pairing at the affected site will result in a change from GC to AT when the uracil base pairs with adenine instead of the original guanine. However, the appearance in DNA of unmethylated thymine (i.e., uracil) is recognized as foreign by uracil-DNA glycosidase. The uracil is excised by uracil-DNA glycosidase (Fig. 15-12) to create an apurinic/apyrimidinic site consisting only of the deoxyribose-phosphate backbone. An apurinic/apyrimidinic endonuclease then nicks the deoxyribose-phosphate backbone, and the deoxyribose-phosphate is removed by a deoxyribose-phosphate lyase. DNA polymerase I then replaces the missing cytosine. DNA ligase finishes the process by sealing the phosphodiester bond.

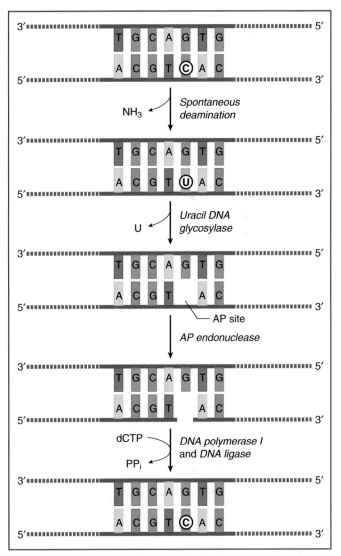

Figure 15-12. Base excision repair. Uracil is recognized as an "incorrect" base in DNA by uracil-DNA glycosidase and removed so that the mistake can be repaired. *AP*, apurinic, apyrimidinic; *dCTP*, deoxycytidine triphosphate; *PP*$_i$, inorganic pyrophosphate.

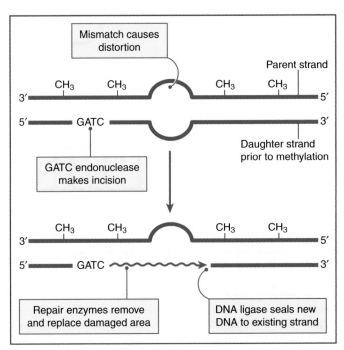

Figure 15-11. Mismatch repair. A guanine, adenine, thymine, and cytosine (*GATC*) sequence directs GATC endonuclease to cut the damaged "new" daughter strand so that it can be repaired.

PATHOLOGY

Hereditary Nonpolyposis Colon Cancer

Hereditary nonpolyposis colon cancer is a relatively common genetic disorder that results from defects in mismatch repair enzymes. This is a dominantly inherited susceptibility with a prevalence of 1 in 400. Patients have one normal allele for the repair protein (hMSH2) and one defective allele.

Nucleotide Excision Repair

DNA can sustain damage greater than just loss or modification of a single base. For example, exposure of DNA to ultraviolet light produces thymine dimers or thymine-cytosine "6-4" photoproducts (Fig. 15-13). Like base-pair mismatching, dimer formation can create distortions in the DNA helix that lead to mutations. These lesions are repaired in a process called nucleotide excision repair (Fig. 15-14). Initially the distortion in the helix is detected by a specialized nuclease called an excision excinuclease. This enzyme nicks the damaged strand on both sides of the lesion and removes the damaged area. Then DNA polymerase I fills in the gap using the undamaged strand as a template. As before, the repair is completed by DNA ligase, which joins the newly synthesized DNA with the original DNA strand.

PATHOLOGY

Xeroderma Pigmentosum

This rare recessive skin disease is caused by a defective excision nuclease in the nucleotide excision repair pathway (one of seven subtypes with different degrees of severity). Ultraviolet irradiation causes pyrimidine dimerization, which usually is repaired by enzymes in the nucleotide excision repair pathway. Patients with xeroderma pigmentosum are extremely sensitive to sunlight. They develop numerous freckles and ulcerative lesions on exposed areas of the body, and they have a 2000 times greater chance of developing skin cancer.

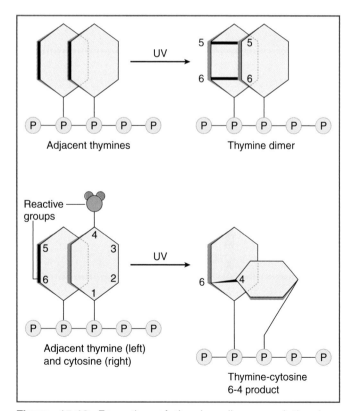

Figure 15-13. Formation of thymine dimers and thymine-cytosine "6-4" photoproducts. *UV*, ultraviolet light.

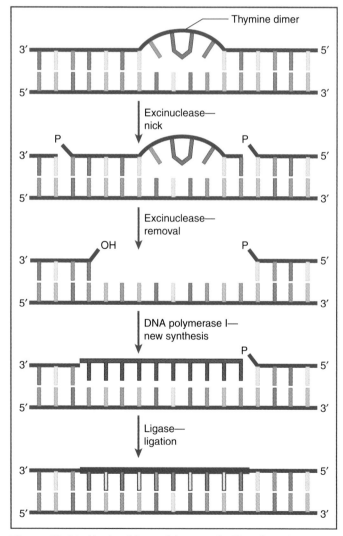

Figure 15-14. Nucleotide excision repair. The dimer is recognized by an excision excinuclease and removed so that the region can be repaired.

PHARMACOLOGY

Anticancer Drug Neutralization

Temozolomide is an oral alkylating agent with demonstrated antitumor activity. However, its effectiveness is limited by MGMT. The temozolomide kills glioblastoma cells by causing point mutations, but it must be administered over a period of 7 weeks to deplete the MGMT enzyme. Because MGMT is a suicide enzyme, it must be resynthesized for continued activity.

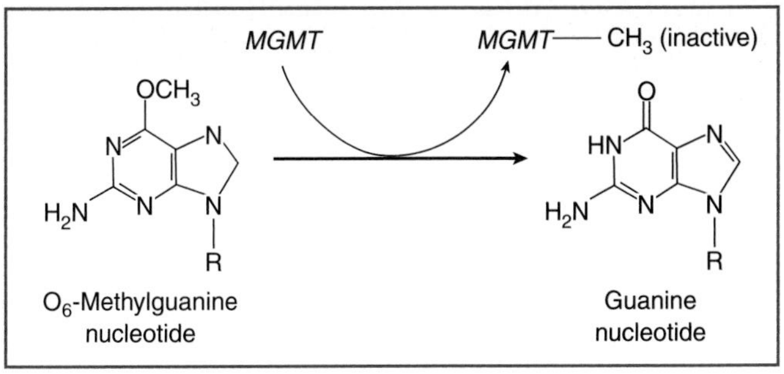

Figure 15-16. Direct repair of guanine by O_6-methylguanine-DNA methyltransferase (*MGMT*).

Direct Repair

Guanine residues in DNA can become methylated when exposed to alkylating agents that are either ingested in the diet or administered as antineoplastic drugs (Fig. 15-15). The methyl group on the guanine ring causes it to mispair with thymine rather than to pair with cytosine, causing a point mutation. The DNA-repair enzyme O_6-methylguanine-DNA methyltransferase (MGMT) acts to repair the altered guanine by removing the methyl group directly (Fig. 15-16), thus avoiding the need for excision and resynthesis. MGMT acts as a suicide enzyme, becoming permanently inactivated upon reaction with the methyl group. To continue its effectiveness, a new enzyme must be produced to replace the inactivated enzyme molecules.

Double-Strand Repair

Exposure to free radical oxidation or ionizing irradiation can cause both strands of the DNA molecule to break; the two ends must be rejoined to avoid cell death. Double-stranded breaks are so lethal to the cell that some chemotherapeutic agents are designed to create this type of DNA damage. Double-stranded breaks are repaired by repair proteins that bring the two ends together and then use helicase activity to unwind both ends to create short, single-stranded ends. The free ends are allowed to base pair with any gaps filled in by normal polymerization and ligase activity.

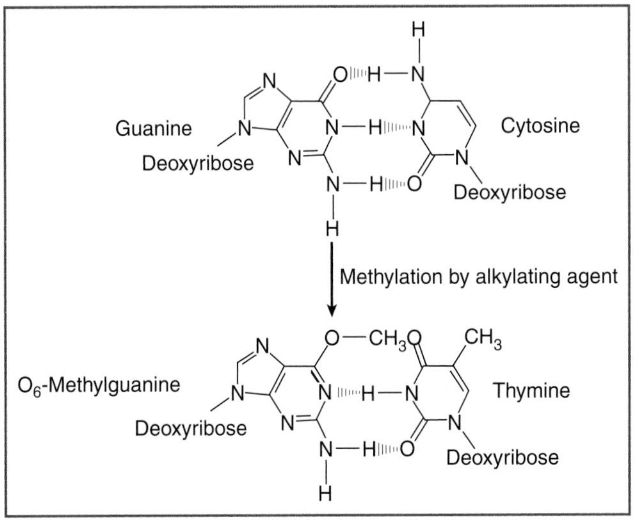

IMMUNOLOGY

Immunoglobulin Gene Rearrangement

Double-strand repair underlies the normal process involved in generating the diversity of the adaptive, or acquired, immune system. The variability in antigen recognition units (e.g., B-cell immunoglobulins and T-cell receptors) is produced by recombination of domains within the antigen receptor genes. Gene segments from larger genes encoding variable and constant regions are reassembled by double-strand repair enzymes to create new genes that recognize unique antigens, thus ensuring a diverse repertoire of antigen-binding specificities.

KEY POINTS ABOUT DNA MUTATION AND REPAIR

■ DNA can be damaged by environmental mutagens such as ultraviolet light, antineoplastic drugs, and oxidizing agents; several systems that can repair this damage include mismatch repair, base excision repair, nucleotide excision repair, direct repair, and double-strand repair.

Figure 15-15. Methylation of guanine by alkylating agents. Methylated guanine will base pair with thymine to create a point mutation.

Self-assessment questions can be accessed at www.StudentConsult.com.

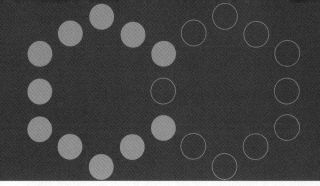

RNA Transcription and Control of Gene Expression

16

●●● RNA CLASSIFICATION

DNA information is first expressed in the form of ribonucleic acid (RNA) in a process that is tightly regulated. This is described in a fundamental biologic principle called the central dogma, which states that all RNA is produced from DNA—except for retroviruses. Three major classes of RNA are produced: one that contains the information needed to synthesize a polypeptide and two that have structural and catalytic functions in the synthesis of those polypeptides.

Messenger RNA

Messenger RNA (mRNA), the blueprint for protein synthesis, is the least abundant of the total RNA species in the cell and is the most heterogeneous. This would be expected of a molecule that is used transiently for synthesis of a wide variety of polypeptides. Eukaryotic mRNA has a 7-methylguanosine attached through a 5′ to 5′ linkage at the 5′ end of the messenger, called the cap, and a 3′ sequence of variable length consisting only of adenine, called the polyA tail. These modifications are added after synthesis of mRNA from the DNA template is completed. The addition of both these features and their function in control of polypeptide synthesis are discussed in the Eukaryotic Transcription of mRNA section.

Ribosomal RNA

Ribosomal RNA (rRNA) self-associates with ribosomal proteins to form the ribosomes, the cellular "workbenches" on which polypeptides are assembled. Different-sized RNA species are produced by the processing of a single transcript. Prokaryotes have three sizes: 23S, 16S, and 5S; eukaryotes have four sizes: 28S, 18S, 5.8S, and 5S (*S* stands for *Svedberg unit,* a measure of molecular size by ultracentrifugation). Ribosomal RNA can account for up to 80% of the total RNA.

Transfer RNA

Transfer RNA (tRNA) is the smallest of the RNA types (around 4S). Because it serves an adaptor function for amino acids in protein synthesis, at least one unique tRNA exists for each of the 20 amino acids typically found in proteins. Transfer RNA has a significant amount of tertiary structure composed of several loops and stems (Fig. 16-1). In addition to adenine, guanine, cytosine, and uracil, several unique bases, such as pseudouracil and dihydrouracil, are also found in tRNA. The structure and function of tRNA are discussed more fully in Chapter 17.

KEY POINTS ABOUT RNA CLASSIFICATION

- mRNA is the blueprint for polypeptide synthesis; tRNA transports amino acids to the ribosome; rRNA provides the structure for the workbench where polypeptides are assembled.

- RNA is transcribed from DNA when RNA polymerase attaches at a promoter site and reads the template strand to produce a messenger; transcription ends at defined termination sequences.

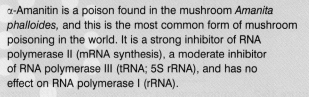

PHARMACOLOGY

Mushroom Poisoning

α-Amanitin is a poison found in the mushroom *Amanita phalloides,* and this is the most common form of mushroom poisoning in the world. It is a strong inhibitor of RNA polymerase II (mRNA synthesis), a moderate inhibitor of RNA polymerase III (tRNA; 5S rRNA), and has no effect on RNA polymerase I (rRNA).

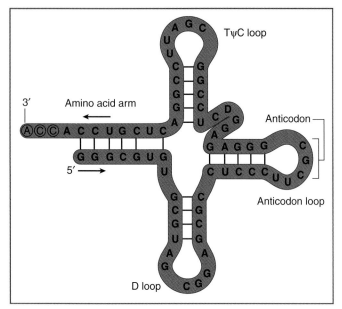

Figure 16-1. Structure of yeast alanine transfer RNA. The structure is opened up to reveal the extensive hydrogen bonding that stabilizes the normally folded tertiary structure.

●●● RNA TRANSCRIPTION

RNA Polymerase

RNA is transcribed from the DNA template by RNA polymerase. Prokaryotic cells have one multisubunit RNA polymerase that transcribes all three major classes of RNA, while eukaryotic cells have a specialized RNA polymerase for transcription of each class of RNA.

- RNA polymerase I makes rRNA.
- RNA polymerase II makes mRNA.
- RNA polymerase III makes tRNA, 5 S RNA, and other small RNAs.

Prokaryotic Transcription of mRNA

The process of synthesizing RNA from a DNA template is called transcription, but not all of the DNA in a gene is transcribed. Prokaryotic genes have regulatory sequences called promoters in addition to the region along the DNA molecule that serves as a template for an RNA molecule called transcription units. DNA sequences within the promoter or the transcription units are often referred to as elements, boxes, sites, or regions.

In a prokaryotic gene, the transcription unit has a promoter on the 5′ end (upstream) of the coding strand and a termination signal on the 3′ end (Fig. 16-2). The coding strand is called the sense strand, and the opposite strand is referred to as the template or antisense strand. There are untranslated regions (UTRs) at both ends of the coding region (genetic code for the polypeptide) representing sequences on the mRNA that serve special functions during polypeptide synthesis (translation). In addition to promoters and termination signals, the prokaryotic 5′ UTR contains a Shine-Dalgarno sequence, which is needed for binding mRNA to the ribosome.

The prokaryotic RNA polymerase is composed of four subunits, known as the core enzyme, that have 5′ to 3′ polymerase activity. It has two associated proteins that help it bind at exactly the right place, transcribe the complete length of DNA into RNA, and then terminate the process before any unwanted sequence becomes transcribed into the new RNA. The σ (sigma) factor is a dissociable protein required for initiation of transcription, and together with the core enzyme, it composes the holoenzyme. The ρ (rho) factor is required in some cases for chain termination when the RNA polymerase core enzyme cannot recognize the termination sequence itself.

The first step in initiation of transcription is binding of RNA polymerase holoenzyme to the promoter region. The promoter contains two sites that bind and precisely position the RNA polymerase: the –10 site (Pribnow box) and

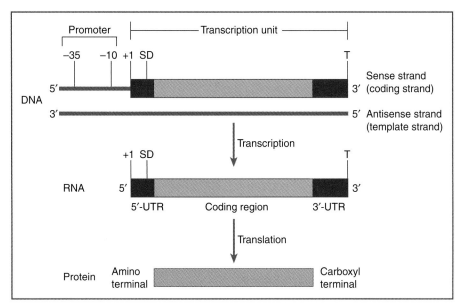

Figure 16-2. Components of a prokaryotic gene. *UTR*, untranslated region; *SD*, Shine-Dalgarno sequence; *T*, termination signal.

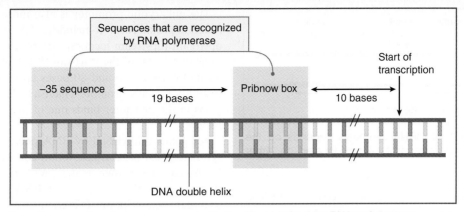

Figure 16-3. The prokaryotic promoter site has sequences that are recognized by RNA polymerase.

the –35 site (Fig. 16-3). The Pribnow box is rich in AT pairs, which melt (separate) easily, allowing the RNA polymerase to open up the helix and begin transcribing it. Initiation of transcription can be inhibited by rifamycin antibiotics that inactivate RNA polymerase.

During elongation, RNA polymerase unwinds and rewinds the DNA helix. As it unwinds DNA almost two full turns (17 bases), RNA polymerase creates a transcription bubble (Fig. 16-4). A supercoiling strain is created ahead of the helix as RNA polymerase spreads it apart to read the template strand, but the strain is relieved when the DNA helix rewinds at the other end of the bubble. The RNA chain is elongated by the addition of 5′ nucleoside triphosphates to the 3′ hydroxyl of the growing RNA chain (Fig. 16-5). Similarly to the polymerization of DNA, transcription of DNA is always in the 5′ to 3′ direction. In contrast to DNA polymerase, RNA

polymerase does not proofread the RNA sequence. Either strand of DNA can serve as the template, but the direction of synthesis is always 5′ to 3′, and thus the template DNA strand is always read 3′ to 5′ (Fig. 16-6). The antibiotic actinomycin D binds strongly to the DNA helical structure and inhibits RNA polymerase.

The prokaryotic chain termination signal is a hairpin structure at the end of every transcription unit (Fig. 16-7). The hairpin structure is created by an inverted hyphenated repeat that allows complementary base pairing to form a double helix. This type of repeat sequence contains a palindrome (a region of DNA where the 5′ to 3′ sequence is the same in both directions, with an interruption that allows the polynucleotide to loop back). There are two classes of chain termination signals:
- The ρ-independent class has a string of T's after the hairpin structure on the coding strand (see Fig. 16-7). This is

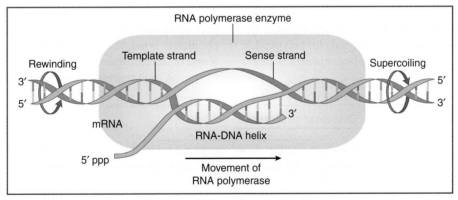

Figure 16-4. The transcription bubble is formed when RNA polymerase separates the helix to read the template strand. The helix re-forms the original base pairing as RNA polymerase moves down the gene.

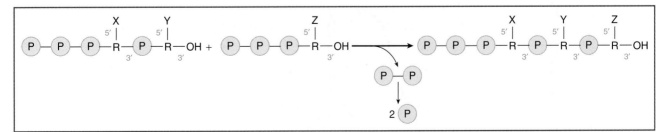

Figure 16-5. Polymerization of "Z" triphosphate with the 3′-hydroxyl of the growing RNA, producing the sequence "XYZ."

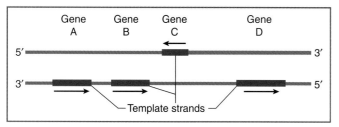

Figure 16-6. Direction of mRNA synthesis depends on the location of the template strand; it can be located on either strand.

transcribed into a series of U's in the nascent (new) RNA, and the weaker hydrogen bonding between AU pairs favors dissociation from the DNA.

• The ρ-dependent chain termination signals lack the string of T's after the hairpin structure; thus RNA polymerase requires the ρ protein for dissociation of the RNA transcript from DNA.

Eukaryotic Transcription of mRNA

Eukaryotic genes have some similarities to prokaryotic genes (Fig. 16-8). The transcription unit has a promoter on the 5' end (upstream) of the coding strand and a termination signal on the 3' end. The coding region is likewise flanked by UTRs. However, the greater complexity of the eukaryotic system also reveals a number of differences. For example, the Shine-Dalgarno sequence is not present; its function in binding the mRNA to the ribosome is assumed by eukaryotic translation initiation proteins. Unlike the continuous sequence in the prokaryotic coding region, the eukaryotic version is divided into segments:

• Exons (expressed sequences) correspond to functional segments in the polypeptide called domains (see Chapter 3).
• Introns (intervening sequences) do not code for polypeptide structure and may actually be much larger in size than the exons.

The eukaryotic promoter is also more complex than that found in prokaryotes. It includes a TATA box about 25 bases upstream (upstream locations are often denoted with minus signs (e.g., –25) of the start site (Fig. 16-9) and a CAAT box located between 70 and 80 bases upstream of the start site. In addition, many promoters have a GC box. Each of these regions in the promoter binds one of the general transcription factors.

For genes transcribed by RNA polymerase II (for mRNA synthesis), the basal transcription complex forms on a short DNA sequence known as the TATA box. RNA polymerase II binds transcription factor for RNA polymerase II (TFII) to initiate transcription. TFII contains the TATA binding protein (TBP), which aligns the basal transcription apparatus with the start site. Other proteins called general transcription factors bind to additional sites in the promoter to form the basal transcription complex. Once an active transcription complex is produced, RNA synthesis proceeds as described for prokaryotes.

Processing of Primary RNA Transcripts

In prokaryotes, the primary mRNA transcript is functional as soon as it is synthesized. This is seen when ribosomes bind to the free 5' end, even before the remainder of the molecule is transcribed. (Remember that synthesis is 5' to 3', so the 5' end of mRNA is synthesized first.) In eukaryotes, however, the RNA transcript must undergo processing before it is a functional mRNA. This processing occurs in the nucleus and involves three steps: 5' capping, 3' polyadenylation (polyA tailing), and exon splicing.

Capping involves the addition of an inverted 7-methylguanosine triphosphate attached to the 5' end of the primary transcript (Fig. 16-10). This produces a 5' to 5' phosphodiester bond, thereby providing a free 3' hydroxyl at the 5' end of the molecule. The polyA tail is attached at the 3' end by polyA polymerase, using adenosine triphosphate as a

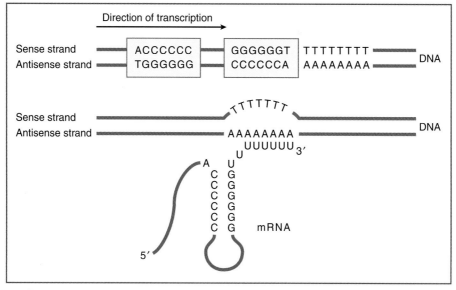

Figure 16-7. Formation of a hairpin structure at the termination signal; looping back allows antiparallel base pairing.

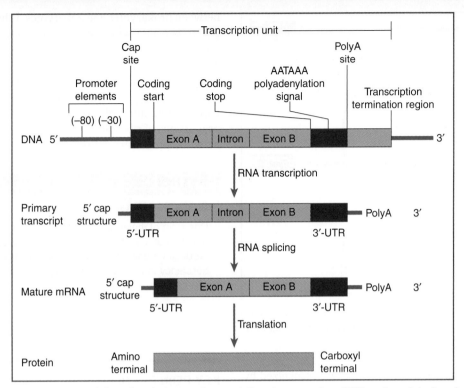

Figure 16-8. A eukaryotic gene containing signals for posttranscriptional processing. *UTR*, untranslated region.

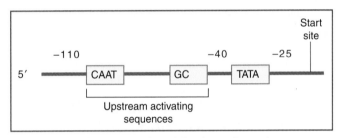

Figure 16-9. Sequences found in the eukaryotic promoter. Each promoter binds a specific transcription factor to form the basal transcription apparatus: the TATA box binds TATA binding protein transcription factor, the CAAT box binds NF-1/CAAT box transcription factor transcription factors, and the GC box binds SP-1 transcription factor.

precursor, and it extends to a length between 20 and 250 bases. Capping and polyadenylation serve a dual purpose. They make the mRNA stable by blocking access to the termini by exonucleases, and they participate in polypeptide chain initiation. Neither of these posttranscriptional elements has a counterpart in the DNA sequence.

Splicing of eukaryotic primary RNA transcripts removes the introns, leaving the exons connected together in a functional message. Primary transcripts are also called heterogeneous nuclear RNA (hnRNA), since they contain from zero to as many as 50 introns of variable length. The introns to be removed are bounded at both ends by specific base sequences called splice sites or splice junctions. Splice junctions usually begin with a consensus sequence GU (the donor site) and end with a consensus sequence AG (the acceptor site). The donor loops over to the acceptor, forming a lariat structure (Fig. 16-11) that is released when the RNA is cleaved at the

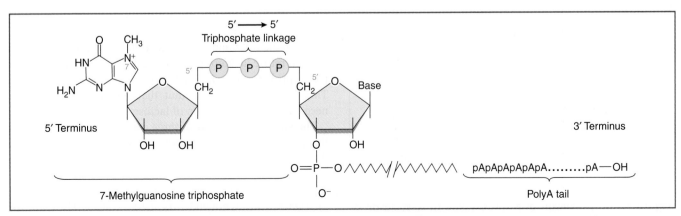

Figure 16-10. Primary RNA transcript with 7-methylguanosine cap and polyA tail.

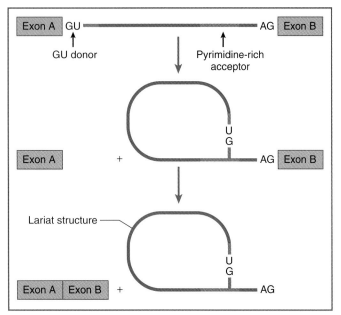
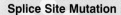

Figure 16-11. Formation of lariat structures during splicing of the eukaryotic primary RNA transcript.

acceptor site. The donor and acceptor sites are recognized by specialized small nuclear RNA particles (Fig. 16-12) that associate with nuclear proteins to form spliceosomes. The small nuclear RNA particles hold onto the 5′ exon and the 3′ exon so both ends can be rejoined.

Primary transcripts of ribosomal and transfer RNA also require processing by nucleases, and there are similarities

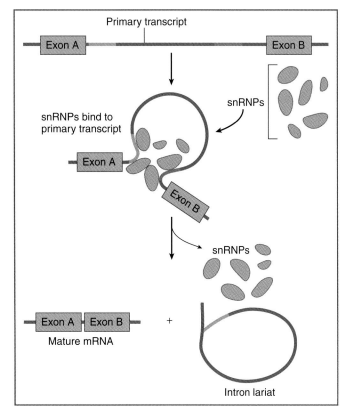

Figure 16-12. Formation of a spliceosome by association of small nuclear RNA particles (*snRNPs*) and intron RNA.

between prokaryotes and eukaryotes. Ribosomal proteins begin to associate with the primary transcript as it undergoes processing. The tRNA precursor is also processed by nuclease cleavage of precursor RNA. An intron is removed from the anticodon loop, and trimming occurs at both ends of the molecule. Processing is completed by modification of selected bases and addition of the -CCA terminal at the 3′ end. The proportions of ribosomal and tRNA species are easily coordinated by processing the precursor transcripts.

PATHOLOGY

Splice Site Mutation

One form of thalassemia (θ-thalassemia) is caused by a mutation at a splice site. Translation of the resulting mRNA produces a polypeptide that is nonfunctional, leaving a deficiency in β-globin synthesis and an excess production of α-globin.

KEY POINTS ABOUT RNA TRANSCRIPTION

- Eukaryotic and prokaryotic transcription are similar, but the attachment of RNA polymerase to the promoter requires a more complex interaction of transcription factors for the former.
- Eukaryotic hnRNA undergoes processing before it is a functional mRNA.

●●● TRANSCRIPTIONAL CONTROL OF GENE EXPRESSION

Because all cells in the body have the same genetic composition, each individual cell type must be able to regulate the expression of necessary genes, while keeping the remainder inactive. Gene expression is controlled at many levels, with transcriptional regulation being the most direct.

Regulation of the Lac Operon

The lack of a nuclear membrane in prokaryotes gives ribosomes direct access to mRNA transcripts, allowing their immediate translation into polypeptides. This makes transcription the rate-limiting step in prokaryotic gene expression and, therefore, a major point of regulation. The classic example of prokaryotic gene regulation is that of the lac operon. This operon is a genetic unit that produces the enzymes necessary for the digestion of lactose (Fig. 16-13).

The lac operon consists of three contiguous structural genes that are transcribed as continuous mRNA by RNA polymerase. An operator sequence located at the 5′ end serves as a binding site for a repressor protein that blocks RNA polymerase. The repressor protein is produced constitutively (continuously) by the *i* gene, which is not under regulatory control. The repressor itself is formed from subunits that self-assemble to form the

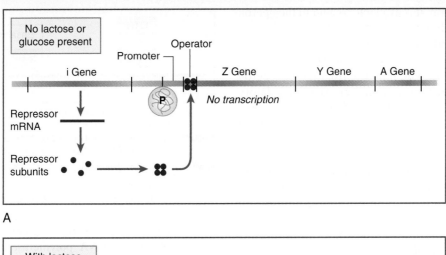

A

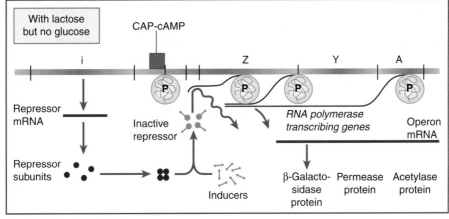

B

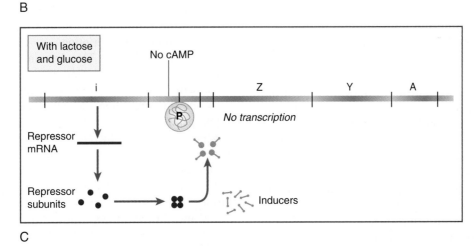

C

Figure 16-13. Expression of the lac operon under different energy sources. *P*, RNA polymerase. *CAP*, catabolite activator protein; *cAMP*, cyclic adenosine monophosphate.

active tetramer. When present, the inducer, allolactose, binds to the repressor subunits, preventing their assembly into an active tetramer. Allolactose is produced from lactose by β-galactosidase at a steady low rate and thus serves as a lactose signal. Another regulatory component is the catabolite activator protein (CAP). CAP forms an active complex with intracellular cyclic adenosine monophosphate (cAMP), which accumulates in the absence of glucose (cAMP is a starvation signal). RNA polymerase binds to the lac promoter effectively only when the CAP-cAMP complex is also bound. This ensures that the lac operon will be expressed only when glucose is absent.

The lac operon exhibits both negative control and positive control. Under negative control, a regulatory factor is needed to prevent expression of the lac operon, whereas under positive control, a regulatory factor is needed to permit expression of the lac operon.

- Negative control (conditions: glucose only; prevent expression of lac operon). If lactose is absent and glucose is present (see Fig. 16-13A), the gene products from the lac operon are not needed. Thus a regulatory factor, the repressor protein, prevents lac operon expression. Since the repressor is produced constitutively and spontaneously assembles as its active tetrameric form, it is available to bind to the operon and prevent transcription.

- Positive control (conditions: lactose only; permit expression of lac operon). If no glucose is present and lactose is present (see Fig. 16-13B), the gene products from the lac operon are needed to use the lactose for energy. Thus a regulatory factor, the CAP-cAMP complex is needed to permit expression of the operon. Because cAMP is a starvation signal indicating an absence of glucose, it is available to form the CAP-cAMP complex and permit transcription.
- Positive control (conditions: lactose and glucose; do not permit expression of the lac operon even if not prevented by repressor). If both lactose and glucose are present (see Fig. 16-13C), the regulatory mechanisms act to avoid wasteful expression of the lac operon. Even though the repressor is inactivated by the presence of lactose, RNA polymerase cannot bind to the promoter, since the CAP-cAMP complex is absent owing to the presence of glucose.

Eukaryotic Transcriptional Control

Eukaryotic transcription is regulated either by controlling physical accessibility of the DNA to RNA polymerase or by controlling the rate of RNA polymerase binding to the promoter.

Physical accessibility to RNA polymerase is determined by the degree to which the DNA is condensed. Condensed chromatin, known as heterochromatin (see Chapter 15), is characterized by having inactive genes. The DNA in heterochromatin is highly methylated, usually on the cytosine residues. This is found in CpG "islands" in or near the promoter. (Note: CpG islands are not the same as the GC box mentioned above.) Methylation is associated with a nearly permanent decrease in transcription of the gene. For example, the cardiac actin gene in heart cells contains little, if any, methylated CpG, whereas the CpG associated with the same gene in nerve cells is heavily methylated. CpG islands are usually found in promoters for housekeeping genes that are needed on a continuous basis and not regulated. Examples of housekeeping genes would be those for the salvage enzyme hypoxanthine-guanine phosphoribosyltransferase and for the ribosomal proteins.

In contrast, euchromatin is highly acetylated, but it is the histones that are modified by the acetylation, not the DNA. Acetylation changes the packing of the nucleosomes to cause local unwinding and exposure of the DNA to the transcription factors that bind to the promoter.

The rate of RNA polymerase binding to the promoter is controlled by the binding of transcription proteins, called transcription factors, to certain DNA sequences (Fig. 16-14). If the DNA sequence is on the same chromosome as the gene being transcribed, it is called a *cis*-acting element. This includes the sequences in the promoter already described: the CAAT box, the TATA box, and the GC box. It can also include enhancer sequences (most common) or silencer sequences that can be more than 1000 bases upstream or downstream from the promoter. These sequences function by binding transcription activator (or repressor) proteins and then folding back to

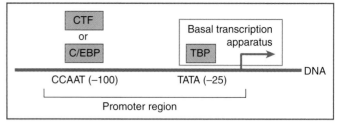

Figure 16-14. Interaction of transcription factors with eukaryotic promoter. *C/EBP*, CAAT enhancer binding protein; *CTF*, CAAT box transcription factor; *TBP*, TATA binding protein.

interact with the basal transcription complex at the promoter (Fig. 16-15). The presence of one or more transcription activator proteins bound to *cis*-acting elements can increase the rate of binding of RNA polymerase and thus the rate of transcription.

Although there are thousands of individual transcription factors and activators, they can be grouped into a relatively small number of families that are classified by common supersecondary structural motifs: the helix-loop-helix family, the leucine zipper family, the helix-turn-helix family, and the zinc finger family. Most transcription factors have three domains:

- *DNA binding domain*: This domain is configured to recognize a base sequence from the arrangement of the functional groups (amino, hydroxyl, and methyl) that project into the major groove and the minor groove of the DNA helix. Thus, they can "read" a sequence without opening up the helix.
- *Activation domain*: This domain interacts with components of the basal transcription complex to accelerate its assembly and initiation of transcription.
- *Dimerization domain*: This domain on an inactive monomer interacts with the dimerization domain on another transcription factor to form an active dimer. The dimers can be the same (homodimer) or different (heterodimer) polypeptides.

Some transcription factors regulate several genes at once. They are produced by master regulatory genes that coordinate all of the genes necessary for the development of a specialized cell. An example of such a gene is myoblast determination protein 1 (MyoD1). When MyoD1 is experimentally introduced into fibroblasts (an undifferentiated cell type), they are converted to myoblasts (Fig. 16-16). This is the result of the MyoD1 transcription activator coordinately stimulating genes that are actively expressed in myoblasts but are not normally active in fibroblasts.

MICROBIOLOGY

The Diauxie Phenomenon

If *Escherichia coli* is grown on a medium containing glucose and lactose, the bacteria exhibit a biphasic growth curve called the diauxie phenomenon. At first, only glucose is metabolized. When the glucose has been consumed, a lag is seen while cAMP levels increase and the CAP-cAMP complex permits expression of the lac operon. Growth resumes as the lactose is consumed.

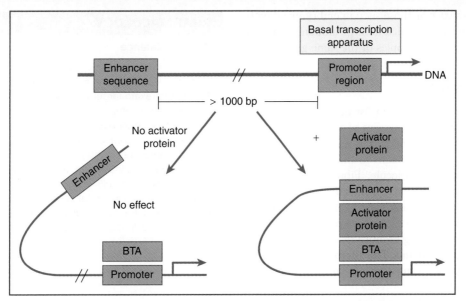

Figure 16-15. Interaction of activated enhancer with promoter region. Enhancers cannot influence transcription rate without activator proteins bound (*left arrow*). Activator proteins interact with the basal transcription apparatus (*BTA*) to increase the rate at which transcription is initiated (*right arrow*).

PATHOLOGY

CpG Islands in Tumor Cells

Loss of tumor suppressor gene function can occur when one allele for the gene is mutated and the other has abnormal methylation of CpG islands. The methylation prevents expression ("gene silencing") of the tumor suppressor gene. An example is loss of the MGMT DNA repair gene (see Chapter 15), which occurs early in the course of colon cancer

Gene Amplification

Gene amplification refers to an increase in the number of copies of the same gene rather than to an increase in its rate of transcription. It results from gene duplication that has been repeated many times over, producing from 100 to 1000 copies of the gene. Examples of gene amplification are the ribosomal genes and histone genes that are found clustered in tandem (end-to-end) arrays in the genome. In actively growing or

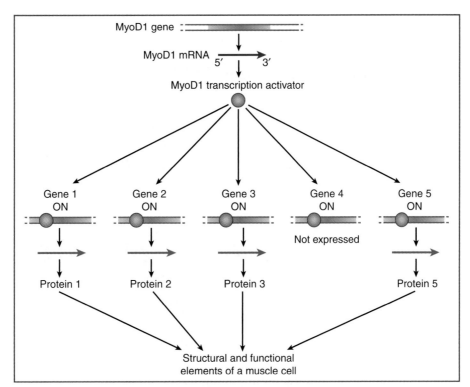

Figure 16-16. The *MyoD1* master regulatory gene. The gene product is a transcription factor that is recognized by the basal transcription apparatus at genes 1, 2, 3, and 5, creating a simultaneous, and thus coordinated, activation.

differentiating tissues such as those seen in embryonic development, ribosomal RNA is needed in large amounts that can only be provided by multiple copies of the same gene.

Alternative Splicing

Alternative splicing is a mechanism for generating multiple protein species from an RNA transcript of a single gene. It involves selective joining of exons during splicing (Fig. 16-17) and can include or exclude domains in the polypeptide. An example is the fibronectin molecule. Fibronectin functions in the binding of cells to the extracellular matrix and exists in three forms: in the extracellular matrix, on the cell surface, or in solution. However, all three forms are produced from the same gene by selective splicing of more than 50 exons to get the final combination of domains. The alternative splicings of these exons are regulated during development to produce the different forms needed.

A special type of alternative splicing is called alternative tailing. This process can anchor or solubilize a membrane protein (see Fig. 16-17) by splicing out the carboxyterminal membrane anchoring domain but retaining the polyA signal. An example is the immunoglobulin G (IgG) heavy chain in B cells. Before antigen stimulation, the last exon in the primary mRNA transcript codes for a transmembrane helix domain that anchors the antibody to the plasma membrane, where it can sense antigen in the extracellular space. Upon binding of antigen and activation of the B cell, the primary RNA transcript is processed to eliminate the anchor domain, converting the IgG to a soluble form, which is excreted by the cell during the immune response.

PHARMACOLOGY

Drug Resistance

Gene amplification is one mechanism by which cancer cells develop resistance to sublethal doses of methotrexate. The methotrexate target enzyme, dihydrofolate reductase (DHFR), can be amplified when its gene number increases either in tandem arrays or as cleaved-out, small "double minute" chromosomes. The increased number of DHFR enzyme molecules in the progeny cells overwhelms the dosage of methotrexate, allowing rapid cell division to continue. Adapted cells survive methotrexate doses 3000 times those that kill normal cells. Adapted cells contain 200 times more DHFR, 200 times more DHFR RNA, and 200 times more DHFR DNA than nonadapted cells.

Messenger RNA Editing

The coding information in a gene can be changed after processing of the primary transcript by RNA editing. The best-known example is the editing of the mRNA for apolipoprotein B (apoB). The full-length mRNA in liver makes apoB-100, which contains a domain for lipoprotein assembly plus a domain for binding to the low-density lipoprotein (LDL) receptor. Since both these domains are needed by the LDL particles that contain apoB-100, the entire mRNA is read during polypeptide synthesis. However, the intestinal mucosa makes chylomicrons that need only an apoprotein with the lipoprotein assembly domain and not the remaining domain for receptor

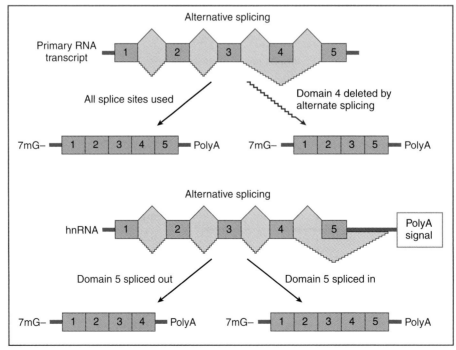

Figure 16-17. Alternative splicing and alternative tailing. Entire domains can be deleted from a polypeptide to alter their function. The exclusion of a membrane-anchoring domain (domain 5) and the splicing of an alternative polyA signal can convert a membrane-bound protein to a soluble protein. *7mG*, 7-methylguanosine.

recognition (see Chapter 20). Thus in the intestine, the mRNA is edited by deamination of a cytosine to uracil. This has the effect of changing a codon from glutamine (CAG) to "stop" (UAG). The truncated protein, called apo-48, contains only the domain for lipoprotein assembly. While it has a role in lipid transport, it is not recognized by LDL receptors in peripheral tissues and does not transport cholesterol to these cells.

RNA editing does not make a completely new apoB protein, just as alternative tailing does not make a completely new IgG. It is noteworthy that in both cases the deleted domains were on the carboxyterminal end.

MICROBIOLOGY AND IMMUNOLOGY

Clonal Selection

A wide variety of B cells are produced, each with its surface covered with thousands of identical copies of a receptor for a specific antigen. Upon binding of a specific antigen (clonal selection), B cells become activated and undergo cell division, which results in the development of a clonal population of B lymphoblasts (clonal expansion). Some of the B lymphoblasts further differentiate into plasma cells that actively secrete the antigen receptors as antibodies.

RNA Interference and "Gene Silencing"

A promising new technology for therapy of human disease called gene silencing is based on a recently discovered process for blocking mRNA translation by RNA interference. The RNA interference components are ubiquitous in eukaryotes and include a "dicer" protein and an RNA-induced silencing complex. The process, which is considered to be a translational regulatory mechanism, uses small hairpin RNA molecules, called microRNAs, as a template to recognize and block the translation of mRNA with complementary sequences. This powerful system needs only a seven base-pair sequence homology with its target to silence the expression of the mRNA for that gene.

KEY POINTS ABOUT TRANSCRIPTIONAL CONTROL OF GENE EXPRESSION

■ The rate of transcription is controlled by feedback from inducers that inhibit the activity of repressors in prokaryotes and enhancers that bind transcription activators; methylation makes promoter sites inaccessible by local induction of heterochromatin.

■ Gene expression also can be regulated by gene amplification, alternative splicing, mRNA editing, and RNA interference.

Self-assessment questions can be accessed at www. StudentConsult.com.

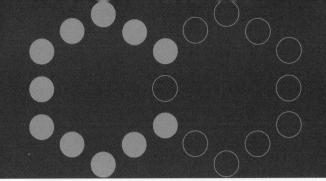

Protein Synthesis and Degradation

17

CONTENTS

●●● THE GENETIC CODE

The general concept underlying the genetic code is that a linear sequence of bases in DNA corresponds to a linear sequence of amino acids in a polypeptide. Therefore the genetic code is contained in the coding region of an mRNA. The genetic code is then translated on the ribosome to direct the polymerization of the proper amino acid sequence into a polypeptide. The genetic code has the following general features:

- *Universality*: The genetic code is the same in all organisms with a few minor exceptions in plants, microorganisms, and mitochondria.
- *Nonoverlapping and commaless sequence*: The genetic code is read in a continuous and contiguous sequence, three bases at a time (Table 17-1). Each group of three bases is referred to as a triplet codon, and there are no combinations of bases that represent spacers between triplets.

- *Specificity*: Only one amino acid is specified for each codon. No amino acid is ever substituted for another during polypeptide synthesis. Each space in Table 17-1 is occupied by only one amino acid.
- *Redundancy (degeneracy)*: Several codons can represent the same amino acid. In Table 17-1, most amino acids appear in more than one space.

Transfer RNA Adaptor Function

The 31 species of transfer RNA (tRNA) differ from each other in two important respects. The most obvious difference is in the different anticodon sequences that match the attached amino acid to the proper codons in mRNA. They also differ in their ability to be recognized by a unique aminoacyl-tRNA synthetase that matches the amino acid to the codon.

All tRNAs have the following common features (see Fig. 16-1):

- *Acceptor arm*: The CCA 3′-hydroxyl terminus is the site for amino acid attachment. It is not specified in the tRNA gene but is added as a posttranscriptional modification.
- *Anticodon loop*: This part of the tRNA contains a triplet of bases that pair with the mRNA codon in standard antiparallel orientation.
- *D arm*: This part of the tRNA is involved in recognition by the proper aminoacyl-tRNA synthetase. The fidelity of translation of the genetic code is totally dependent on the simultaneous recognition of an amino acid and its corresponding tRNA. This arm is named for its dihydrouracil content.
- *TψC arm*: This part of the tRNA is involved in a functional binding to the ribosome. It is named for thymine and pseudouracil bases.

Aminoacyl-tRNA Synthetases

The enzymes that covalently link the correct amino acid to the correct tRNA are called aminoacyl-tRNA synthetases. This process, often referred to as charging the tRNA, occurs in two reaction steps: amino acid activation and tRNA acylation (Fig. 17-1). The amino acid activation step uses adenosine triphosphate to produce an aminoacyl–adenosine monophosphate. The acylation step then transfers the amino acid from

TABLE 17-1. The Genetic Code

5′-OH TERMINAL BASE					3′-OH TERMINAL BASE
	U	**C**	**A**	**G**	
U	Phe	Ser	Tyr	Cys	U
	Phe	Ser	Tyr	Cys	C
	Leu	Ser	Term	Term	A
	Leu	Ser	Term	Trp	G
C	Leu	Pro	His	Arg	U
	Leu	Pro	His	Arg	C
	Leu	Pro	Gln	Arg	A
	Leu	Pro	Gln	Arg	G
A	Ile	Thr	Asn	Ser	U
	Ile	Thr	Asn	Ser	C
	Ile	Thr	Lys	Arg	A
	Met	Thr	Lys	Arg	G
G	Val	Ala	Asp	Gly	U
	Val	Ala	Asp	Gly	C
	Val	Ala	Glu	Gly	A
	Val	Ala	Glu	Gly	G

Each amino acid is represented by three bases: a 5′ base, a middle base, and a 3′ base. *Term* refers to termination (nonsense) codons. Data from Pelley JW: *Ace the boards: Biochemistry*, St Louis, 1997, Mosby.

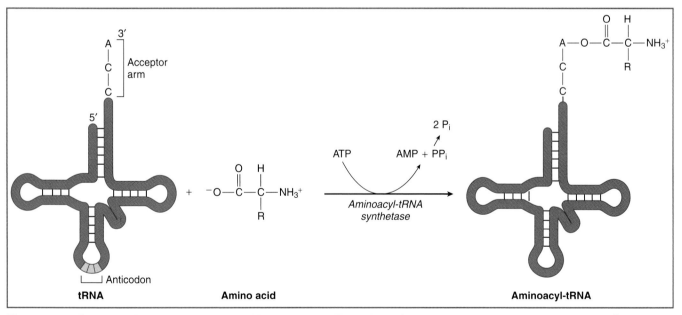

Figure 17-1. Charging of tRNA by aminoacyl-tRNA synthetase. The amino acid is linked by a high-energy bond to the 3′-adenylate residue on the acceptor arm.

the adenylate of adenosine monophosphate to the terminal 3′-adenylate of the acceptor arm on tRNA.

The aminoacyl-tRNA synthetase is the only point in nature at which the genetic code and a corresponding amino acid are recognized simultaneously. Once the tRNA is charged, the amino acid attached to it will be inserted into the polypeptide based on the information in the anticodon, not on recognition

of the amino acid. Because the tRNA is an amino acid adaptor, this principle has been referred to as the adaptor hypothesis.

Proof of the adaptor hypothesis was obtained in a classic experiment in which the amino acid was modified after charging of the tRNA. First, cysteinyl-tRNA was charged with cysteine and then treated with a catalyst that removed the thiol from the cysteine side chain to produce alanine. When this modified

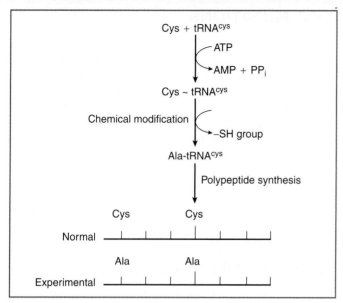

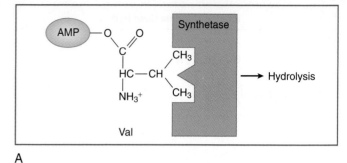

A

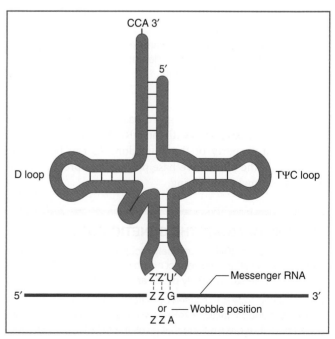

B

Figure 17-2. Effect of conversion of cysteinyl tRNA^{-cys} to alanyl tRNA^{cys}. The new aminoacyl-tRNA directed alanine rather than cysteine into the polypeptide, showing that the tRNA anticodon controls the amino acid that is inserted; the amino acid itself is not recognized during protein synthesis. *PP$_i$*, inorganic pyrophosphate.

Figure 17-3. Proofreading by isoleucyl-tRNA synthetase. Valine fits the hydrolytic site and is removed (**A**); isoleucine is not affected (**B**). *AMP*, adenosine monophosphate.

aminoacyl-tRNA was used in polypeptide synthesis, sequence analysis showed the alanine was incorporated at the cysteine positions. Thus polypeptide synthesis was guided exclusively by correct base pairing between the codon in the mRNA and the anticodon in the tRNA (Fig. 17-2).

Aminoacyl-tRNA Synthetase Proofreading

Any mistake by the aminoacyl-tRNA synthetase would have the same effect as a point mutation because the wrong amino acid would be joined to the tRNA. To prevent the introduction of these errors, the synthetase can proofread the attached amino acid and hydrolyze it if it is incorrect. The aminoacyl-tRNA synthetases contain hydrolytic sites that remove incorrect matches (Fig. 17-3). For example, correctly activated isoleucyl-tRNA will not allow the isoleucine to fit into the hydrolytic site, and it is released from the enzyme to be used in polypeptide synthesis. However, if the isoleucyl-tRNA is incorrectly charged with valine, the valine will fit into the hydrolytic site, leading to its hydrolysis from the incorrect tRNA.

Wobble in Anticodon Base-Pairing

Although 61 different codons specify amino acids in a polypeptide (3 of the 64 are termination codons), there are only 31 species of tRNA. This imposes a requirement on most of the tRNA molecules to recognize more than one codon for the same amino acid. The ability of one tRNA molecule to accomplish this task explains the redundancy in the genetic code.

The ability of one tRNA to base pair with more than one codon specifying the same amino acid is due to nonstandard

base pairing called wobble. Wobble occurs between the base in the first (5′) position of the anticodon and the third (3′) position of mRNA codon (Fig. 17-4). The bases adopt an alternative hydrogen bonding according to the following rules:

- U in the anticodon can base pair with A or G on the mRNA.
- G in the anticodon can base pair with C or U on the mRNA.
- I (inosine) in the anticodon can base pair with U, C, or A on the mRNA (Fig. 17-5).

Figure 17-4. The wobble position in the anticodon. Note that the anticodon can base pair with two different codons.

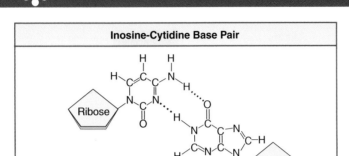

Figure 17-5. Base pairing between inosine in the anticodon wobble position and cytosine, adenine, or uracil in the codon on mRNA. Inosine is on the right.

The ability of each of the given bases in the anticodon to adopt alternate base pairs with the mRNA codons means that wobble is a property of the anticodon. As can be seen in Figure 17-5, the alternative base pairing is as precise and as strong as normal base pairing.

KEY POINTS ABOUT THE GENETIC CODE

- The structure of tRNA is uniquely recognized by the synthetase enzymes that attach the correct amino acid; this gives the genetic code its universal specificity of one amino acid for a given codon.

- The genetic code is translated by matching the anticodon in tRNA to the codons contained in mRNA; wobble in the anticodon allows the alternative base pairing that gives the genetic code its property of degeneracy.

●●● MUTATIONS

Although proofreading and repair of DNA are designed to prevent mutation, a small number of lesions remain unrepaired at cell division. Once the lesion is replicated during DNA synthesis, it becomes a permanent, heritable change called a mutation. That is why continuously proliferating cells are more susceptible to mutagenesis than quiescent cells. The three major categories of mutation are the following:

- Base change (substitution) mutation—a change from one base to another.
- Frameshift mutation—an alteration of the normal codon reading frame by addition or deletion of a base.
- Recombination mutation—an exchange between two DNA molecules.

Base Change Mutations

Base change (point) mutations are produced by chemical modifications to existing bases, or by incorporation of base analogs that masquerade as normal bases. Base analogs can become incorporated in place of a normal base and then cause an incorrect base to be incorporated during DNA synthesis. A transition mutation involves the substitution of one type of base with the same type (e.g., a pyrimidine for a pyrimidine), whereas a transversion mutation substitutes one type of base with its opposite type.

Not all base change mutations are harmful (Fig. 17-6). They can lead to no change in the protein if the new codon specifies the same amino acid (silent mutation). They can also specify a change from one amino acid to a similar amino acid (missense mutation) and thus have a minimal effect on the protein tertiary structure. However, base change mutations can destroy a protein if they produce a missense mutation for an amino acid with a significantly different side chain (e.g., leucine [hydrophobic] to serine [hydrophilic] or glutamate [negative charge] to lysine [positive charge]). In addition, when a termination codon appears within the polypeptide (nonsense mutation), a truncated polypeptide will be produced. The closer a nonsense mutation is located to the amino terminus, the shorter the protein product.

Frameshift Mutations

Frameshift mutations are produced by molecules that can insert (intercalate) between the normal bases to create mistakes during DNA synthesis. These are usually flat molecules, such

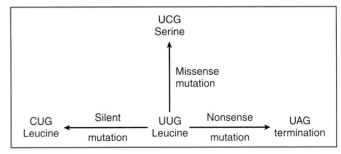

Figure 17-6. Effects of base change mutation range from silent to termination.

Normal							
mRNA	AUG	GGG	GCC	AAA	AGU	UAG	UUUG...
polypeptide	Met -	Gly -	Ala -	Lys -	Ser	Stop	

Insertion +U
↓

mRNA	AUG	GGC	GCC	AAA	UAG	UUAGUUUG...
polypeptide	Met -	Gly -	Ala -	Lys -	Stop	

Deletion −G
↓

mRNA	AUG	GGC	CCA	AAA	GUU	AGU	UUG
polypeptide	Met -	Gly -	Pro -	Lys -	Val -	Ser -	Leu

Random

Figure 17-7. Effect of frameshift mutations. The new sequence can produce a stop codon or a random sequence of amino acids.

as the acridine dyes, that have a hydrophobic nature (remember that hydrophobic base stacking is a contributing force in the structure of the helix). A frameshift mutation is produced either by insertion or deletion of one or more new bases. Because the reading frame begins at the start site, any mRNA produced from a mutated DNA sequence will be read out of frame after the point of the insertion or deletion, yielding a nonsense protein. Similarly to a point mutation, a frameshift mutation can produce a termination codon (Fig. 17-7). In addition, frameshift mutations, like point mutations, are less deleterious if they are close to the carboxyl terminal.

HISTOLOGY

Continuously Dividing Cells

Cells undergoing continuous cell division are either differentiating mitotic cells or vegetative intermitotic cells (stem cells) that replicate both to replace themselves and to provide precursors for specialized cells. Examples of stem cells are basal cells in the epidermis, regenerative cells in the intestines, and bone marrow stem cells. Examples of differentiating mitotic cells are the prickle cells in the stratum spinosum of the epidermis and fibroblasts in the connective tissue during wound healing.

Recombination Mutations

Recombination is a normal process through which chromosomes exchange gene alleles (alternative forms of the same gene). When it occurs during meiosis, it is referred to as crossing over. During this process, genes are not created or destroyed, but if a misalignment occurs (Fig. 17-8), then an unequal distribution of DNA results. This creates a deletion from the affected gene on one strand accompanied by a partial duplication on the other strand. When this type of unequal crossover occurs during meiosis, the new chromosomal arrangement becomes a heritable change. An example of such an unequal crossover is the Lepore thalassemia variant allele (Fig. 17-9). The similarity between the β-globin gene and the adjacent δ-globin gene led to a misalignment and an unequal crossover within the gene. Since the δ-globin protein has normal function in forming active hemoglobin tetramers, there is no loss of function from this mutation. Instead, the defect is in the fact that the hybrid δ-β globin, which is the same length as the normal β-globin, is produced by the slower δ-globin promoter, thus classifying the mutation as a thalassemia (reduced production of a globin leading to altered hemoglobin tetramers).

KEY POINT ABOUT MUTATION

- The effect of a mutation can range from silence to destruction of the polypeptide or deletion of the gene; the effect of the mutation is determined by where in the mRNA the change occurred and what the new codon specifies (e.g., a termination codon vs. an amino acid change).

●●● PROTEIN SYNTHESIS

Protein synthesis is the process of assembly of a peptide on a ribosome workbench using an mRNA blueprint from tRNA parts. Proteins may also need posttranslational modification before they are functional.

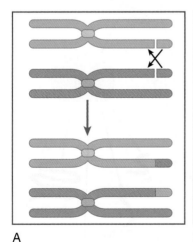
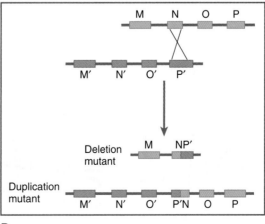

A   B

Figure 17-8. Normal versus nonaligned (unequal) recombination between chromosomes. When genes are misaligned **(A)**, one chromosome receives a duplication, while the other receives a deletion **(B)**.

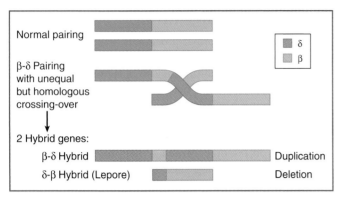

Figure 17-9. Formation of a Lepore hemoglobin gene by unequal crossing over between the β-globin gene and the δ-globin gene. The 5′ end of the deletion mutant (Lepore mutant) contains the slower promoter of the δ-globin gene, thus reducing the amount of globin produced (thalassemia).

TABLE 17-2. Protein Factors Required for Polypeptide Synthesis in Prokaryotes and Eukaryotes

STAGE OF POLYPEPTIDE	PROKARYOTE	EUKARYOTE
Initiation factors	IF-1 IF-2 IF-3	eIF-1 through eIF-10
Elongation factors	EF-Tu EF-Ts EF-G	eEF-1α eEF-1β eEF-2
Termination factors	RF-1 RF-2	eRF

Data from Pelley JW: *Ace the boards: Biochemistry,* St Louis, 1997, Mosby.

The Ribosome

The ribosome is a ribonucleoprotein particle (Fig. 17-10) that is similar in composition for both prokaryotes and eukaryotes. Ribosomal proteins and RNA will spontaneously self-assemble into two subunits when mixed. A complete ribosome is assembled only during the process of polypeptide chain initiation. Protein translation factors (Table 17-2) coordinate the initiation, elongation, and termination steps in the synthesis of a polypeptide. A completely assembled ribosome contains three sites for binding of tRNA: the A (aminoacyl) site, which binds the new aminoacyl-tRNA; the P (peptidyl) site, which binds the growing peptide that remains attached to the most recently bound tRNA; and the E (exit) site that contains deacylated tRNA. The growing peptide is attached to the ribosome by a tRNA at all times during elongation

and is not released until the termination codon appears. Since both eukaryotic and prokaryotic protein synthesis are similar in their general features, the prokaryotic is described here, with important differences noted.

Polypeptide Chain Elongation

It is easier to understand the events occurring during chain initiation by first understanding the process of elongation. This is a three-step cyclic process that incorporates new amino acids into the growing polypeptide chain. Polypeptides are synthesized in the amino to carboxyl terminal direction; thus new amino acids are inserted at the carboxyl terminal of the growing polypeptide. The three steps in elongation are aminoacyl-tRNA binding, peptide bond formation, and peptidyl-tRNA translocation (Fig. 17-11).

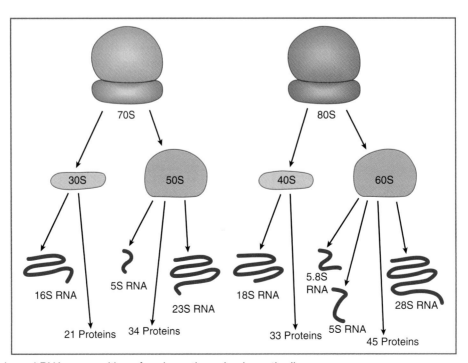

Figure 17-10. Protein and RNA composition of prokaryotic and eukaryotic ribosomes.

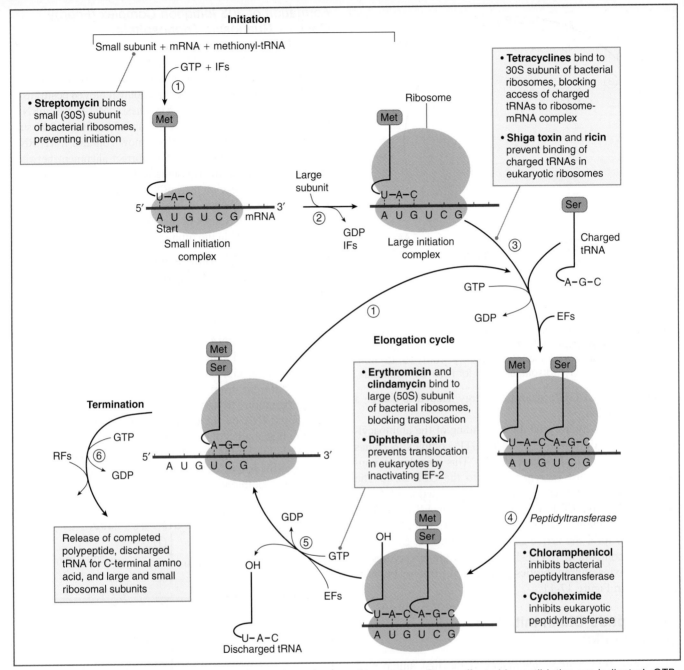

Figure 17-11. Overview of initiation, elongation, and termination of translation. Steps affected by antibiotics are indicated. *GTP*, guanosine triphosphate; *GDP*, guanosine diphosphate; *IF*, initiation factor; *EF*, elongation factor.

Aminoacyl-tRNA Binding (Energy Cost = 1 Guanosine Triphosphate)

An aminoacyl-tRNA cannot bind until a binding complex is formed with the elongation factor (EF)-Tu and guanosine triphosphate (GTP). Binding of this complex leads to ejection of the deacylated tRNA from the E site.

Peptide Bond Formation (Energy Cost = 0 Guanosine Triphosphate)

The new aminoacyl-tRNA binds to the A site and is aligned with the peptidyl-tRNA at the P site, and a peptide bond is formed by the action of peptidyltransferase. Peptidyltransferase activity is catalyzed by 23S ribosomal RNA (a ribozyme). The formation of the peptide bond attaches the growing polypeptide to the newly bound aminoacyl-tRNA, which is now a peptidyl-tRNA.

Peptidyl tRNA Translocation (Energy Cost = 1 Guanosine Triphosphate)

Since the A site must be open for binding of the next aminoacyl-tRNA, the peptidyl-tRNA must be moved over to the P site. EF-G uses one GTP to catalyze this process, and both the mRNA and peptidyl-tRNA move the distance of one codon. The deacylated tRNA moves to the E site.

The energy cost of incorporating one aminoacyl-tRNA into a protein is 2 GTP, but the total cost of incorporating one amino acid into a protein is four high-energy bonds (2′ adenosine

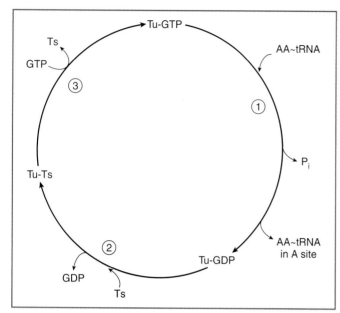

Figure 17-12. Regeneration of prokaryotic Tu–guanosine triphosphate (*GTP*) complex by Ts translation factor. Step 1: Tu-GTP binds aminoacyl-tRNA to A site on ribosome; 2: Ts displaces guanosine diphosphate (*GDP*) from Tu to form Tu-Ts complex; 3: GTP displaces Ts to form Tu-GTP complex.

triphosphate + 2 GTP) when the energy needed to charge a tRNA is included.

When GTP is hydrolyzed during binding of the aminoacyl-tRNA to the ribosome, the EF-Tu-GTP complex becomes EF-Tu–guanosine diphosphate (GDP). This complex is nonfunctional and must be regenerated to the GTP form. The EF-Tu-GDP complex is regenerated by the action of EF-Ts (Fig. 17-12). First, EF-Ts displaces GDP from EF-Tu to form an EF-Tu-Ts complex. Then GTP displaces Ts from the Tu-Ts complex to form the active EF-Tu-GTP complex. EF-Tu and EF-Ts are comparable to eEF-1α and eEF-1β in eukaryotes.

Some toxins and antibiotics that disrupt protein synthesis are listed in Figure 17-11.

Polypeptide Chain Initiation (Prokaryotic)

Chain initiation requires alignment of the first amino acid with the initiation codon and association of the subunits into a complete ribosome. It is also critical that the first amino acid be located in the P site on the ribosome to make the A site available for a new aminoacyl-tRNA. This process occurs in two stages: formation of the 30S initiation complex and formation of the 70S initiation complex.

MICROBIOLOGY

Virulence Factors for Diphtheria

For *Corynebacterium diphtheriae* to cause diphtheria, it must produce two virulence factors: diphtherial cord factor and diphtheria toxin. The cord factor allows the bacteria to grow in ropelike lateral aggregates to colonize in the upper respiratory tract. The toxin kills host cells by permanently inactivating EF-2 (translocase) through adenosine diphosphate ribosylation.

Formation of 30S Initiation Complex (Energy Cost = 1 Guanosine Triphosphate)

N-formylmethionine (fMet) is the amino acid coded by the AUG codon, which is the start codon for protein synthesis. Therefore, fMet is the N-terminal amino acid of nearly all proteins in prokaryotic systems; however, it is commonly removed posttranslationally. For initiation of protein synthesis, fMet-tRNA, mRNA, GTP, and the initiation factors (IF)-1, and -3 bind to the 30 S subunit (Fig. 17-13). The future P site now contains fMet-tRNA aligned with the AUG codon. The correct alignment between the AUG codon and the ribosome is due to a special upstream (noncoding) sequence on the mRNA called the Shine-Dalgarno sequence. This sequence of base pairs with a complementary sequence in the 16 S RNA of the 30 S subunit results in precise positioning of AUG in the future P site.

Formation of 70S Initiation Complex (Energy Cost = 0 Guanosine Triphosphate)

The 70S initiation complex is formed as the 50 S subunit binds and GTP is hydrolyzed. This initiation complex is a complete ribosome containing fMet tRNA in the P site, aligned with the AUG codon on mRNA, and the ribosomal A site is ready to receive the second aminoacyl-tRNA.

There is a special initiator tRNA specific for methionine that is different from normal methionyl-tRNA; it carries the designation tRNAf. fMet tRNA is produced from methionyl-tRNA by the enzyme transformylase, which uses *N*-formyltetrahydrofolate as the carbon donor. Tu will not form a binding complex with fMet-tRNA, preventing it from binding to the A site. Methionine insertion at interior sites uses unmodified methionyl-tRNA bound by Tu.

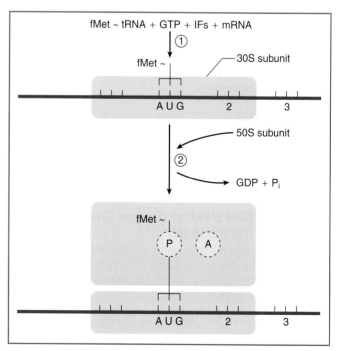

Figure 17-13. Prokaryotic polypeptide chain initiation. Step 1: Binding of *N*-formylmethionine (*fMet*)-tRNA, guanosine triphosphate (*GTP*), three initiation factors (*IF-1, IF-2, IF-3*), and mRNA to the 30S subunit forms the 30S initiation complex. Step 2: binding of the 50S subunit to the 30S initiation complex completes the initiation process. *GDP*, guanosine diphosphate.

PHARMACOLOGY

Streptomycin Versus Erythromycin

Streptomycin blocks polypeptide chain initiation in prokaryotes by binding to the 30 S subunit. It also causes misreading during translation. It is usually reserved for use in tuberculosis or other antibiotic-resistant infections, since it can cause hearing loss. Erythromycin can be used instead, since it has less serious side effects. Erythromycin inhibits translocation by binding to the prokaryotic 50 S ribosomal subunit.

Polypeptide Chain Initiation (Eukaryotic)

Eukaryotes follow a similar initiation process but use more proteins. An initiation complex is formed with the 40S subunit, but the Shine-Dalgarno function in prokaryotes is assumed by cap-binding proteins that recognize the methylguanosine cap on the mRNA. In addition, a specialized initiator tRNA that is specific for methionine is used, but the methionine is not formylated. The AUG codon is aligned with the methionyl-tRNA by the initiation factor eIF-3 (the "e" signifies eukaryotic). Binding of the 60 S subunit creates the 80 S initiation complex (see Fig. 17-11).

Polypeptide Chain Termination

Polypeptide chain termination is less complicated than either initiation or elongation because no tRNA is bound to the A site; no tRNA exists with a "stop" anticodon. Instead a polypeptide release factor complexed with GTP binds to the stop codon and uncouples the activity of peptidyltransferase. This causes the peptide chain to be transferred to water, releasing it from the ribosome (energy cost = 1 GTP). Upon release of the polypeptide, the ribosome dissociates into subunits and cannot reassemble until the chain initiation step. Eukaryotes have one release factor; prokaryotes have two.

Polyribosomes

Polyribosomes, also known as polysomes, are mRNAs with multiple ribosomes attached. This happens when new initiation complexes form sequentially on the same mRNA (Fig. 17-14). Polysomes allow for the synthesis of several polypeptides concurrently on the same mRNA molecule. Both prokaryotes and eukaryotes form polyribosomes.

Posttranslational Modification

Polypeptides undergo a variety of modifications after their release from the ribosome to become biologically active.

Trimming
The amino-terminal methionine and the carboxyterminal amino acids are often removed in both eukaryotes and prokaryotes.

Proteolytic Processing
Specialized proteases convert inactive, stored precursor forms into an active form. This is seen in the conversion of prohormones and proenzymes to their active forms.

Signal Sequences (Targeting Sequences)
Specialized amino acid sequences direct (target) newly synthesized proteins to their ultimate location, such as in membranes, organelles, or extracellular secretion, and are then removed by special peptidases (see below).

Prenylation
Isoprenyl groups are attached to specific cysteine side chains, providing a lipid anchor for some proteins.

Glycosylation
One or more carbohydrates or oligosaccharides are added to specific amino acid side chains of secreted proteins. When linked to serine or threonine, they are called O-linked carbohydrates; and when added to the amide nitrogen of asparagine, they are called N linked. One protein may contain multiple sites of glycosylation with different linkages and structures.

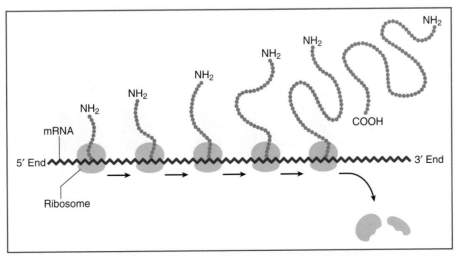

Figure 17-14. Polyribosomes form when ribosomes continue to initiate new polypeptides as soon as the 5′ end of the mRNA is physically available.

Formation of Disulfide Bonds

Protein disulfide isomerase catalyzes the formation of disulfide bonds after formation of the tertiary structure of protein. This is common for secreted proteins.

Prosthetic Group Attachment

Prosthetic groups are nonprotein modifications that are joined by covalent attachment or by hydrophobic association in a protected pocket.

Phosphorylation

Many enzymes are reversibly phosphorylated as a result of cell signaling after hormone binding. In addition, phosphorylation of serine on milk casein creates calcium-binding sites, providing a rich source of calcium for nursing infants.

Hydroxylation

Hydroxylysine and hydroxyproline are formed during the maturation of functional collagen; the hydroxylases require ascorbic acid as a cofactor.

Carboxylation

γ-Carboxylation of glutamic acid residues in prothrombin requires vitamin K. The γ-carboxyglutamate residues bind Ca^{++} during the blood clotting cascade.

Acetylation

Many amino-terminal residues in eukaryotic proteins are acetylated.

Cellular Sorting of Proteins

Cells produce proteins for secretion and for functions in various subcellular organelles. There are several mechanisms for delivering proteins to their final destination: signal sequences for secreted proteins, mannose phosphate tagging for lysosomal enzymes, translocase presequences for mitochondrial proteins, and nuclear localization sequences for nuclear proteins.

Secreted Proteins

A signal sequence at the amino terminus of a protein targets a polypeptide to the lumen of the endoplasmic reticulum (Fig. 17-15). When the signal sequence is exposed during the early stages of the synthesis of the polypeptide, it is recognized and bound by a ribonucleoprotein signal recognition particle that causes polymerization to stop. The signal recognition particle then guides the ribosome to a membrane receptor on the endoplasmic reticulum, and polymerization resumes. The growing polypeptide is directed through a translocon channel in the membrane into the lumen of the endoplasmic reticulum, and the signal sequence is removed by proteolytic cleavage.

Lysosomal Enzymes

Enzymes destined for the lysosome are tagged by a phosphotransferase enzyme (Fig. 17-16). In a two-step reaction, phosphate is attached to terminal mannose residues on oligosaccharides of mannose-rich glycoproteins. Mannose 6-phosphate binds to a receptor in the Golgi membrane. Vesicles containing the receptor-bound enzymes bud off of the Golgi apparatus to fuse with lysosomes.

Mitochondrial Proteins

The mitochondrial genome codes for only a small number of the total proteins in the mitochondrion. Mitochondrial proteins that are synthesized in the cytoplasm from nuclear genes are imported by translocation through translocation complexes in the mitochondrial membrane. Mitochondrial proteins must be unfolded and passed through the membrane in a single strand, followed by refolding when they reach the matrix.

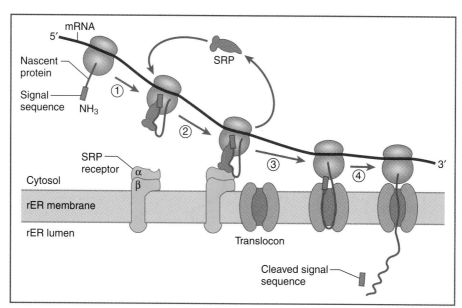

Figure 17-15. Targeting of a polypeptide into the lumen of rough endoplasmic reticulum (*rER*). The signal sequence directs the binding of the ribosome to the membrane, and the growing polypeptide passes through a translocon to the lumen, where it is glycosylated to increase its solubility. *SRP*, signal recognition particle.

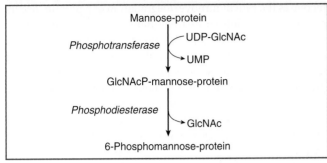

Figure 17-16. Formation of mannose 6-phosphate on a lysosomal enzyme directs it to the lysosome instead of to secretion in the blood. A defect in this process leads to I-cell disease, which is characterized by an appearance of lysosomal enzymes in the blood but not in the lysosomes. *UDP*, uridine diphosphate; *UMP*, uridine monophosphate.

PATHOLOGY

I-Cell Disease (Mucolipidosis II)

When the phosphotransferase enzyme is genetically deficient, the mannose 6-phosphate tag is missing from enzymes destined to be located in the lysosome. Instead they are routed into secretory vacuoles and released into the serum. This creates a lysosomal storage disease with the accumulation of sphingolipids and glycosaminoglycans in the lysosomes. Patients have skeletal deformities and mental deterioration.

Nuclear Proteins

Proteins destined for the nucleus, including histones, contain a nuclear localization signal that is rich in positively charged amino acids (Lys and Arg). A carrier protein, called an importin, associates with the nuclear protein and forms a complex that is transported through the nuclear pores. In contrast to mitochondrial proteins that must be unfolded before translocation, nuclear proteins are transported while folded into their native conformation.

Translational Repression

Messenger RNA (mRNA) is not always translated as soon as it appears in the cytoplasm. Translation repressor proteins exist that can bind to stem-loop structures near the 5' end of the mRNA, preventing formation of the initiation complex.

Ferritin

Ferritin is an iron storage protein that is needed only when iron is present in large quantities. A ferritin mRNA repressor protein remains bound to the mRNA during iron deficiency (Fig. 17-17). When iron levels are restored, excess iron binds to the repressor protein, causing it to dissociate and allow synthesis of ferritin for storage of the excess iron.

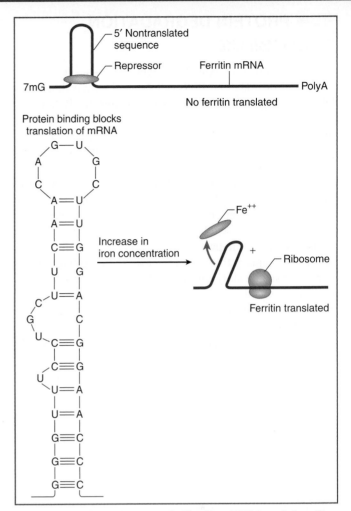

Figure 17-17. Negative control of ferritin mRNA translation. The repressor represses the mRNA until ferrous ions cause its removal, followed by initiation of ferritin synthesis.

Unfertilized Ovum

Before fertilization, the ovum is filled with ribosomes and with mRNA needed for proteins associated with early development, but since the mRNA is repressed, no polyribosomes are present. Upon fertilization, the mRNA forms polyribosomes for synthesis of the necessary proteins.

KEY POINTS ABOUT POLYPEPTIDE ELONGATION

- Polypeptide elongation is a cyclic three-step process involving binding of the new aminoacyl-tRNA to the ribosome, formation of a peptide bond when the growing polypeptide is moved over and attached to the new amino acid, and translocation of the new peptidyl-tRNA to a holding site so a new aminoacyl-tRNA can bind.

- The initiation of a new polypeptide requires special initiation factors that help recognize sites on the ribosome for precise alignment of the mRNA so that it can be read "in frame."

- Proteins are modified and transported to specific cellular locations after they are released from the ribosome. The genetic code in the mRNA specifies the signals for cellular localization, while the post-translational modifications are carried out by cellular enzymes.

●●● PROTEIN DEGRADATION

Protein Half-Life

All cellular processes exhibit turnover cycles—a cycle of synthesis and degradation. Both cellular and extracellular proteins are degraded to produce free amino acids that are available for use in synthesis of new proteins. Extracellular proteins are taken up by endocytosis and degraded in lysosomes, but cellular proteins have a different pathway: the ubiquitin-proteasome system.

Proteins destined for degradation are labeled with ubiquitin through covalent attachment to a lysine side chain. The amino acid composition at the amino terminus determines how quickly the protein will be ubiquinated and thus the half-life of the protein. Some proteins have very long half-lives, such as the crystallins in the lens of the eye; these proteins do not turn over significantly during the human life span. Because they were synthesized largely in utero, about half the crystallins in the adult lens are older than the person. Other proteins have half-lives of 4 months (proteins such as hemoglobin that last as long as the red blood cell), or the half-life can be very short, such as for ornithine decarboxylase, which has a half-life of 11 minutes. Polyubiquination, which increases the rate of turnover/degradation of a protein, occurs by successive addition of free ubiquitin to that which is already bound to the protein. The polyubiquinated protein then enters a large, barrel-shaped, multisubunit complex called a proteasome, a multicatalytic protease complex that cuts the protein into small peptide fragments, typically octapeptides to decapeptides, as it passes through. These peptide fragments are further digested to amino acids by proteases. Proteasome digestion is an energy-requiring process unlike lysosomal hydrolysis.

KEY POINT ABOUT PROTEIN DEGRADATION

- Proteins must also be degraded for the cell to maintain control over normal functions; proteasomes degrade proteins that are tagged with ubiquitin, and the amino acids are recovered for new polypeptide synthesis.

Self-assessment questions can be accessed at www. StudentConsult.com.

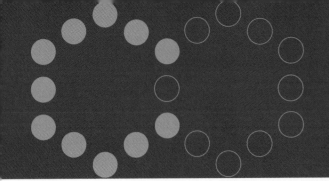

Recombinant DNA and Biotechnology 18

●●● THE NEW GENETICS

Before the use of restriction enzymes in the early 1970s to produce recombinant DNA, the concept of biotechnology did not exist. Science was limited to extraction and purification of biologic molecules, and our understanding of human genetics had to be deduced from classic mendelian genetics. When it became possible to manipulate and sequence DNA, an understanding of the entire human genome at the molecular level became possible. The elucidation of the entire sequence of the human genome was completed in 2003 as one of the goals of the Human Genome Project. This 13-year project identified approximately 20,000 to 25,000 genes and determined the complete sequence in human DNA. Work on the human genome continues as we now look forward to understanding, and curing, disease at the molecular level.

●●● RESTRICTION ENZYMES

The discovery of restriction endonucleases made it possible to "cut" DNA at specific locations whose base sequence is known. They are not digestive enzymes but instead serve as a primitive immune system in prokaryotes. These enzymes recognize unique sites in foreign DNA, such as plasmids and viruses, that can infect the bacterial cell. Instead of cleaving the DNA randomly, they are highly specific for the sites where they act. These sites are called restriction sites, and the enzymes are named for their function in "restricting" the invasion by foreign DNA. These restriction enzymes can recognize "self" from "non-self," like the human immune system, by recognizing DNA methylation. The bacterial cell methylates its own DNA shortly after it is synthesized, thus protecting it from attack by restriction endonucleases. Foreign DNA is not methylated, resulting in its cleavage and subsequent degradation.

Restriction enzymes act by wrapping around the DNA molecule. They "read" the bases by detecting the functional groups that extend from their rings into the major and minor grooves (like reading Braille). Each base has a unique topography of functional groups so the sequence can be read without opening up the helix. The restriction site is recognized by its characteristic palindrome structure (Fig. 18-1). Most restriction enzymes make staggered cuts on opposite strands, although some cut straight across the helix (blunt cuts). Staggered cuts produce complementary single-stranded ends called "sticky ends." Sticky ends are cohesive and can reanneal, not only with themselves but also with other DNA molecules, called vectors, that have also been cut by the same restriction enzyme (Fig. 18-2).

Restriction enzymes are named for their bacterial source. For example, PstI is obtained from *Providencia stuartii* and EcoR1 is obtained from *Escherichia coli*.

●●● RECOMBINANT DNA

When a fragment of DNA is recombined into a larger carrier DNA molecule, called a vector, it has become recombinant DNA. Recombinant DNA may be a gene or part of a gene, or it may be noncoding DNA that is to be studied. The target DNA of interest is often called the insert DNA, since it is inserted into a vector to be cloned, a process that involves replicating the vector in a host such as a bacterium, a yeast cell, or a mammalian cell. Cloning amplifies the quantity of the insert DNA so that it can be analyzed. Once the vector has been amplified, the insert DNA can be released by means of restriction enzymes.

Insert DNA can be obtained from two different sources: mRNA and genomic DNA.

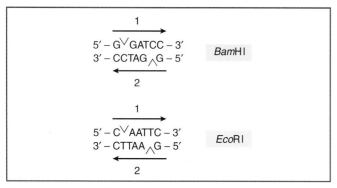

Figure 18-1. Palindromic restriction sites.

Complementary DNA

Complementary DNA (cDNA) is synthesized in the laboratory from messenger RNA (Fig. 18-3). cDNA is not genomic DNA, because the transcript of genomic RNA has been processed (i.e., it lacks promoters and introns). The enzyme reverse transcriptase (see Chapter 15) is used to synthesize double-stranded DNA that is a complementary copy of the mRNA. The addition of linker sequences to the end of this DNA, which contain the restriction site, followed by treatment with a restriction enzyme, produces a cDNA preparation with cohesive ends ready for insertion into a vector. A preparation of cDNA represents the genes that were actively being expressed in a cell, an organ, or a whole organism at the time of harvesting and is called a cDNA library.

Genomic DNA

As the name suggests, a genomic DNA preparation is obtained by digesting extracted DNA that represents the entire genome. Since restriction enzymes cleave only at specific nucleotide sequences, an approximate size range of the fragments produced can be estimated statistically. Larger fragments increase the likelihood of finding a complete target gene sequence (Fig. 18-4, fragment 2 from restriction enzyme B). All of the fragments produced will be bounded by identical cohesive ends, so the recombinant vector will contain inserts representing the entire genome. This is called a genomic library, and it will contain intact genes, noncoding DNA, and portions of genes that were cut by the restriction enzyme.

KEY POINTS ABOUT RESTRICTION ENZYMES AND RECOMBINANT DNA

- Restriction enzymes are endonucleases that act at unique sites that have palindromic sequences; they generally cut asymmetrically so that the ends of the DNA are staggered and always have the same sequence (even from different DNA samples), thus permitting reannealing.

- Fragments of DNA can be inserted into the genome of a vector by reannealing and ligation to produce a molecule that can grow in a host and thus amplify the recombinant DNA.

●●●● CLONING VECTORS

A cloning vector is a genome that can accept the target DNA and increase the number of copies through its own autonomous replication. It can be a plasmid, a bacteriophage, or yeast artificial chromosome. Cloning vectors usually are selected on the basis of differences in their capacity for the size of the insert DNA.

Plasmids are small, circular, extrachromosomal DNA molecules that normally invade bacteria and undergo autonomous replication in host cells. They characteristically do not

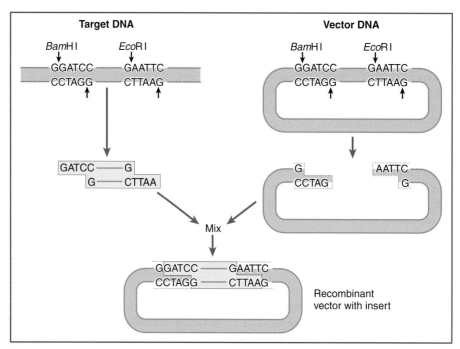

Figure 18-2. Treatment target DNA and vector DNA with restriction enzymes. Both target DNA and vector DNA have complementary "sticky" ends that can reanneal.

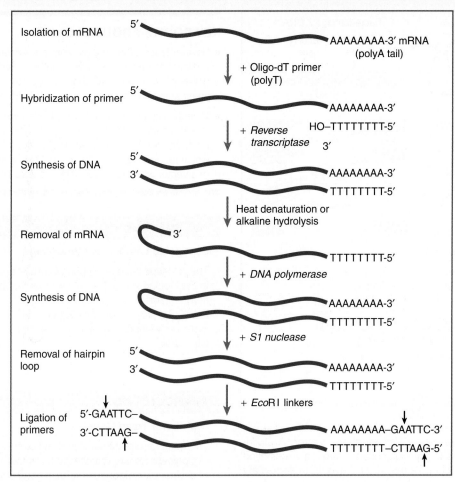

Figure 18-3. Preparation of cDNA from mRNA. The polyA tail on eukaryotic mRNA allows synthesis to start with a polyT primer. The addition of linker sequences to cDNA allows insertion into vectors.

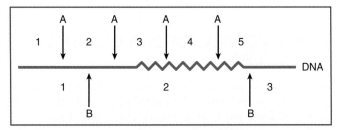

Figure 18-4. Preparation of genomic DNA. More frequent cutting by enzyme A produces smaller fragments. The target sequence is obtained with enzyme B owing to the larger fragments produced. Fragment 2 from enzyme B contains the target sequence.

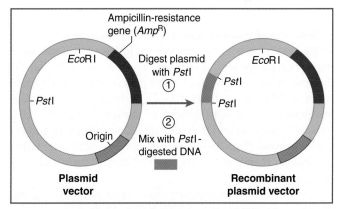

Figure 18-5. Structure of a plasmid and its chimeric recombinant form after insertion of the target DNA. The ampicillin resistance gene allows any host bacterium that contains the plasmid to grow on ampicillin-containing medium. The origin of replication allows the plasmid to replicate as the bacterial culture grows.

kill the host, and if a plasmid carries a gene for antibiotic resistance, it will confer that property to the host bacterium, allowing it to acquire resistance to that specific antibiotic (Fig. 18-5). Plasmids used as vectors maintain a modified origin of replication that allows their replication within the host, and they contain a gene for antibiotic resistance which ensures that, following treatment with a high dose of antibiotic, all viable bacterial colonies will contain several copies of the plasmid. They also contain an insertion site that is cleaved by known restriction enzymes and a reporter gene within the insertion site that identifies bacterial colonies that have

received a DNA insert. The reporter gene can confer antibiotic resistance or produce a visible color reaction, both of which are lost in bacterial colonies that have received a DNA insert. Plasmids have the smallest capacity for DNA inserts, with a maximum capacity of 5 kb (kilobases).

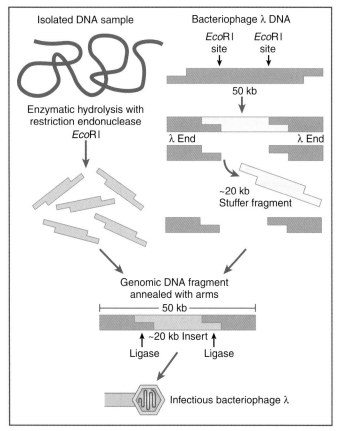

Figure 18-6. Structure of a γ bacteriophage vector. A stuffer fragment is removed by digestion with a restriction endonuclease, producing "arms" that have complementary sticky ends with the target DNA. Mixing of both preparations, treatment with ligase, and spontaneous reassembly with phage coat proteins produces infectious phage particles that can be grown on a bacterial host culture.

A bacteriophage is a bacterial virus that multiplies within the cell and kills the host by causing lysis, followed by dispersal of the progeny phage to reinfect new hosts. Lambda (λ) bacteriophage vectors have been genetically engineered to carry a DNA insert from 9 to 25 kb in size. They contain restriction sites at both ends of a "stuffer" fragment that is replaced by the insert DNA after digestion with the restriction endonuclease (Fig. 18-6). In addition to accepting larger fragments, these vectors are more efficient than plasmids in infecting the host.

Yeast artificial chromosomes have been genetically modified to carry inserts up to 1000 kb (Fig. 18-7).

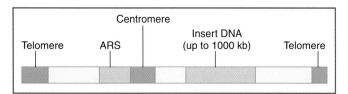

Figure 18-7. Components of a yeast artificial chromosome. Typical features required for replication of a chromosome are a centromere and telomeres and a replication origin, called the autonomous replicating sequence (*ARS*).

KEY POINTS ABOUT CLONING

■ Several types of cloning vectors are available: plasmids, which grow in bacteria and hold the smallest inserts; λ bacteriophages, which grow in bacteria and destroy them in the process; and yeast artificial chromosomes, which hold the largest inserts.

■ Both the vector and a DNA sample are digested with the same restriction enzyme and then recombined so they can be grown in a host; vectors contain selectable markers in order to determine which recombinant has the insert DNA of interest. A pure culture of a vector with the target DNA allows unlimited amplification.

MICROBIOLOGY

Lysogenic Lambda Bacteriophage

The wild-type lambda (λ) phage contains genes which are not in the cloning vector that allow it to integrate with the host chromosome and express its genes. The incorporated phage is called a prophage, and it remains in this state until an inducing agent causes it to exit the chromosome and enter a lytic cycle.

MICROBIOLOGY

Diphtheria Toxin Gene

The gene for diphtheria toxin is not contained in the genome of *Corynebacterium diphtheriae* but rather in the genome of several bacteriophages (e.g., β-corynephage) that infect it. The diphtheria toxin gene within the prophage of β-corynephage is regulated to be expressed in the late stages of the bacterial life cycle.

●●● OVERVIEW OF DNA CLONING STEPS

The purpose of cloning is to amplify the DNA of interest so that it can be analyzed. The following general steps apply to both plasmid and lambda phage vectors (Fig. 18-8).

1. Both vector DNA and insert DNA are treated with the same restriction enzyme. This produces matching ends on both insert DNA and vector DNA, allowing them to reanneal with each other.
2. The restriction digests of the vector and insert DNA are mixed and allowed to reanneal.
3. After the DNA ends are sealed with DNA ligase, the vector is propagated in a host (bacterium) that has been modified for this purpose.
4. After propagation is complete, the bacterial culture or the λ phage lysate constitutes a recombinant DNA library.

Screening Libraries with Probes

A probe is a short piece of labeled DNA with a sequence complementary to the target DNA of interest. The label can be radioactive, but fluorescent probes are more commonly used

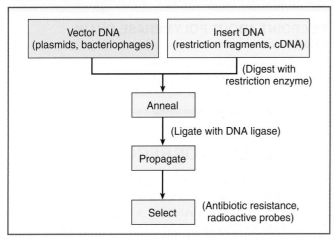

Figure 18-8. Overview of cloning procedure. Insertion of target DNA is followed by propagation of the vector and selection of the recombinant clone from a library.

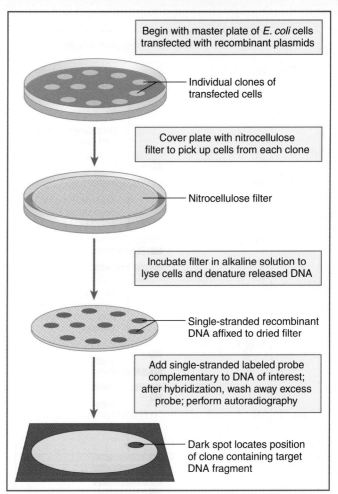

Figure 18-9. Identification of a clone carrying the target DNA. Colonies containing recombinant DNA are blotted with a nitrocellulose filter paper, allowing them to adhere. DNA that also adheres after lysis of the cells is then denatured and hybridized (reannealed) with probes of known sequence to identify the colony (or colonies) containing the target DNA.

now because of the cost of disposing of radioactive waste. A probe is used to visualize target DNA after separation by blotting. The simplest blot is used to identify a bacterial colony grown from a library on a Petri dish (Fig. 18-9). A nitrocellulose filter paper is overlaid on the surface so that each colony binds to the filter paper in a mirror image pattern. When the filter paper is treated to lyse the cells and denature the DNA, a probe can be used to identify one or more colonies that have DNA complementary to the probe. The original colony can then be sampled and cultured to amplify the target DNA. Similarly, a lambda phage library can be applied to a bacterial lawn, which then develops plaques, each containing the recombinant DNA from only one phage particle. The blotting procedure then identifies the plaques that are cultured to amplify the target DNA.

●●● POLYMERASE CHAIN REACTION

The polymerase chain reaction (PCR) (Fig. 18-10) is an alternative method for in vitro amplification of DNA. It does not depend on propagation of either bacteria (for plasmid vectors) or viruses (for bacteriophage vectors). Instead, it relies on oligonucleotide primers to initiate DNA synthesis of sequences from 50 to 10,000 bases in length that are bounded by the primers (see Fig. 18-10). As its name suggests, the amplification is accomplished by repeated cycles of synthesis by the enzyme DNA polymerase. This method can amplify a target sequence 10^9-fold after just 30 cycles within a few hours. The sensitivity of primers for their complementary sequence allows detection of a target sequence from the DNA of a single cell. PCR is used for DNA fingerprinting, prenatal diagnosis, tissue typing, and early detection of infectious agents.

The PCR method involves repeating 4- to 5-minute cycles of denaturation and synthesis:

1. DNA is heat-denatured in the presence of a large excess of short primers (20 to 35 bases) that represent sequences on both ends of the target DNA.
2. The mixture is allowed to cool, and the primers reanneal with the denatured strands at the 3′ end of the target DNA (remember that antiparallel base pairing places the 5′ end of the primer toward the 3′ end of the target DNA).
3. The primers are then extended by DNA polymerase in the 5′ to 3′ direction. This doubles the amount of target sequences.
4. A new cycle begins when the mixture is heated again to denature (melt) the DNA. The DNA polymerase is heat stable and does not have to be replaced during successive cycles. Each cycle doubles the amount of the target sequence.

The PCR method has some limitations but also some major advantages. One important limitation is that some knowledge of the target sequence must be known to construct the primers. Its extreme sensitivity makes it vulnerable to false-positive results by contamination with another DNA molecule that contains the target sequence. A major advantage is the speed with which DNA can be amplified. This simple procedure uses a single stable enzyme and synthetic primers with minimal manipulation to produce a final product in just a few hours, as compared with the cloning method, which requires vector preparation and propagation.

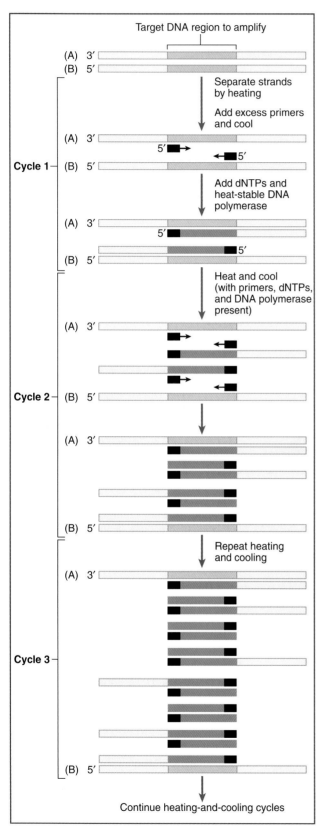

Figure 18-10. The polymerase chain reaction. Repeating cycles of heating and cooling create single-stranded templates to which primers can reanneal and initiate DNA synthesis. Each round of heating and cooling results in doubling of the target sequence, producing 10^9 molecules after 30 cycles. *dNTP*, deoxyribonucleoside triphosphate.

KEY POINT ABOUT POLYMERASE CHAIN REACTION

■ The PCR can amplify any DNA sequence that lies between two primers by means of a heat-resistant DNA polymerase, nucleotide precursors, and an excess of primers.

●●● ANALYSIS OF RECOMBINANT DNA

Once a target DNA has been amplified by either cloning or PCR, a number of questions need to be answered.

1. Are there landmarks that create a map of the target DNA?
2. Are there landmarks that help identify mutations?
3. Are there landmarks that help determine, or eliminate, genetic identity?
4. What is its base sequence?

Restriction Maps

Once target DNA has been obtained by cloning or PCR, the first task is to develop a physical map called a restriction map (Fig. 18-11). If the target DNA is digested with several different restriction enzymes, and then subjected to gel electrophoresis, different patterns of bands are obtained. Because DNA separates in gel electrophoresis based on its size, each band represents a given molecular weight and, therefore,

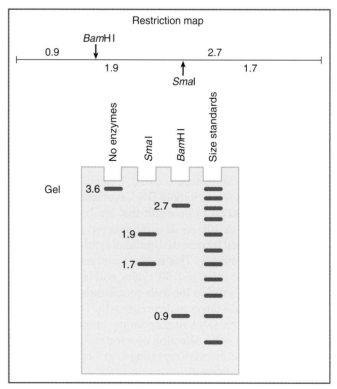

Figure 18-11. Determination of a restriction map by gel electrophoresis. Treatment of the DNA sample with two different enzymes, followed by separation of the digest on electrophoresis, allows deduction of the relative locations and distance of the restriction sites from each other.

a given length. By deducing the correct sequence of overlapping restriction fragments so that all restriction enzyme digests give consistent distances, a restriction map is established. Knowledge of the restriction map for a target DNA allows removal and analysis of specific segments. Thus restriction sites within the target DNA serve as landmarks.

A restriction enzyme digest is analyzed by a process called Southern blotting. There are several different blotting procedures that are similar in methodology and differ primarily in the type of molecule being detected (Fig. 18-12).

- Southern blotting detects DNA by using labeled DNA probes.
- Northern blotting detects RNA by using labeled DNA probes.
- Western blotting detects proteins by using labeled antibodies.

Restriction Fragment Length Polymorphisms

If a mutation alters a restriction site within a gene, the restriction enzyme will cease to recognize that site and it will not be cut during a restriction digest. This produces a larger fragment of DNA containing the mutated site. When a restriction digest of the mutated DNA is analyzed by gel electrophoresis, it will produce a different electrophoretic pattern than that of normal DNA. Since any normal variation (as opposed to a deleterious mutation) in a gene in the same population is referred to as a polymorphism, the appearance of a variant electrophoretic pattern for restriction fragments of a gene is called a restriction fragment length polymorphism. Most

polymorphisms occur in introns and do not affect the protein composition of the cell.

There are two types of polymorphisms: single nucleotide and tandem repeats. The single nucleotide polymorphisms (SNPs; known as "snips") are useful in identifying deleterious mutations, and tandem repeats are useful in DNA fingerprinting.

- SNPs occur in more than 1% of the human genome, but because only about 3% to 5% of the genome codes for proteins, most SNPs are found outside genes. If an SNP occurs within an exon, it can represent a deleterious point mutation and can be detected on a Southern blot. The mutation that is responsible for sickle cell anemia lies within the restriction site for the *Mst*II restriction enzyme. When patients from an affected family are subjected to restriction fragment length polymorphism analysis, a pedigree can be constructed to show the inheritance of the mutation (Fig. 18-13).

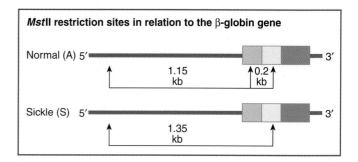

A

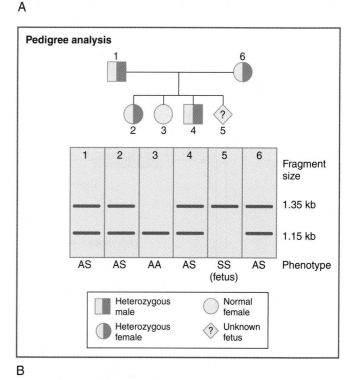

B

Figure 18-12. Comparison of blotting procedures for nucleic acids and proteins. A gel containing the sample after electrophoresis is placed on a nitrocellulose filter (blotting), allowing the sample to transfer and bind to the filter. The filter is then treated with nucleic acid probes or antibodies containing either radioactive or fluorescent tags.

Figure 18-13. Restriction fragment length polymorphism analysis of sickle cell hemoglobin. **A,** A restriction map of a portion of the β-globin gene and an adjacent upstream sequence reveals that the sickle mutation causes removal of one of the three sites for the *Mst*II endonuclease. This allows interpretation of a Southern blot **(B)** comparing restriction digests from each family member.

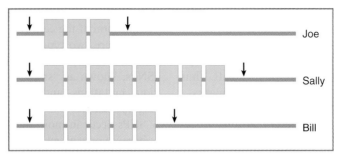

Figure 18-14. Polymorphism among three subjects for a specific DNA sequence. Joe, Sally, and Bill can be distinguished from one another by the number of repeats found in their DNA. Each box represents the six-base sequence GATTCC, and the arrows represent restriction sites that are located on either side of the repeat sequences. These tandem repeat sequences were generated by unequal recombination and inherited by subsequent generations. Since each fragment has a different number of repeats, they will migrate differently on electrophoresis (see Fig. 18-15).

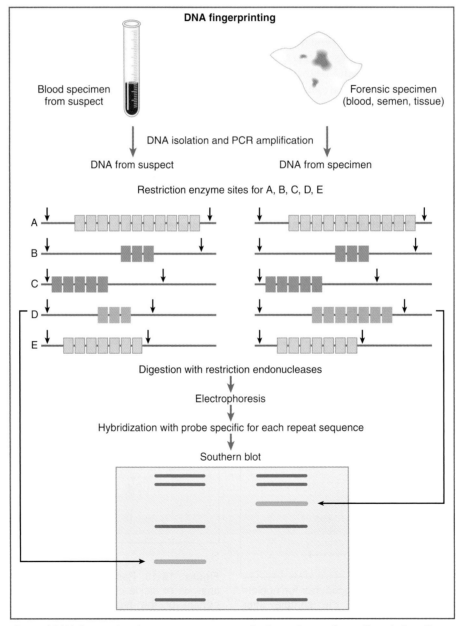

Figure 18-15. Comparison of DNA fingerprints between a suspect and a forensic specimen. Restriction digests *(arrows)* of DNA from both samples are amplified to produce samples from selected polymorphic regions *(boxes* indicate repeated sequences). Electrophoresis of samples reveals a match or confirms innocence.

- Tandem repeat polymorphisms are due to the appearance of dinucleotide or trinucleotide (or longer) sequences that are connected in tandem but with the number of repeats being variable from person to person (Fig. 18-14). Repetitive DNA in humans is highly polymorphic with respect to the number of copies of repetitive sequences. The variable number of tandem repeats produces restriction fragments of different lengths that can be detected on a Southern blot, referred to as a DNA fingerprint (Fig. 18-15). This method is 100% effective in eliminating genetic identity if a match between a reference DNA sample and an individual does not occur. However, proof of identity relies on an estimate of statistical probability of the frequency of a given polymorphism in the population (e.g., the number of false positives).

DNA Sequencing

The sequence of any DNA fragment can be determined with the Sanger dideoxy method. This procedure, which has been automated for large scale use in the Human Genome Project, relies on the use of dideoxynucleotides to interrupt DNA synthesis using the unknown DNA as the template. When the dideoxynucleotides are placed in separate incubation tubes along with DNA polymerase, a primer, and all four deoxynucleotide precursors, fragments of unequal length are obtained representing a random interruption of DNA synthesis at each point that a dideoxynucleotide is inserted in place of the normal precursor. The absence of a 3′-hydroxyl group at the 3′ terminal nucleotide prevents further extension of the new strand. Since incorporation of a dideoxy precursor in place of a normal precursor is random, a mixture of products of different lengths is obtained. Separation of each incubation mixture on gel electrophoresis sorts out DNA fragments based on their size and produces a set of bands that reveal the sequence by their physical position.

KEY POINTS ABOUT ANALYSIS OF RECOMBINANT DNA

- Recombinant DNA can be analyzed by determining its sequence and then digesting it with multiple restriction enzymes; the analysis of restriction digests with Southern blotting allows a calculation of the distances between each restriction site.
- Individuals usually differ with respect to the size of certain restriction fragments in their genome—a polymorphism of restriction fragments; the polymorphism can be caused by mutations in restriction sites or by a variation in the number of certain characteristic tandem connected repeat sequences.

Self-assessment questions can be accessed at www. StudentConsult.com.

Nutrition

●●● NUTRIENT AND ENERGY REQUIREMENTS

The dietary requirements for protein, vitamins, minerals, and trace elements are specified in terms of the recommended daily allowance (RDA). RDA represents an optimal dietary intake of nutrients that will maintain a healthy population. RDA varies with age, sex, body weight, and physiologic status; it increases during pregnancy and lactation and during childhood.

Basal Metabolic Rate

The basal metabolic rate (BMR) is the rate of energy expenditure of a person at rest; it eliminates the variable effect of physical activity. The BMR accounts for approximately 60% of the daily energy expenditure. Thus it includes energy used for normal body cellular homeostasis, cardiac function, brain and other nerve function, and so on. It is related to body weight by the calculation:

$$\text{BMR (Cal/d)} = 24 \times \text{Body weight (kg)}$$

A passive increase in energy expenditure occurs during digestion of food. This is referred to as the thermic effect or, in the older literature, specific dynamic action of food; it accounts for about 10% of the daily energy expenditure.

The total daily energy expenditure is calculated from knowledge of the BMR and a physical activity factor. The physical activity factor is a function of the type of activity for an individual (e.g., 1.3 for sedentary, 1.5 for moderately active, and 1.7 for extremely active). When multiplied by the BMR, an estimate of the daily energy expenditure is obtained.

Example: A 220 lb (220/2.2 = 100 kg) person with moderate energy expenditure (e.g., a cabinet maker):

$$\text{BMR} = 24 \times 100 = 2400 \text{ kcal/day}$$
$$\text{Energy expenditure} = 2400 \times 1.5 = 3600 \text{ kcal/day}$$

Body Mass Index

The body mass index (BMI) is used as an index of a healthy body weight. It assumes a normal distribution between muscular and adipose tissue and thus would not be appropriate for muscular individuals such as athletes. The BMI is calculated by

$$\text{BMI (kg/m}^2) = \text{Weight (kg)/height (m}^2)$$

A BMI between 20 and 25 is considered a healthy body weight, 25 to 30 is considered overweight, and 30 to 40 is obesity. Higher BMI values are morbidly obese weights.

KEY POINT ABOUT NUTRIENT AND ENERGY REQUIREMENTS

■ The BMR represents the energy expenditure of a person at rest and includes energy needed to digest food, called the thermic effect of food; the BMI represents a ratio between height and weight that can indicate different stages of obesity when it exceeds a healthy index value.

●●● CARBOHYDRATE DIGESTION AND ABSORPTION

For dietary carbohydrates to be used by the body, they must be converted during digestion to monosaccharides. In addition to starch, the other major dietary carbohydrates are the disaccharides lactose and sucrose, and the monosaccharide fructose. The monosaccharides produced by complete digestion

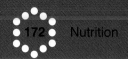
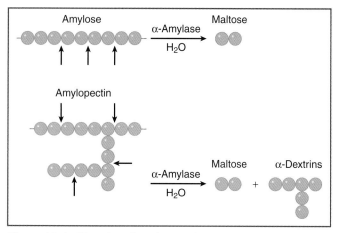

Figure 19-1. Digestion of amylose and amylopectin by α-amylase.

of these dietary carbohydrates are glucose, galactose, and fructose.

The digestive process begins with salivary amylase, which randomly cleaves the α-1,4 linkages of starch. Although amylase digestion begins in the saliva, pancreatic α-amylase is more important to the complete digestion of starch (Fig. 19-1). Starch is degraded first to dextrins and then to a mixture of glucose, maltose, and isomaltose (containing the α-1,6 linkages that are not digested by amylase).

The major disaccharidases, located in the brush border of the intestinal lumen, are

- Maltase—hydrolyzes maltose
- Sucrase-isomaltase—hydrolyzes sucrose and isomaltose
- Lactase—hydrolyzes lactose

Whenever lactose goes undigested, it is not absorbed and passes into the large intestine. Here lactose is acted on by the intestinal flora that ferment it, producing large quantities of CO_2, hydrogen gas, methane, and organic acids; the latter irritate the intestines, increasing intestinal motility. All these products have only one way out. Thus the symptoms that characterize lactose intolerance are bloating and flatulence and, in extreme cases, a frothy diarrhea. Lactose intolerance is least common in Northern Europeans and their descendants, and most common in descendants of Asian, African, and South American origin.

Cellulose and other polysaccharides of plant origin with β-1,4 linkages are not digested by humans owing to the lack of β-1,4 glucosidase. They constitute the fiber in the human diet. During early stages following a meal, the concentration of monosaccharides in intestinal fluids may exceed that in the body; thus sugar transport may be passive and facilitated. At later stages and for most of the digestive process, transport of monosaccharides from the gut into the bloodstream occurs against a concentration gradient; carbohydrate absorption is primarily an active process. Glucose and galactose are transported by an Na^+/K^+-adenosine triphosphatase from the lumen into epithelial cells. As the concentration of glucose builds up in the epithelial cell, it moves downhill into blood by passive, facilitated transport. Fructose, which is not normally present at significant concentrations in blood, is transported by facilitated diffusion.

HISTOLOGY

Brush Border Dynamics

The unstirred brush border of the intestinal lumen consists of fingerlike processes, known as microvilli, of the surface absorptive cells. Many enzymes associated with the process of digestion and absorption are located on the surface of these microvilli. This allows the products of digestion, such as free fatty acids, amino acids, and monoglycerides, to be absorbed by the cells rather than to be swept into the lumen itself.

●●● LIPID DIGESTION AND ABSORPTION

The major dietary lipids are triglycerides, cholesterol, and phospholipids. Plant sources supply fats that are primarily unsaturated, whereas animal sources are primarily saturated.

- Saturated fats are predominant in coconut oil and palm oil, and in animal dairy products and lard.
- Polyunsaturated fats are predominant in soybean oil and corn oil.
- Monounsaturated fats are enriched in canola oil and olive oil.

Emulsification of lipids by bile salts increases the surface area of lipid particles for interaction with intestinal lipases and increases their rate of digestion. There are several different types of lipases:

- Pancreatic α-lipase hydrolyzes ester linkages at the 1- and 3-positions in triacylglycerols. The free fatty acids and 2-monoglycerides then enter the mucosal epithelial cell by passive diffusion. A concentration gradient is maintained by rapid resynthesis of triacylglycerols in the mucosal cell (Fig. 19-2).
- Phospholipase A_2 hydrolyzes the carbon-2 (β) fatty acid from lecithin, forming lysolecithin.
- Cholesterol esters are hydrolyzed to cholesterol plus fatty acids by cholesterol esterase.

KEY POINTS ABOUT CARBOHYDRATE AND LIPID DIGESTION AND ABSORPTION

- Digestion of carbohydrate requires amylases to break down starch to disaccharides, which are further digested to monosaccharides; carbohydrate absorption is largely an active process.

- To be absorbed, fats must first be emulsified and then enzymatically digested to fatty acids and monoglycerides; triglycerides are reassembled after absorption.

MICROBIOLOGY

Apparent Lactose Intolerance

Although lactase is gradually lost in adolescence, lactose digestion can remain normal in people who continue to consume sufficient amounts of dairy products. The constant supply of lactose provides a growth medium that maintains a favorable lactose-using bacterial culture in the gut.

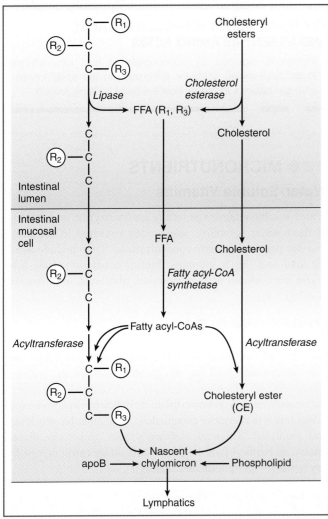

Figure 19-2. Digestion and absorption of dietary lipids and assembly of nascent (new) chylomicrons. Cholesterol and 2-monoglycerides are reesterified and packaged into chylomicrons. *FFA*, free fatty acid; *CoA*, coenzyme A; *apoB*, apolipoprotein B.

ANATOMY

Secretion of Lipases and Bile

The secretion of lipases from the pancreas and of bile from the liver is coordinated anatomically. The common bile duct joins the main pancreatic duct to form the hepatopancreatic ampulla, which empties into the second part of the duodenum. This allows digestion of fats to begin immediately in the more favorable alkaline environment of the small intestine.

HISTOLOGY

Pepsin Secretion

Pepsin is produced in the zymogenic cells (also known as chief cells) that line the gastric glands. Pepsin precursors are stored in the apical secretory granules as the inactive pepsinogen until its secretion is stimulated by gastrin, a hormone released into the connective tissue of the stomach.

●●● PROTEIN DIGESTION AND ABSORPTION

For dietary protein to be used by the body, it must be hydrolyzed to amino acids for absorption. This process begins in the stomach and is aided by the low pH. Although stomach acid is not sufficiently concentrated to hydrolyze proteins, it causes their denaturation, allowing easier access by the proteolytic enzyme pepsin. Pepsin has a broad specificity but preferentially attacks peptide bonds of aromatic amino acids, as well as leucine and methionine, to yield small peptides but relatively few free amino acids. In the small intestine, stomach acid is neutralized by pancreatic juice, which is rich in bicarbonate, and the peptic digest is further hydrolyzed by the pancreatic alkaline proteases—trypsin and chymotrypsin—and peptidases to release free amino acids. Trypsin cleaves on the carboxyl side of arginine and lysine, and chymotrypsin cleaves on the carboxyl side of aromatic amino acids. The peptidase carboxypeptidase A is an exopeptidase that removes amino acids, one at a time, from the carboxyl end of a peptide.

The absorption of amino acids from the intestinal lumen and their release into the portal circulation is energy dependent.

●●● NITROGEN BALANCE AND ESSENTIAL AMINO ACIDS

Protein nutrition is based on the balance of the nine essential amino acids (see Table 12-1). Since these cannot be synthesized by the body, they must be supplied in amounts needed to sustain the continuous turnover and resynthesis of proteins in the body. The biologic value of a protein source is determined by its limiting amino acid (i.e., the essential amino acid present in the lowest amount). The highest biologic value is in protein supplied by eggs, beef, fish, and dairy products. In contrast, protein supplied by most common plant sources (e.g., wheat, corn, rice, and beans) is of low biologic value. For example, corn is deficient in lysine, and beans are deficient in methionine. Cultural diets compensate for these deficiencies by combining plant proteins that provide amino acid complementation. An example is the Latin American diet of corn and beans: the corn is deficient in lysine, which is supplied by the beans, and the beans are deficient in methionine, which is supplied by the corn. An inexpensive vegetarian diet is thereby increased in biologic value.

Nitrogen balance defines how well the body is using dietary protein. When the amount of protein (nitrogen) consumed is equal to the amount excreted, the body is considered to be in nitrogen balance.

Positive Nitrogen Balance

More nitrogen is consumed than excreted during positive nitrogen balance. This indicates active synthesis of new protein as a result of growth, as seen in pregnancy, in growing children, and in recovery from severe wounds or extreme starvation.

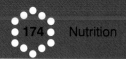

Negative Nitrogen Balance

More nitrogen is excreted than consumed during negative nitrogen balance. During periods of starvation, protein is mobilized to maintain normal blood sugar concentrations. Negative nitrogen balance also develops on artificially restricted, low-protein diets, with protein of low biologic value, and during breakdown of damaged tissue during normal wound healing following physical trauma, surgery, or burns.

Since the carbon skeletons from amino acids can be metabolized for energy, dietary carbohydrate has a protein-sparing effect.

Marasmus

This starvation syndrome is general protein-calorie malnutrition. The total lack of fuel from foods is characterized by tissue wasting as a result of breakdown of muscle protein for energy.

Kwashiorkor

This starvation syndrome involves only protein malnutrition in the presence of adequate carbohydrate and is characterized by edema, skin lesions, and liver malfunction. There is no muscle breakdown, but reduced albumin production by the liver leads to edema and slow wound healing. This disease is more common in regions where carbohydrate is plentiful but protein is limited, and it illustrates the muscle protein-sparing effect of carbohydrate.

KEY POINT ABOUT NITROGEN BALANCE AND ESSENTIAL AMINO ACIDS

- Protein is digested by endopeptidases and exopeptidases to produce amino acids for absorption in the small intestine; nitrogen balance indicates how the body is using protein.

●●● MICRONUTRIENTS

Water-Soluble Vitamins

Water-soluble vitamins generally are coenzymes and, because of their water solubility, are readily excreted in the urine, thereby preventing toxic concentrations. They include ascorbic acid and the B vitamins, biotin, cobalamin, folic acid, niacin, pantothenic acid, pyridoxine, riboflavin, and thiamine (Table 19-1).

Thiamine (Vitamin B₁)

The active form of thiamine is thiamine pyrophosphate. It functions in oxidative decarboxylation (e.g., α-ketoacid dehydrogenase complexes) and in the pentose phosphate pathway (transketolase). Thiamine deficiency occurs early during general malnourishment. A common thiamine deficiency syndrome seen in alcoholics is Wernicke encephalopathy (dementia, weakness, and paralysis). Thiamine deficiency also causes the disease known as beriberi (wet beriberi—congestive cardiomyopathy, dry beriberi—peripheral neuropathy).

TABLE 19-1. Water-Soluble Vitamins

VITAMINS	FUNCTION	DIETARY SOURCE	DEFICIENCY SYMPTOMS
Thiamine (B₁)	Cofactor for oxidative decarboxylation, transketolase	Whole grains and legumes	Beriberi (polyneuritis, tachycardia, edema)
Riboflavin (B₂)	Redox cofactor in FAD	Dairy products, green leafy vegetables	Glossitis (loss of tongue papillae), dermatitis
Niacin (B₃)	Redox cofactor in NAD⁺ and NADP⁺	Whole grains, liver	Pellagra (diarrhea, dermatitis, and dementia), glossitis
Pyridoxine (B₆)	Cofactor for transamination, transsulfuration	Wheat, corn, liver, beef	Deficiency rare; overdose produces neurologic symptoms
Biotin (H)	Cofactor for carboxylases	Liver, milk, egg yolk	Dermatitis, nausea, anorexia
Folic acid (B₉)	Cofactor for 1-carbon	Green leafy vegetables, liver, whole grains	Megaloblastic anemia transfers (most common in pregnant women) without nerve degeneration; sprue, glossitis
Cobalamin (B₁₂)	Cofactor for methionine methylmalonyl-CoA mutase	Liver, milk, eggs, meat	Megaloblastic anemia synthesis from homocysteine, *and* nerve degeneration
Ascorbic acid (C)	Cofactor for hydroxylation reactions (e.g., lysine and proline in collagen)	Citrus fruits, potato skins, tomatoes, green vegetables	Scurvy (blood vessel fragility, impaired wound healing)
Pantothenic acid (B₅)	Transfer of acyl groups (component of CoA)	Eggs, liver, yeast	Not described in humans

CoA, coenzyme A; *FAD*, flavin adenine dinucleotide; *NAD*, nicotinamide adenine dinucleotide; *NADP*, nicotinamide adenine dinucleotide phosphate.
Data from Pelley JW: *Ace the boards: Biochemistry*, St Louis, 1997, Mosby, p 306.

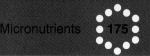

Riboflavin (Vitamin B₂)

The active form of riboflavin is either flavin adenine dinucleotide or flavin mononucleotide. It functions in reduction-oxidation reactions (e.g., citric acid cycle, electron transport chain, peroxisomal enzymes). Riboflavin deficiency is caused by its sensitivity to visible light or by a diet low in dairy products, such as a pure vegetarian diet. Riboflavin deficiency is characterized by glossitis and dermatitis.

Niacin (Vitamin B₃)

The active form of niacin is either nicotinamide adenine dinucleotide or nicotinamide adenine dinucleotide phosphate. It functions, like riboflavin, in reduction-oxidation reactions (e.g., dehydrogenases, reductive biosynthesis). Niacin deficiency is caused by diets deficient in both niacin and tryptophan or in conditions such as Hartnup disease, an amino acid transport deficiency disease in which tryptophan is lost in the urine and feces. Although niacin can be produced from tryptophan, it supplies only 10% of the RDA. Niacin deficiency produces pellagra and glossitis. Niacin is used pharmacologically to reduce serum cholesterol concentration, but at elevated concentrations it can produce flushing from vasodilation.

Pantothenic Acid (Vitamin B₅)

The active form of pantothenic acid is either as coenzyme A or as a prosthetic group for the acyl carrier protein in fatty acid synthase. It functions in the citric acid cycle (citrate synthase) and in fat synthesis. Pantothenic acid deficiency is rare.

Pyridoxine (Vitamin B₆)

The active form of pyridoxine is pyridoxal phosphate. Its functions are among the most diverse of any vitamin:

- Transamination reactions
- Alanine synthetase (heme synthesis)
- Decarboxylation of histidine to histamine
- Deamination of serine to pyruvate
- Glycogen phosphorylase action
- Conversion of tryptophan to niacin
- Synthesis of several neurotransmitters

Approximately one half of the total pyridoxine is bound to muscle glycogen phosphorylase. Pyridoxine deficiency is caused by isoniazid therapy for tuberculosis and by alcoholism. Deficiencies in pyridoxine are rare, producing a peripheral neuropathy, but overdosage can also present with neurologic symptoms.

Biotin (Vitamin H)

Biotin is the coenzyme for carboxylation reactions (e.g., pyruvate and acetyl–coenzyme A carboxylase. The active form of biotin is bound as a prosthetic group through an amide linkage with the lysine side chain of its apoenzyme. Biotin deficiency is rare, since it is supplied by the gut flora, but its absorption can be blocked by eating raw egg whites, which contain avidin, a biotin-binding protein. Symptoms of biotin deficiency are dermatitis, alopecia, and lactic acidosis.

Folic Acid (Vitamin B₉)

The active form of folic acid is tetrahydrofolate modified by a string of glutamate (polyglutamate) residues that form a "tail." Tetrahydrofolate functions in single-carbon transfers (e.g., thymidylate synthesis). The polyglutamate form of folate remains trapped in the cell, prolonging its half-life. Folate is easily destroyed by cooking (and canning). Folate is present as the polyglutamylated form in foods and must be converted to the monoglutamate in the jejunum, where it is absorbed. Folate deficiency may develop on diets low in fruits and vegetables and in pregnancy (increased requirement), cancer (increased use), celiac disease (reduced absorption), and alcoholism. Symptoms of folate deficiency are megaloblastic anemia and spina bifida in affected newborn children.

Cobalamin (Vitamin B₁₂)

The active form of cobalamin is deoxyadenosylcobalamin. It functions in single-carbon transfers (e.g., conversion of homocysteine to methionine). Cobalamin has the lowest RDA of any vitamin because it is highly conserved in the enterohepatic circulation (secretion in the bile and reabsorption from the gut into the hepatic portal vein). It forms a complex with intrinsic factor, a gastric mucosal glycoprotein that is required for absorption from the gut. Cobalamin is transported on transcobalamin in plasma and delivered to cells or stored in the liver, which usually contains a 6- to 9-year supply. Cobalamin deficiency is caused by autoimmune destruction of the parietal cells in the stomach, producing pernicious anemia. Other causes of deficiency are a pure vegetarian diet, chronic pancreatitis, tapeworm, and terminal ileal disease. Symptoms are megaloblastic anemia and neurologic degeneration.

Ascorbic Acid (Vitamin C)

The active form of vitamin C is ascorbate (reduced form); it is converted to dehydroascorbate (oxidized form) during enzymatic reaction or antioxidant activity, and then recycled back to ascorbate by dehydroascorbate reductase. Ascorbate functions as a cofactor in hydroxylation reactions and also serves an antioxidant role in the body, maintaining vitamin E in the reduced, active state. Absorption of iron is also facilitated by ascorbate. Deficiency is produced by diets lacking in fruits and vegetables. Symptoms of ascorbate deficiency include scurvy (bleeding gums, impaired wound healing), as a result of deficient hydroxylation of lysine and decreased cross-linking of collagen. Large amounts (>4 g/day) of ascorbate are slowly oxidized to oxalate, which combines with Ca^{++} to form oxalate stones.

Fat-Soluble Vitamins

The fat-soluble vitamins are vitamins A, D, E, and K. They function as hormones, cofactors, and antioxidants (Table 19-2). They are absorbed with fats and transported in chylomicrons. As a result of their ability to dissolve in body fat stores, several fat-soluble vitamins can accumulate to toxic levels in tissues.

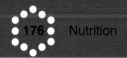

TABLE 19-2. Fat-Soluble Vitamins

VITAMIN	FUNCTION	DIETARY SOURCE	DEFICIENCY SYMPTOMS
Vitamin A (retinol)	Components of visual pigments	Liver, egg yolk, yellow and green vegetables	Night blindness, dry eye (xerophthalmia), dry skin
Vitamin D (calcitriol)	Regulation of calcium and phosphorus metabolism	Fortified milk, 7-dehydrocholesterol in skin (sunlight activated)	Rickets (soft pliable bones) in children; osteomalacia (demineralization of bones) in adults
Vitamin E (tocopherol)	Antioxidant in membranes	Vegetable oils, liver, eggs	Erythrocyte hemolysis, especially in newborns
Vitamin K	Synthesis of prothrombin and clotting factors (γ-carboxylation of glutamate)	Gut flora, cauliflower, egg yolk, liver	Prolonged coagulation time; deficiency rare (oral antibiotics produce temporary deficiency)

Data from Pelley JW: *Ace the boards: Biochemistry,* St Louis, 1997, Mosby, p 306.

Retinol (Vitamin A)

The active forms of vitamin A are retinol, retinal, and retinoic acid. β-Carotene in the diet is hydrolyzed to produce two molecules of retinal. Retinal is absorbed, esterified, and transported in chylomicrons to the liver and stored. Retinal is transported from the liver to the tissues on retinol-binding protein. Retinol and retinal are interconverted during the visual cycle (Fig. 19-3). Retinol and retinal play a role in male and female reproductive tissues and are essential for fertility. Retinol also functions in normal development of bones and teeth. Retinoic acid is produced from retinal and acts like a steroid to activate genes needed for cell differentiation. Vitamin A deficiency results from fat malabsorption and develops in diets deficient in green leafy and yellow vegetables. Symptoms of vitamin A deficiency are night blindness, dermatologic abnormalities, and poor wound healing. Vitamin A overdosage produces pain in the long bones, liver toxicity, and increased intracranial pressure.

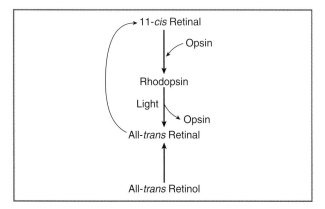

Figure 19-3. The visual cycle in the retina. The form that combines with opsin to form rhodopsin is 11-*cis* retinal. On exposure to light, the 11-*cis* form is converted to the all-*trans* form, which must be subsequently converted back to the 11-*cis* form.

HISTOLOGY

Source of Intrinsic Factor

The parietal (also known as oxyntic) cells that line the gastric glands in the body and fundus of the stomach make gastric intrinsic factor; parietal cells also secrete HCl.

Calcitriol (Vitamin D)

The active form of vitamin D is a steroid hormone, calcitriol (1,25-dihydroxycholecalciferol). Calcitriol maintains adequate levels of calcium in serum. It regulates bone resorption, calcium uptake from the gut, and reabsorption of calcium from the glomerular filtrate of the kidney. Vitamin D, cholecalciferol, is converted to calcitriol by two hydroxylation reactions (Fig. 19-4). It is first obtained as preformed cholecalciferol in the form of dietary ergocalciferol or 7-dehydrocholesterol in skin exposed to sunlight. After undergoing one hydroxylation in the liver, it is hydroxylated again in the kidney to produce 1,25-dihydroxycholecalciferol (calcitriol). When the parathyroid hormone is present, calcitriol stimulates mobilization of calcium and phosphate from bone; calcitonin prevents bone resorption when serum calcium is elevated. The parathyroid hormone stimulates the production of calcitriol when serum calcium levels are low. Vitamin D deficiency is caused by renal failure (most common), fat malabsorption, chronic liver disease (failure to hydroxylate), and inadequate exposure to sunlight. Symptoms of vitamin D deficiency are rickets (soft pliable bones) in children and osteomalacia (demineralization of bone) in adults. Vitamin D toxicity is characterized by deposition of calcium and phosphorus in soft tissues, with damage to the heart, blood vessels, and kidneys.

Tocopherol (Vitamin E)

The active forms of vitamin E are a family of tocopherols and tocotrienols; α-tocopherol has the highest biologic activity. Vitamin E functions as an antioxidant to protect

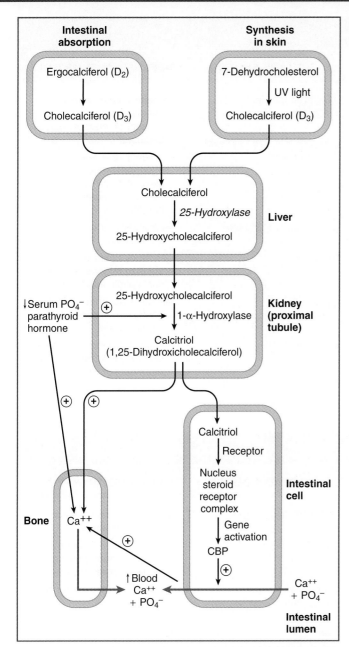

Figure 19-4. Formation of calcitriol, the active form of vitamin D, and its action in calcium homeostasis. Note that the key role of calcitriol is to mineralize bone using calcium and phosphorus. Additionally, in combination with parathyroid hormone, calcitriol maintains serum calcium levels. *CBP*, calcium-binding protein; *UV*, ultraviolet.

polyunsaturated fatty acids in membranes from oxidation. It helps prevent premature hemolysis by stabilizing the red cell membrane. Vitamin E also protects against oxidation of polyunsaturated fatty acids in low and very low density lipoproteins, limiting vascular inflammation and development of atherosclerosis. Vitamin E deficiency is uncommon and primarily occurs in fat malabsorption syndromes.

Vitamin K

Vitamin K does not require conversion to an active form; it is absorbed from the gut as menaquinone, which is produced by bacteria, or as phylloquinone, which is found in vegetables

(menadione is the synthetic form of the vitamin). Vitamin K functions in the γ-carboxylation of glutamate residues in several clotting factors. When these factors are γ-carboxylated, they are able to bind calcium, which is necessary to their function in the clotting cascade. Deficiencies in vitamin K are rare but can be caused by broad-spectrum antibiotics that reduce the primary source, the intestinal flora. Newborns are most vulnerable to a deficiency. Other causes of deficiency are fat malabsorption and pharmacologic treatment with coumarin blood thinners (relative deficiency due to increased requirement). Symptoms of vitamin K deficiency are prolonged clotting time.

Minerals and Electrolytes

The body relies on minerals obtained from the diet for a wide range of biologic functions (Table 19-3).

Sodium and Potassium

Sodium is the most abundant cation in the extracellular fluid, and potassium is the most abundant cation in the intracellular fluid. They function in the regulation of osmotic pressure (i.e., water movement between compartments) and maintenance of membrane potential required for neurotransmission and muscle activity. They can be depleted by excessive perspiration, vomiting and diarrhea, thiazide and loop diuretics, and oversecretion of antidiuretic hormone.

Calcium

Calcium has a wide range of functions, including formation of bones and teeth, transmission of nerve impulses, muscle contraction, blood coagulation, and intracellular signaling. It is regulated by calcitonin, calcitriol (from vitamin D), and parathyroid hormone. Deficiencies are most commonly the result of vitamin D deficiency, hypomagnesemia (most common pathologic cause), hypoalbuminemia (most common non-pathologic cause), and inadequate consumption in the diet. Alkalosis can lower ionized serum Ca^{++} by increasing its binding to serum albumin; this leads to tetany.

Phosphate

Phosphate is the most abundant intracellular anion (chloride is the most abundant extracellular anion) and functions primarily as a counter-ion to Ca^{++} in mineralization and as a transferable functional group on nucleotide triphosphates. It is also an important buffer in the blood. The most common cause of phosphate depletion is alkalosis.

Magnesium

Magnesium functions in bone structure, nerve impulse transmission, muscle contraction, calcium regulation (parathyroid synthesis and release), and as an enzyme cofactor, especially for adenosine triphosphatase. It can be depleted by diuretics and in alcoholism as a result of renal excretion.

Trace Elements

Most trace elements are metals that are required in the diet, since they play a role in the function of many proteins (Table 19-4). However, most trace elements are toxic at

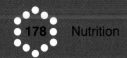

TABLE 19-3. Major Minerals and Electrolytes

MINERAL	FUNCTION	DIETARY SOURCE	DEFICIENCY SYMPTOMS
Calcium	Constituent of bones and teeth, muscle and nerve function	Dairy products, leafy vegetables, beans	Paresthesias (pins and needles), muscular excitability, cramps, bone fractures
Phosphorus	Constituent of bones and teeth, phosphorylation of proteins and metabolic intermediates	Dairy products	Deficiency rare; secondary hypophosphatemia leads to skeletal deformities, muscle weakness, increased hemolysis
Magnesium	Constituent of bones and teeth, enzyme cofactor	Leafy green vegetables	Neuromuscular excitability, paresthesia
Sodium	Plasma volume, nerve and muscle function, extracellular cation	Table salt	Deficiency unknown; excess leads to hypertension in susceptible individuals
Potassium	Nerve and muscle function, extracellular cation	Fruits, nuts	Muscular weakness, mental confusion; excess leads to cardiac arrest
Chloride	Fluid and electrolyte balance, gastric fluid	Table salt	Primary deficiency unknown; secondary deficiency due to diarrhea, vomiting

Data from Pelley JW: *Ace the boards: Biochemistry,* St Louis, 1997, Mosby, p 309.

TABLE 19-4. Trace Elements

MINERAL	FUNCTION	DIETARY SOURCE	DEFICIENCY SYMPTOMS
Iron	Component of heme, iron-sulfur proteins	Red meat, liver, eggs	Anemia; excess leads to hemochromatosis
Zinc	Enzyme cofactor	Meat, liver, eggs	Hypogonadism; impairment in growth, wound healing, sense of taste and smell
Chromium	Component of glucose tolerance factor (from yeast); works with insulin	Cheese, whole grains, nuts, yeast	Impaired glucose tolerance
Copper	Component of oxidase enzymes	Liver	Anemia
Iodine	Component of thyroid hormones	Iodized salt, seafood	Thyrotoxicosis, goiter
Manganese	Enzyme cofactor, especially superoxide dismutase	Plant foods, tea	Deficiency unknown
Selenium	Component of glutathione peroxidase as selenomethionine	Liver	Reduced glutathione peroxidase, Keshan disease

Data from Pelley JW: *Ace the boards: Biochemistry,* St Louis, 1997, Mosby, p 309.

higher than trace doses. To prevent these unwanted side reactions, most metals are bound by specific proteins.

Iron

Since excess iron is toxic, iron uptake from the gut is tightly regulated. This is accomplished by regulating the amount of the iron-binding protein apoferritin (called ferritin when iron is bound) that is synthesized in the intestinal mucosa.

Apoferritin also traps excess iron from the bloodstream by binding over 4000 molecules of iron per ferritin molecule (Fig. 19-5). During iron depletion, apoferritin synthesis is reduced, releasing more iron into the bloodstream. Any iron bound to ferritin and not used is sloughed off with normal shedding of mucosal cells. Sloughing of intestinal mucosal cells is the only iron elimination mechanism in the body. Normal menstruation eliminates some body stores in

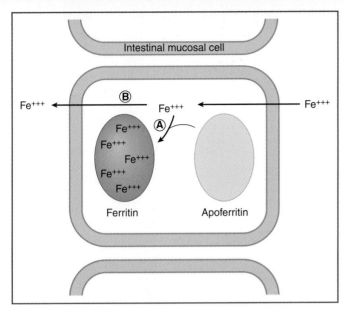

Figure 19-5. Storage of ferritin in the intestinal mucosa. A, Adequate body stores of iron; apoferritin binds iron for storage. B, Depleted body stores of iron; apoferritin levels drop, allowing iron to pass through to the bloodstream.

premenopausal women; other mechanisms that reduce excess iron are blood donation and occult bleeding (e.g., from an ulcer). Iron is stored in the liver as either ferritin or hemosiderin (denatured ferritin that is saturated with iron); excess hemosiderin in tissues is toxic (hemosiderosis).

Iron is transported in the bloodstream by the serum protein transferrin. Each molecule of transferrin binds two iron molecules; the transferrin pool is normally about one third saturated in plasma. Since it is the oxidized (ferric; Fe^{+++}) form that binds to transferrin, a serum enzyme, ferroxidase II (ceruloplasmin), oxidizes any iron so it can be transported. Iron functions as a component of heme, as nonheme iron in the electron transport chain, and as a cofactor for enzymes (e.g., catalase). Iron deficiency can be caused by inadequate intake, chronic loss of blood (usually occult), or excessive menstruation. The earliest sign of iron deficiency is anemia.

Zinc

Zinc functions as a cofactor for metalloenzymes such as super-oxide dismutase, collagenase, and alcohol dehydrogenase. It also has an important function in spermatogenesis and growth in children. Deficiencies are caused by inadequate intake, alcoholism, chronic diarrhea, and inflammatory disease. Symptoms of zinc deficiency include poor wound healing, hypogonadism, and growth impairment.

Copper

Copper functions as a cofactor for metalloenzymes such as ferroxidase (ceruloplasmin), lysyl, superoxide dismutase (antioxidant enzyme), tyrosinase (melanin synthesis), and oxidase (cross-links collagen), cytochrome-c oxidase, and other oxidases. It is transported on the serum protein ceruloplasmin. Deficiencies are usually due to total parenteral nutrition. Wilson disease is characterized by an excess of free copper, resulting from defective secretion in the bile. Patients experience dementia and deposition of copper in the lens (Kayser-Fleischer rings).

Iodine

Iodine functions in the synthesis of thyroid hormones. Deficiencies are due to inadequate intake and are characterized by goiter.

Manganese

Manganese functions as an enzyme cofactor, primarily in mitochondria. There are no well-described deficiencies.

Selenium

Selenium functions as a component of glutathione peroxidase, in which it substitutes for sulfur in the amino acid selenocysteine. Selenium deficiency is rare, usually resulting from total parenteral nutrition.

Chromium

Chromium functions in the "glucose tolerance factor," an organic complex found in yeast and wheat germ that is believed to play a postreceptor role in insulin action. Chromium deficiency may develop during total parenteral nutrition.

Fluoride

Fluoride is not an essential trace element, functioning primarily in strengthening the calcium phosphate matrix of teeth and bones when it is incorporated into their crystal matrix. Excesses of fluoride in geographic locations where it occurs in the drinking water produces fluorosis (mottling of teeth, calcification of ligaments).

KEY POINTS ABOUT MICRONUTRIENTS

- The water-soluble vitamins are usually coenzymes. Because they are not stored and are readily excreted in urine, they are required as part of a balanced diet.

- The fat-soluble vitamins are absorbed with fats and transported in chylomicrons to function as hormones, cofactors, and antioxidants; since they can dissolve in body fat stores, some can accumulate to toxic levels.

- Several inorganic minerals, such as calcium, are required in large amounts to maintain bone structure, whereas other metal ions are toxic at high levels but are needed at trace levels for proper metalloenzyme function.

Self-assessment questions can be accessed at www. StudentConsult.com.

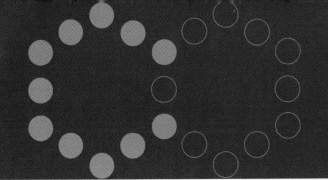

Tissue Biochemistry 20

●●●● MUSCLE CONTRACTION AND ENERGY SOURCES

Much of the adenosine triphosphate (ATP) energy from fuel oxidation is used in the contraction of muscle. Muscle is designed to use this chemical energy to create mechanical energy. This is accomplished through conformational changes within the muscle myosin protein and changes in the association between muscle actin and myosin that occur during the binding of ATP. To sustain a constant source of energy for this process, creatine phosphate is created to act as an energy battery.

Contraction Mechanism

At the anatomic level, muscle contraction creates movement at a joint by bringing two bones closer together. Similarly at the tissue level, coordinated contraction of muscle cells is due to contraction of its myofibrils. At the cellular level, the fundamental unit for the coordinated contraction of the myofibrils is the sarcomere, a unit containing overlapping filaments that slide past each other during contraction (Fig. 20-1). This causes all sarcomeres in the myofibril to decrease in length during contraction. At the biochemical level, the overlapping filaments are composed of actin and myosin that interact in a consistent fashion and move with respect to one another in response to changes in Ca^{++} and ATP.

Two types of filaments overlap and interact in the sarcomere—F-actin (thin filaments) and myosin (thick filaments). Additional proteins—tropomyosin and troponin—regulate the interaction between actin and myosin (Fig. 20-2).

F-actin filaments are produced when G-actin, a globular protein, polymerizes. While ATP is required for G-actin polymerization, it remains bound to each G-actin monomer within the F-actin polymer and does not participate in contraction. Tropomyosin and troponin associate with F-actin filaments.

Rod-shaped myosin monomers polymerize to form thick myosin filaments. Myosin monomers are composed of six subunits that associate to form globular head groups and a rod-shaped tail. The globular ends have adenosine triphosphatase (ATPase) activity and interact with F-actin to form cross-bridges.

The movement of myosin relative to actin produces sliding filaments that shorten the sarcomere. This movement occurs through a change in the shape, or flexing, of the myosin head groups. The myosin head groups alternate between a charged, high-energy form with ATP bound and a discharged, low-energy form with adenosine diphosphate (ADP) bound. The steps in a contraction cycle involve the development of a high-energy myosin head followed by a release of energy as it associates with and pulls the actin filament (the power stroke).

1. ATP binds to the myosin head group in the relaxation phase after a power stroke. Myosin-ATP has a low affinity for actin and thus releases it.
2. While still in the relaxation phase, myosin adopts the high-energy state by hydrolyzing ATP to ADP and inorganic phosphate (P_i), but both ADP and P_i remain bound to the head group. The head group remains in this energized state, and if it could bind to actin it would spontaneously undergo a power stroke with release of the P_i and a concomitant release of energy.
3. The interaction between the high-energy myosin-ADP-P_i complex and actin is blocked by tropomyosin. Until the tropomyosin is moved, the power stroke is prevented.
   - Tropomyosin can be moved to expose the actin filament only by the action of troponin, which cannot act until a nerve impulse arrives.
   - Troponin is active only when it forms a complex with Ca^{++}, but between nerve impulses continuous active pumping it maintains the intracellular concentration of Ca^{++} very low (at ~ 100 nmol).
   - Ca^{++} concentrations in the sarcoplasmic reticulum are 10,000 times greater than in the cytoplasm.
   - When a nerve impulse depolarizes the muscle plasma membrane, a Ca^{++} influx increases the concentration 100-fold, and Ca^{++} complexes with troponin.

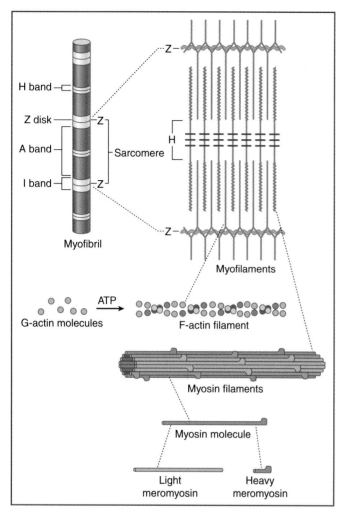

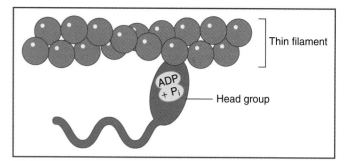

A

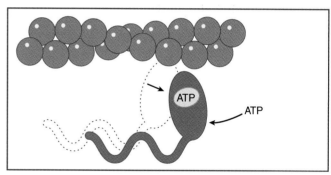

B

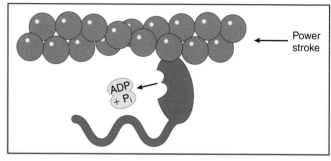

C

Figure 20-1. Actin and myosin components of a sarcomere. A single multinucleate muscle fiber contains many individual myofibrils, which give it a striated appearance. *ATP*, adenosine triphosphate.

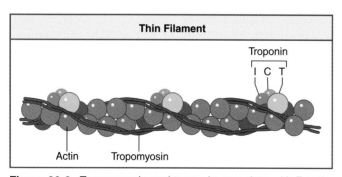

Figure 20-2. Tropomyosin and troponin associate with F-actin to regulate its interaction with myosin.

4. The movement of tropomyosin by the troponin-Ca^{++} complex allows an association between the high-energy myosin-ADP-P$_i$ complex and actin, and the initiation of the power stroke (Fig. 20-3). Upon completion of the conformational change in the group, the myosin head group is in the low-energy state, ADP and P$_i$ have been released, and the power stroke is completed. All that remains is for ATP to bind to myosin and release the head group from the actin.

Figure 20-3. The power stroke involves a change in the orientation of the myosin head group that results in a physical movement relative to the tail. **A,** The head group gains access to the actin filament when troponin moves the tropomyosin block (not shown). **B,** Both adenosine diphosphate (*ADP*) and inorganic phosphate (*P$_i$*) are released as the head group moves during the power stroke. **C,** Adenosine triphosphate (*ATP*) binds during the relaxed state following the power stroke. "Before" and "after" in the last frame are superimposed for comparison.

HISTOLOGY

Sarcoplasmic Reticulum

To provide simultaneous access of Ca^{++} to troponin throughout the muscle fiber, a modified smooth ER called the sarcoplasmic reticulum is arranged in such a fashion that it surrounds each myofibril. The lumen of the sarcoplasmic reticulum is isolated from the cytosol and serves as the Ca^{++} reservoir between nerve impulses. Upon depolarization, Ca^{++} is released in the immediate vicinity of the myofibril rather than being limited to the sarcolemma (plasma membrane).

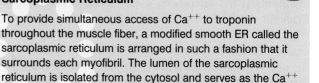

Energy Sources

Because muscular contraction can become quite intense, the short-term demands of the muscle cell can exceed the energy provided by normal fuel metabolism. Two main enzymes create short-term supplies of ATP: creatine kinase and adenylate kinase (myokinase).

Creatine phosphate is formed by phosphorylation of creatine with ATP catalyzed by creatine kinase (Fig. 20-4). This reaction is reversible, allowing rapid generation of ATP from creatine phosphate and ADP. During normal metabolism, the ample supply of ATP favors the formation of creatine phosphate, which then acts as a storage battery, ready to regenerate ATP when ADP accumulates.

Adenylate kinase can combine two ADP molecules to produce one ATP and one adenosine monophosphate. This squeezes all the energy available from ADP supplies once the creatine phosphate has been depleted. During normal metabolism, the ample supply of ATP favors the restoration of ADP, which then undergoes oxidative phosphorylation to ATP.

Lactate dehydrogenase (LDH) isoenzymes are different in heart and skeletal muscle, reflecting their different metabolic requirements. Heart is an aerobic tissue and is adapted to use lactate as a fuel, whereas skeletal muscle can experience temporary anaerobic conditions and is adapted to produce lactate under those conditions. LDH is a tetramer of four catalytic subunits; there are two types of subunits: heart (H) and muscle (M). The five possible LDH isoenzyme tetramer combinations are H_4, H_3M, H_2M_2, HM_3, and M_4H.

Skeletal muscle has more M subunits expressed, which produces more HM_3 and M_4 tetramers. The M subunit has a high affinity for pyruvate, favoring the production of lactate (pyruvate $\rightarrow$ lactate) under anaerobic conditions. Some lactate is produced, even at rest.

Heart muscle has more H subunit expressed, which produces more H_4 and H_3M tetramers. The H subunit has a higher affinity for lactate and is inhibited by pyruvate, favoring production of pyruvate (lactate $\rightarrow$ pyruvate) for aerobic metabolism.

PATHOLOGY

Rigor Mortis

Subsequent to a person's death, metabolism becomes anaerobic with the depletion of ATP. Since ATP is needed to bind to myosin and release it from the actin filament, the myosin remains bound in the contracted state. When this final state occurs in all of the myofibrils, the muscle fiber enters a state of constant contraction.

KEY POINTS ABOUT MUSCLE CONTRACTION AND ENERGY SOURCES

- Muscle contraction involves a change in the physical relationship between actin filaments and myosin-ADP-P_i complexes; the power stroke involves a conformational change in the myosin head groups when ADP dissociates.

- Muscle contraction relies on creatine phosphate and adenylate kinase to maintain ATP concentrations; the energy needs of heart and skeletal muscle are reflected in their LDH isozyme composition.

●●● CONNECTIVE TISSUE PROTEINS

Unlike the softer tissues such as brain and liver, connective tissue is a firmer, fibrous material needed for mechanical function in the body. The fibrous proteins that compose the extracellular matrix of a tissue determine whether it will have structural rigidity (bone), tensile strength (tendon), or elasticity (blood vessels, skin, lungs). They are embedded in an amorphous ground substance composed of hyaluronic acid, nonfibrous glycoproteins, and proteoglycans.

Fibrous Proteins

Collagen and elastin represent the two major fibrous proteins in connective tissue. Collagen is the more abundant and represents about 25% of the protein in the body. It is found in tissues with tensile strength and rigidity (e.g., tendons). Elastin, although a fibrous protein like collagen, serves a stretch and recoil function in connective tissues (e.g., in the arterial wall).

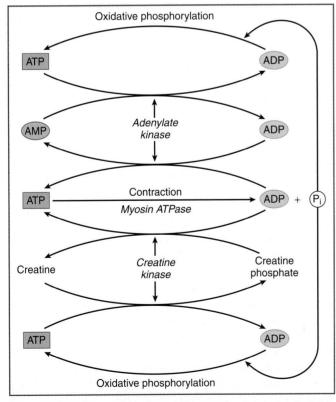

Figure 20-4. The contribution of creatine kinase and adenylate kinase in maintaining cellular concentrations of adenosine triphosphate (*ATP*) in muscle fibers. *ADP*, adenosine diphosphate; *AMP*, adenosine monophosphate; *ATPase*, adenosine triphosphatase.

Collagen

Structure

Collagen is a long triple helix of peptide chains, known as α-chains (Fig. 20-5). Each individual collagen polypeptide is an α-chain of about 1400 residues. Every third amino acid is glycine (-Gly-X-Y-) with a very high proportion of proline and lysine in the other two positions. Many proline and lysine residues are hydroxylated to hydroxyproline and hydroxylysine after synthesis of the α-chain. The hydroxylation reactions require ascorbic acid and iron (Fig. 20-6). To pack the three α-chains into a triple helix, the repeating glycine occupies one side along the axis of the helix. The absence of side chains allows the tight packing of α-chains in a triple helical array.

Classification

The several different types, or superfamilies, of collagen differ in their composition of α-chains, which determines their function and thus their location. For example, type I collagen is composed of two α_1 chains plus one α_2 chain ($\alpha1_2\alpha2$).

- Type I collagen: found in most connective tissues including bone (Fig. 20-7)
- Type II collagen: found in cartilage and vitreous humor
- Type III collagen: found in skin, lung, and blood vessels
- Type IV collagen: found in basement membranes and forms networks by assembling into a flexible, sheetlike, multilayered network

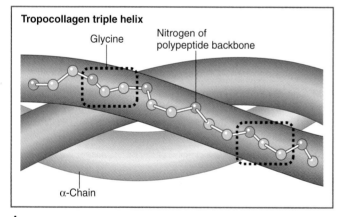

Tropocollagen triple helix

Glycine

Nitrogen of polypeptide backbone

α-Chain

A

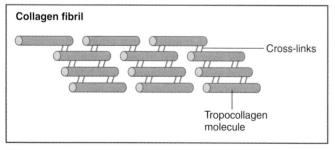

Collagen fibril

Cross-links

Tropocollagen molecule

B

Figure 20-5. Collagen structure. **A,** Triple-stranded helix of tropocollagen, the structural unit of collagen. The three chains are able to pack closely because glycine, which lacks a side chain, is present where the helices touch each other. **B,** A typical staggered array of tropocollagen units cross-linked to increase the tensile strength of connective tissue.

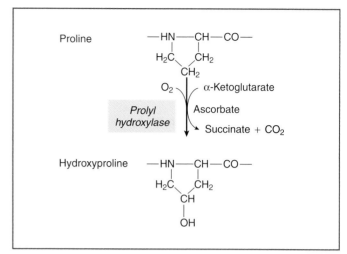

Proline

O_2 α-Ketoglutarate

Prolyl hydroxylase

Ascorbate

Succinate + CO_2

Hydroxyproline

Figure 20-6. Formation of hydroxyproline by prolyl hydroxylase. Ascorbate is required as a cofactor.

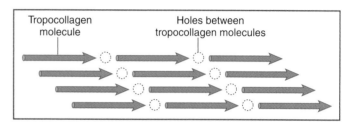

Tropocollagen molecule

Holes between tropocollagen molecules

Figure 20-7. Type I collagen has holes between the tropocollagen units as sites for deposition of the calcium phosphate mineral, hydroxyapatite.

Synthesis and Degradation

Collagen will spontaneously assemble into fibrils. To avoid premature assembly of fibers within the cell, a precursor form, procollagen, is synthesized. Synthesis of procollagen involves (1) extensive posttranslational modification of the α-chain polypeptide, and (2) α-chain assembly into procollagen (Fig. 20-8).

The α-chain (preprocollagen) is first targeted to the endoplasmic reticulum (ER) with a signal sequence that is immediately removed in the ER. Selected proline and lysine residues are then hydroxylated in the ER.

Selected hydroxylysine residues are glycosylated by galactosyltransferase and glucosyltransferase.

The pro-α-chains spontaneously assemble into procollagen triple helices within the ER. The resulting molecule has propeptide extensions on both ends, still preventing spontaneous assembly into collagen fibrils. The procollagen is translocated from the ER into the Golgi apparatus and packaged in secretory vesicles.

Procollagen is secreted into the extracellular matrix by exocytosis (fusion with the plasma membrane), and procollagen peptidases remove the propeptide ends. Procollagen then forms units called tropocollagen, which spontaneously assemble into collagen fibrils (see Fig. 20-5).

The collagen fibrils are strengthened further by cross-linking between adjacent lysine side chains by the enzyme

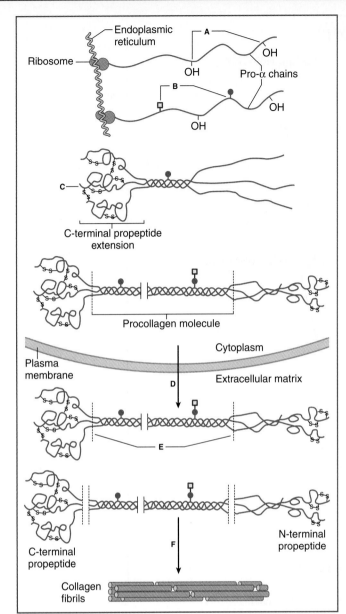

Figure 20-8. Synthesis and assembly of the collagen fiber. *A,* The individual helices assemble in the lumen of the endoplasmic reticulum endoplasmic reticulum to form procollagen. Hydroxylation of proline and lysine also occurs here. *B,* Glucose and galactose are added to hydroxylysine residues. *C,* The propeptide extensions prevent premature assembly of collagen in the endoplasmic reticulum. *D,* Exocytosis of procollagen is followed by (*E*) removal of the propeptide ends by peptidases. *F,* The tropocollagen units then spontaneously assemble to form collagen fibrils.

lysyl oxidase. This is a slow, continuous process throughout an individual's life. Cross-linking permits scar tissue to strengthen long after a wound has healed, but it also causes collagen to stiffen, contributing to the decline in vascular elasticity with age.

Collagen can be remodeled by degradation with metalloproteinases. The action of these digestive enzymes is balanced by a tissue inhibitor of metalloproteinases. Patients with osteoarthritis have an imbalance between metalloproteinases and their tissue inhibitor, allowing degradation to exceed reconstruction.

Diseases Related to Collagen

Osteogenesis imperfecta is caused by unstable type I collagen molecules. They form an abnormal matrix and lead to the formation of weakened bones. One form of the disease is lethal in utero; in a less severe form, the patient has easily fractured bones ("brittle bones") and retarded wound healing. Patients with the less severe disease, Ehlers-Danlos syndrome, have defective, poorly cross-linked collagen molecules producing stretchy skin and loose joints.

Elastin
Structure

Elastin is similar to collagen and also is assembled spontaneously from monomers (tropoelastin). However, tropoelastin has much less hydroxyproline and no hydroxylysine, and its content of alanine and valine are high; it is among the most hydrophobic of the body's proteins. Its elasticity results from the deformability of desmosine cross-links (Fig. 20-9), which produces an interconnected network of fibrils with the properties of rubber. The desmosine cross-links are catalyzed by lysyl oxidase, the same enzyme that forms cross-links in collagen.

Diseases Related to Elastin

Destruction of elastin by neutrophils would lead to emphysema were it not for α_1-antitrypsin. Neutrophils patrol the lungs to detect and fight off environmental insults. One of their weapons is elastase, a protease with specificity for small hydrophobic residues, such as alanine and valine. However, if left unchecked, elastase will also digest elastin in the alveolar walls, causing them to break down, creating enlarged alveoli with a reduced surface area; this condition is known as emphysema. This damage to the lungs is prevented by the proteinase inhibitor α_1-antitrypsin (also called α_1-antiprotease for its broad specificity), which is present in the blood (and elevated during infections). Patients with inherited defects in α_1-antitrypsin are at serious risk for emphysema; intravenous administration of α_1-antitrypsin is an effective treatment. Smoking also can cause emphysema, since a methionine residue in α_1-antitrypsin essential for binding to elastase is vulnerable to oxidization by cigarette smoke.

Amorphous Ground Substance

Amorphous "ground substance" participates in tissue cohesion by interacting with both connective tissue fibers and cell surfaces. The ground substance is flexible also, contributing to tissue resiliency and deformability. Major components of the ground substance are the glycosaminoglycans (GAGs) and proteoglycans (which contain GAGs).

Glycosaminoglycans

GAGs are unbranched polysaccharides that consist of repeating disaccharide units. One of the sugars is always acetylated or sulfated, and the other is almost always uronic acid

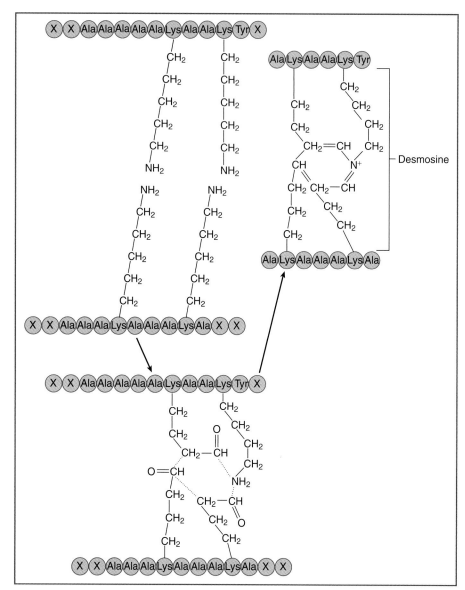

Figure 20-9. Formation of desmosine cross-links between lysine residues in elastin.

(produced from uridine diphosphate glucose in the uronic acid pathway). Hyaluronic acid is a GAG consisting of repeating glucuronic acid/N-acetylglucosamine disaccharide units. It has a mucoid consistency and is found in synovial fluid and the vitreous fluid of the eye.

Proteoglycans

All other GAGs are sulfated and bound to a core protein to form a proteoglycan. There are many different proteoglycans (also called mucopolysaccharides) serving a variety of roles:

- They are major components of the amorphous ground substance.
- They are components of mucus.
- Heparin, an anticoagulant proteoglycan, prevents excessive clotting along the vascular wall during an inflammatory response.

- They provide the cell surface with a smooth hydrophilic coat, the glycocalyx.
- Aggrecan, a large proteoglycan, forms large aggregates to give cartilage its resilience and elasticity.

PATHOLOGY

Mucopolysaccharidoses

Defects in the degradation of proteoglycans cause accumulation within lysosomes of various stages of degradation. Hurler syndrome is due to a deficiency of α-iduronidase, which is needed to hydrolyze terminal α-iduronic acid residues from GAGs. Patients are normal at birth but soon develop hepatosplenomegaly, mental retardation, and coarse facial features owing to accumulation of GAGs in parenchymal cells. These patients also excrete undigested GAGs.

KEY POINTS ABOUT CONNECTIVE TISSUE PROTEINS

■ There are at least 19 collagen types that differ in α-chain compositions, with types I, II, and III comprising about 70% of the total; tropocollagen is a right-handed triple helix of left-handed α-chains. Procollagen synthesis prevents premature assembly of collagen fibrils inside the cell.

■ Elastin is a connective tissue that is similar in composition to collagen, but with properties that allow it to bend and stretch like rubber. Destruction of elastin by neutrophils could lead to emphysema, if it were not for α₁-antitrypsin. The glycosaminoglycans and proteoglycans (which contain GAGs) make up much of the amorphous ground substance that functions in cell adhesion, mucus formation, the vitreous fluid of the eye, and support for bone.

●●● BLOOD—CLOTTING FACTORS AND LIPOPROTEINS

Two of the major protein classes in blood are the clotting factors and the lipoproteins.

Clotting Factors

Blood clotting is actually a balance between two processes occurring simultaneously: clot polymerization and clot dissolution. Blood clotting in response to a wound consists of four overlapping phases:

● The smooth muscle in the wall of the damaged vessel constricts, restricting blood loss from the injury.
● Platelets aggregate at the wound and form a platelet plug. They bind to collagen exposed by the injury with the help of von Willebrand factor and become activated by either thrombin or ATP to release clotting factors.
● The clotting cascade produces a fibrin mesh that provides a stable physical structure for development of a stable clot.
● Clot dissolution by plasmin begins during formation of the fibrin mesh to control the ultimate size of the clot.

The size and shape of the clot are a result of the dynamic interplay between clot formation and clot dissolution.

Fibrinogen, a large fibrous plasma protein, is kept water soluble by highly charged fibrinopeptides located at the center of the fibrinogen molecule (Fig. 20-10). Thrombin, the terminal enzyme of the clotting cascade, converts the soluble plasma fibrinogen into the insoluble polymerized fibrin through limited proteolytic digestion and removal of the fibrinopeptides (Fig. 20-11). Thrombin also activates transglutaminase, a fibrin cross-linking enzyme that strengthens the fibrin mesh (Fig. 20-12).

Thrombin is synthesized by the liver as prothrombin, an inactive zymogen that is found in the plasma. Prothrombin remains inactive until it binds to a complex produced by the clotting cascade called the Va-Xa complex that is located on the platelet membrane. The Va-Xa complex cleaves a prothrombin amino-terminal fragment to produce active thrombin (mnemonic: Activate your prothrombin at the five [V]

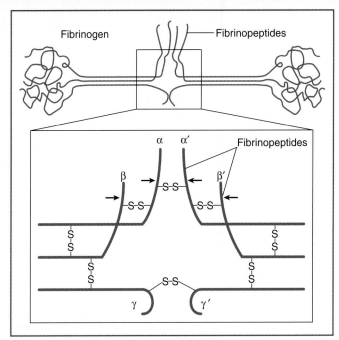

Figure 20-10. Structure of fibrinogen. The fibrinopeptides at the center of the molecule are highly charged, serving to make fibrinogen highly soluble and to prevent it from aggregating.

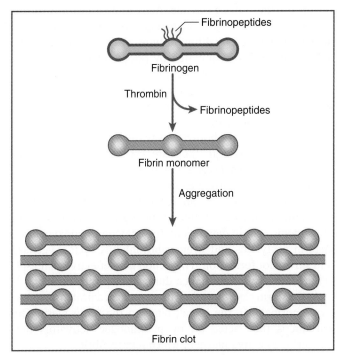

Figure 20-11. Thrombin digests away the fibrinopeptides, causing fibrinogen to aggregate into fibrin, forming a fibrin clot.

and dime [X]). Prothrombin binding to the Va-Xa complex requires Ca^{++}, which binds to γ-carboxyglutamate at the amino terminus of prothrombin. Vitamin K is required for carboxylation of glutamate, so prothrombin activation can be blocked by dicumarol (warfarin), a vitamin K analog and inhibitor. In the presence of dicumarol, an abnormal prothrombin is produced that cannot be activated.

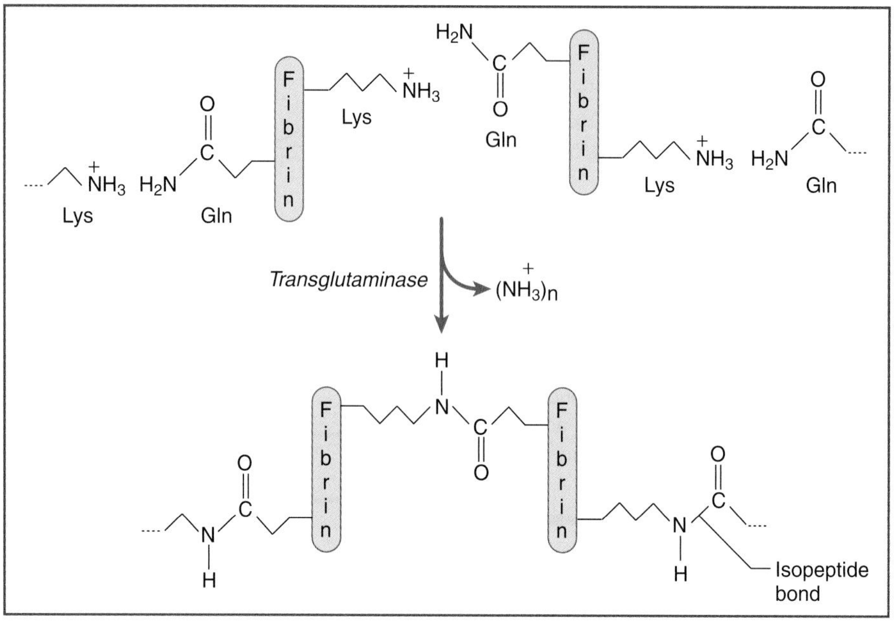

Figure 20-12. Transglutaminase cross-links fibrin monomers by linking lysine and glutamine residues.

Both factor Va and factor Xa are produced by the clotting cascade. Like fibrinogen and prothrombin, they are normally present in the blood as proenzymes, along with the other components of the clotting cascade. Activation of factor X to factor Xa occurs at the convergence of two pathways of activation initiated by different types of injury (Fig. 20-13).

- Extrinsic pathway: initiated by release of tissue factor, a transmembrane glycoprotein on the surface of cell types not normally in contact with blood.
- Intrinsic pathway: initiated by exposure of clotting factors in blood to collagen.
- Clotting factors for both pathways also bind Ca^{++} for their activity. In addition, they are carboxylated in vitamin K–dependent reactions in the liver.

The eicosanoid, thromboxane A_2, is needed for release of the platelet granules containing the clotting factors to initiate the clotting cascade. Thromboxane A_2 is synthesized from arachidonic acid in platelets by the enzyme cyclooxygenase. Aspirin acetylates and irreversibly inhibits cyclooxygenase and slows clot formation. This action is so effective that aspirin enhances survival if taken during a heart attack.

As the fibrin clot is forming, plasminogen, a protease proenzyme normally in the blood, binds to the fibrin mesh. The plasmin is then acted on by plasminogen activators that convert it to active plasmin, which digests fibrin.

Tissue-type plasminogen activator is found in endothelial cells. Recombinant tissue plasminogen activator has been used clinically to decrease tissue damage produced by coronary thrombosis.

Urokinase-like plasminogen activator, found in kidney tubular epithelia, and streptokinase, obtained from bacteria, are also used clinically to accelerate clot dissolution.

Hemophilia

Hemophilia, the tendency toward uncontrolled bleeding, is caused by a genetic deficiency in the clotting cascade.

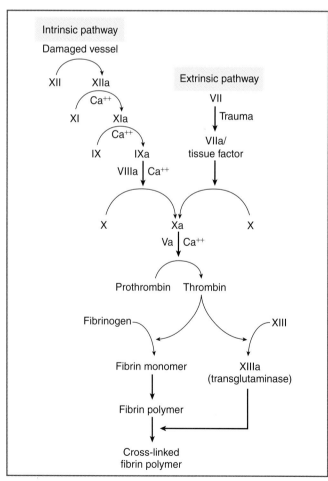

Figure 20-13. The blood clotting cascade. The extrinsic and intrinsic pathways converge to form factor Xa, which can complex with factor Va and Ca^{++} to activate prothrombin. Thrombin then creates fibrin monomers that assemble into the fibrin clot; its activation of transglutaminase ensures that the fibrin clot becomes cross-linked.

Hemophilia A, accounting for about 85% of cases, results from an X-linked deficiency of factor VIII. Although factor VIII is not directly in the clotting cascade, it serves to stimulate activation of factor X by factor IXa.

Hemophilia B is due to a deficiency in factor IX and presents an almost identical picture to hemophilia A.

PHARMACOLOGY

Other Antiplatelet Drugs

In addition to aspirin, the drug clopidogrel interferes with prostaglandin synthesis in the platelet but via a different mechanism of action. By blocking the ADP receptor on the surface of the platelet, clopidogrel causes a reduction in the activity of platelet membrane lipases, leading to a reduction in the release of arachidonic acid, the precursor to prostaglandin synthesis. The overall effect is to stabilize the platelet and prevent activation.

Lipoproteins

Serum lipoproteins are spherical particles that resemble a micelle because they have a hydrophobic core containing triglycerides and cholesterol esters, and a hydrophilic surface consisting of phospholipids and free cholesterol. Their function is to transport cholesterol and other lipids between tissues.

Their protein components package the lipids in a form that can be transported in blood and include recognition elements that interact with receptors in peripheral tissues. Following endocytosis and lysosomal degradation of the protein, the lipids are used for biosynthesis of tissue lipids. The functions of several apolipoproteins are summarized in Table 20-1. The size and density of the lipoprotein particles are inversely related, since the larger particles have a lower percentage of protein, which is denser than fat.

Four classes of lipoprotein particles found in the plasma have differing amounts of fat and protein (Table 20-2).

Chylomicrons

Chylomicrons (Fig. 20-14) are formed in the intestinal epithelium to transport long-chain triglycerides to the tissues. Medium- and short-chain fats are transported directly to the liver through the portal circulation without packaging into lipoprotein particles. Chylomicrons pick up apolipoprotein C-II (apoC-II) from high-density lipoprotein particles and circulate through the tissues. Lipoprotein lipase on the endothelial surface is activated by apoC-II and releases much of the triglyceride that is taken up by the tissues (adipose, muscle, heart); the glycerol is recycled to liver. A degraded chylomicron remnant is eventually removed by the liver and digested for repackaging in very low-density lipoprotein particles. The liver recognizes chylomicron remnants because they contain apoE, which is also obtained from high-density lipoprotein particles.

TABLE 20-1. Apolipoprotein Characteristics

APOLIPOPROTEIN	LIPOPROTEIN ASSOCIATION	SOURCE	BIOLOGIC ROLE
A-I	HDL, chylomicrons	Liver, intestine	Activates lecithin-cholesterol acyltransferase in HDL
B-48	Chylomicrons	Intestine	Serves as structural protein for chylomicrons
B-100	VLDL, LDL	Liver	Serves as structural protein for VLDL and LDL; contains LDL receptor-binding domain
C-II	HDL, VLDL, chylomicrons	Liver	Activates extrahepatic lipoprotein lipase
E	VLDL, chylomicrons	Liver	Mediates uptake of chylomicron remnants by the liver

HDL, high-density lipoprotein; *LDL*, low-density lipoprotein; *VLDL*, very-low-density lipoprotein.

TABLE 20-2. Composition of Serum Lipoproteins

LIPOPROTEIN	SOURCE	PROTEIN (%)	TG	PHOSPHOLIPID	CHOLESTEROL + CHOLESTEROL ESTERS
Chylomicrons	Intestine	2	85	8	5
VLDL	Liver	10	55	18	17
LDL	VLDL	22	9	20	49
HDL	Liver, intestine	50	4	30	16

Values are approximate.
HDL, high-density lipoprotein; *LDL*, low-density lipoprotein; *TG*, triglyceride; *VLDL*, very-low-density lipoprotein.

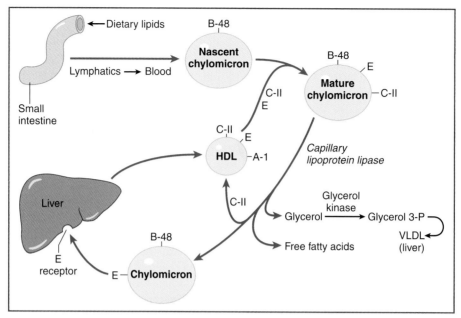

Figure 20-14. Transport of dietary lipids via chylomicrons. Chylomicrons release most of their triglyceride in the tissues through lipoprotein lipase action. The chylomicron remnants return to the liver to be reprocessed. Chylomicrons interchange apolipoproteins with high-density lipoprotein (*HDL*). *VLDL*, very-low-density lipoprotein.

Very-Low-Density Lipoproteins

Very-low-density lipoproteins (VLDLs) (Fig. 20-15) are formed in the liver to transport hepatic lipids to peripheral tissue. Like chylomicrons, they acquire apoC-II and apoE from high-density lipoprotein (HDL), and release much of their triglyceride to fat and muscle tissue. As they lose triglycerides, VLDLs mature into LDL particles. The difference between chylomicron remnants and LDL is the presence of apoB-48 in chylomicrons and apoB-100 in LDL.

ANATOMY

Lymphatics—The Other "Portal"

All dietary components, except for long-chain fats, are taken directly to the liver through the hepatic portal vein before they enter the general circulation. However, the route for chylomicrons, which carry the long-chain fats (in addition to fat-soluble vitamins), is through the lymphatics, where they enter the junction of the left subclavian and left internal jugular veins through the thoracic duct.

Low-Density Lipoproteins

LDLs (see Fig. 20-15) lose apoC and apoE, and contain primarily apoB-100. This apoprotein has a domain that recognizes the LDL receptor in peripheral tissues where it binds. Binding of the LDL particle to its receptor is followed by endocytosis and digestion of the lipoprotein in lysosomes. The cholesterol is released into the cell to be used for membrane synthesis, or it is stored as cholesterol ester.

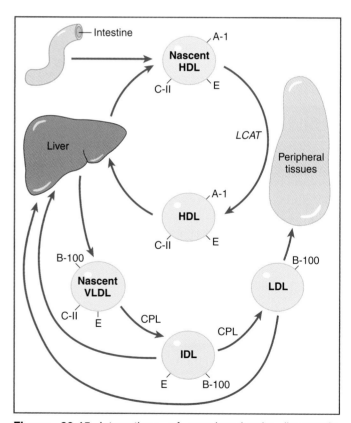

Figure 20-15. Interactions of very-low-density lipoprotein (*VLDL*), low-density lipoprotein (*LDL*), and high-density lipoprotein (*HDL*). VLDLs produced in the liver distribute their triglyceride to the tissues (not shown) and mature into LDLs, which then transport cholesterol to the tissues. HDLs receive cholesterol from the tissues and carry it back to the liver. HDLs also interchange apolipoproteins with VLDLs and LDLs. *CPL*, capillary lipoprotein lipase; *LCAT*, lecithin-cholesterol acyltransferase; *IDL*, intermediate-density lipoprotein.

High-Density Lipoproteins

HDLs (see Fig. 20-15) are apoprotein storage depots. In addition to their cholesterol transport function, they are the source of several apoproteins for the other lipoprotein particles. HDL is considered a scavenger lipoprotein. In the peripheral tissues, HDL picks up excess cholesterol and phospholipids; it esterifies the cholesterol through the action of one of its enzyme components, lecithin-cholesterol acyltransferase, forming mainly cholesterol linoleate. The cholesterol esters are then transferred to LDL and chylomicron remnants by another HDL protein, cholesterol ester transfer protein. The remnants then transport the cholesterol esters back to the liver, completing their tissues-to-liver journey.

KEY POINTS ABOUT BLOOD CLOTTING FACTORS AND LIPOPROTEINS

- The clotting cascade is actually two pathways that converge to produce an activated factor V–factor X complex (Va-Xa complex) that activates prothrombin; the extrinsic pathway initiates with tissue factor, while the intrinsic pathway initiates with clotting factors.
- Blood clotting involves simultaneous polymerization and dissolution of a fibrin clot.
- Apolipoproteins activate enzymes that metabolize lipoproteins, provide structure for lipoprotein particles, and serve as receptor recognition proteins.
- There are four major classes of lipoproteins: chylomicrons (diet) and VLDL (liver) are similar in composition and function in delivering triglyceride to tissues; LDL delivers cholesterol to the tissues; and HDL carries lipids from the tissues back to the liver.

PATHOLOGY

Macrophage Scavenger Receptors

Macrophages serve a phagocytic function in removing foreign antigens from the body. They will also phagocytose oxidized LDL particles that bind to their "scavenger" receptors. They cannot digest the altered LDL, so the cytoplasm fills with lysosomes that give the appearance of foam; thus these cells are called "foam cells."

●●● LIVER METABOLISM OF XENOBIOTICS AND ETHANOL

The diet contains a number of nonnutritive chemicals, called xenobiotics, from both a plant and animal origin that must be detoxified and eliminated. Those that are water soluble can be excreted in urine or in bile. Instead of using a separate route for eliminating the fat-soluble xenobiotics, the body converts them to a water-soluble form and excretes them in urine and bile also. The primary organs of xenobiotic metabolism are (1) the liver, which is directly exposed to dietary chemicals transported through the hepatic portal vein, and (2) the lungs, which are directly exposed to airborne chemicals. Xenobiotics are metabolized in two phases: oxidation (usually as hydroxylation; phase 1 reactions) and conjugation (phase 2 reactions).

Phase 1 Reactions

The most common type of phase 1 reaction is hydroxylation by cytochrome P450. This same enzyme participates in hydroxylation and side-chain cleavage of steroid hormones. Cytochrome P450 is a term for a large family of heme-containing oxidative enzymes that are located in the ER and in the mitochondrion. They act by transferring an electron from nicotinamide adenine dinucleotide phosphate (NADPH) to molecular O_2, creating an active O_2 species (Fig. 20-16). By their very nature, nearly all pharmaceuticals are metabolized by the liver. Since cytochrome P450 enzymes are inducible, many patients can develop a tolerance for some drugs, necessitating an increase in dosage with time.

Phase 2 Reactions

Conjugation with glucuronic acid, sulfate, glutamine, glycine, or glutathione increases the water solubility of the xenobiotic and decreases its biologic activity (Fig. 20-17). This is the true detoxification step, since phase 1 reactions often can convert inactive xenobiotics to toxic products.

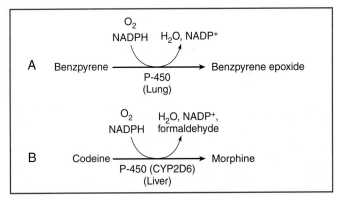

Figure 20-16. A, Phase 1 conversion of benzpyrene (cigarette smoke, charcoal-grilled meat) to benzpyrene epoxide. **B,** Phase 1 conversion of codeine to morphine with removal of single-carbon formaldehyde (O-demethylation). *NADP,* nicotinamide adenine diphosphate; *NADPH,* reduced NADP.

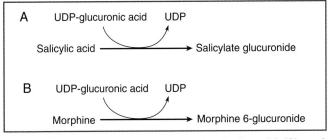

Figure 20-17. Phase 2 conversion of salicylic acid **(A)** and morphine **(B)** to their water-soluble glucuronides. *UDP,* uridine diphosphate.

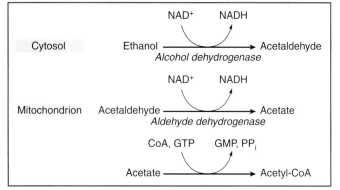

Figure 20-18. Production of acetyl-coenzyme A (*CoA*) from ethanol. This pathway increases the amount of nicotinamide adenine dinucleotide (*NAD*) in the liver cell. *NADH*, reduced NAD; *GMP*, guanosine monophosphate; *GTP*, guanosine triphosphate; *PP$_i$*, inorganic pyrophosphate.

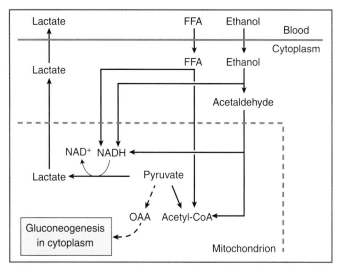

Figure 20-19. Shunting of pyruvate to lactate in the metabolism of ethanol in the fasting state. Nicotinamide adenine dinucleotide (*NAD*) is produced from free fatty acid (*FFA*) mobilization and ethanol metabolism, causing a shunt of pyruvate away from oxaloacetate (*OAA*) and gluconeogenesis and into the production of lactate. *NADH*, reduced NAD; *CoA*, coenzyme A.

Ethanol is either a metabolite or a xenobiotic, depending on the amount consumed. When consumed in excess, ethanol is detoxified by the cytochrome P450 microsomal ethanol oxidizing system. However, when consumed in lower amounts, ethanol can enter normal metabolic pathways. In this case,

it is metabolized as if it were fat. Two enzymes, alcohol dehydrogenase (cytosol) and acetaldehyde dehydrogenase (mitochondrion), convert ethanol to acetate (Fig. 20-18). This increases the NADH to NAD$^+$ ratio in the cytosol and the mitochondrion, which becomes a significant problem in the chronic alcoholic who neglects carbohydrate intake. The shift to fasting metabolism mobilizes free fatty acids to the liver, adding to the acetyl-coenzyme A (CoA) already produced from ethanol metabolism. As is the case in starvation and untreated diabetes, when acetyl-CoA reaches very high levels for a sustained period, acetyl-CoA is shunted into production of ketones with resulting ketoacidosis. The situation is further complicated by the effect of the high NADH to NAD$^+$ ratio on pyruvate. Pyruvate would normally be routed to oxaloacetate for gluconeogenesis during inadequate carbohydrate intake, but instead it is shunted into lactate (Fig. 20-19). This not only produces lactic acidosis, but it leads to hypoglycemia as well.

PHARMACOLOGY

First-Pass Effect

Drugs that are administered orally (as opposed to intravenously, intramuscularly, sublingually, or transdermally) must first pass from the intestine to the liver before reaching the general circulation. Thus for many drugs, much of the dose is reduced by xenobiotic metabolism before reaching the tissues. Since some drugs are metabolized by gut flora or digestive enzymes, the first-pass effect refers to the combined effect of metabolism by the liver and in the gut.

KEY POINT ABOUT LIVER METABOLISM OF XENOBIOTICS AND ETHANOL

- Xenobiotics are nonnutritive chemicals that are metabolized in the liver in two phases: In phase 1 cytochrome P450 adds a hydroxyl group to the foreign molecule, and in phase 2 conjugation enzymes add a water-soluble molecule such as glycine that allows excretion in the urine or bile; xenobiotics include not only toxins and poisons but therapeutic drugs and ethanol.

Self-assessment questions can be accessed at www. StudentConsult.com.

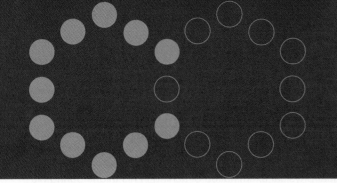

Case Studies

CHAPTER 1: ACID-BASE CONCEPTS

A 28-year-old female medical student is brought to the emergency room unconscious. Her blood pressure is 75/40, pulse 120, respiration rate 32. She demonstrates rapid, deep breathing and has a fruity odor to her breath. Her mother reports that she was studying for a biochemistry examination and that she had been very anxious about this examination for several days. She has taken daily insulin shots since the diagnosis of diabetes at the age of 15 with no prior complications. Blood tests showed pH 7.2 (normal 7.35 to 7.45), glucose 700 mg/dL, bicarbonate 10.1 mEq/L (normal 21 to 30 mEq/L), pCO_2 22 mm Hg (normal 35 to 40 mm Hg), and increased anion gap.

1. **What is the cause of her acidosis (lowered pH)?**

2. **How can her acidosis best be reversed?**

3. **How are her increased pulse and respiration related to ketoacidosis?**

CHAPTER 2: STRUCTURE AND PROPERTIES OF BIOLOGIC MOLECULES

A 7-day-old female full-term infant was brought to the emergency room with an enlarged liver, jaundice, failure to thrive, and urinary excretion of reducing sugars and albumin. Labor and delivery were normal, and her birth weight of 3.7 kg was normal. She was increasingly indolent and difficult to feed from the first day after birth. At the time of admission, her weight had dropped to 15% below normal. Blood analysis showed a normal hemoglobin level and elevated serum aspartate transaminase (AST) and alanine transaminase (ALT). Urinalysis with glucose oxidase was negative. She tolerated feeding with sucrose, maltose, glucose, and fructose at doses of 2 g/kg, but she vomited after lactose feeding.

1. **What is the reducing sugar that was found in the urine?**

2. **What other tissues will be affected by this disease?**

3. **Which substance causes the damage mentioned in question 2?**

CHAPTER 3: PROTEIN STRUCTURE AND FUNCTION

A 40-year-old woman developed dementia, myoclonus, weakness, and spasticity. Cerebellar ataxia was present. She became comatose, with decerebrate posturing, several months after the onset of neurologic signs. Postmortem brain biopsy showed spongiform encephalopathy consistent with Creutzfeldt-Jakob disease. Several encephalopathies including Creutzfeldt-Jakob disease are thought to be caused by prions.

1. **What is the composition of the prion that caused her encephalopathy?**

2. **What is the mechanism of infection for prions?**

3. **Draw an analogy between prion infections and cooperativity in hemoglobin.**

CHAPTER 4: ENZYMES AND ENERGETICS

A 30-year-old male scheduled an appointment with his physician because of tightness and discomfort in his chest. He experienced these symptoms while working in his yard, and they subsided after about 20 minutes of rest. At a previous appointment, his blood cholesterol was found to be greater than 400 mg/dL, but he did not follow the physician's advice concerning a cholesterol reduction diet. The physical examination revealed no abnormalities; however, his fasting cholesterol was measured at 436 mg/dL (normal < 200 mg/dL). He was started on simvastatin, 20 mg each evening, and was prescribed a cholesterol-lowering diet.

1. **What category of drugs does simvastatin belong to, and how do they work?**

2. **Simvastatin is effective in the range of 1 nmol/L, which is three orders of magnitude below the affinity for substrate. A portion of the simvastatin molecule bears a close resemblance to an intermediate in the formation of mevalonate from HMG-CoA. What is the likely mechanism of action of this drug?**

3. **Why can drugs of this category produce rhabdomyolysis with myoglobinuria?**

CHAPTER 5: MEMBRANES AND INTRACELLULAR SIGNAL TRANSDUCTION

A 42-year-old female medical student has returned from a medical missionary trip to a tropical rain forest in South America. She has developed watery diarrhea, nausea, and light-headedness. Upon admission to the hospital, she was experiencing faint heart sounds and orthostatic hypotension, and her diarrhea in large amounts of clear liquid continued. She recovered after treatment with oral antibiotics and fluid and electrolyte replacement.

1. **Which microorganisms are most likely to be found in the stool?**

2. **What is the biochemical mechanism for the watery diarrhea?**

3. **What is the cause of the faint heart sounds and orthostatic hypotension?**

CHAPTER 6: GLYCOLYSIS AND PYRUVATE OXIDATION

A 9-year-old boy was brought to the clinic with the complaint that he was acting and talking strangely, "as if he were drunk." His mother reported that this had occurred occasionally since he was 1 year of age. These episodes occurred after stressful periods such as a febrile illness or fatigue. On examination, the boy showed rapid breathing and rapid heart rate. He walked with an unsteady, wide-based gait and had generalized weakness of the extremities. Laboratory analysis showed elevated blood lactate (3.8 mmol/L; normal 0.5 to 2.2 mmol/L) and blood pyruvate (0.36 mmol/L; normal 0.03 to 0.08 mmol/L), although the lactate-to-pyruvate ratio was normal. A similar elevation with a normal lactate-to-pyruvate ratio was observed in the cerebrospinal fluid. Alanine was elevated (855 μmol/L; normal 338–472 μmol/L). Blood pH was slightly acid at 7.30 (normal 7.35 to 7.45). Blood glucose and ketones were normal. No ragged red fibers were observed in a skeletal muscle biopsy.

1. **What is the most likely enzyme deficiency?**

2. **How would you determine if this was a high anion gap acidosis?**

3. **What is the underlying cause of the neurologic observations for this patient?**

CHAPTER 7: CITRIC ACID CYCLE, ELECTRON TRANSPORT CHAIN, AND OXIDATIVE PHOSPHORYLATION

A 53-year-old physiology professor complained during an annual physical examination of aching in his thighs during his 4-mile morning run. No significant changes had been made in the length or speed of the running schedule. The aching occurs only during the last part of a run and subsides upon cessation. He has been running 20 to 25 miles per week since age 35 without significant complications. He has a history of elevated blood lipids and has been taking a standard daily dose of a statin drug for the past 2 years. A routine laboratory profile was normal, but the creatine phosphokinase (CPK) value was 250 IU/L (normal 20 to 200 IU/L).

1. **How could the action of the statin drug be correlated with his symptoms?**

2. **What other potential complications does this patient need to be aware of?**

3. **What cellular compartment(s) contain coenzyme Q?**

CHAPTER 8: GLUCONEOGENESIS AND GLYCOGEN METABOLISM

A 6-year-old male is examined by his family physician for episodic fatigue, nausea, and light-headedness brought on when meals are skipped. He has marked hepatomegaly on physical examination. Laboratory results indicate lactic acidosis, hyperlipidemia, elevated serum uric acid, and marked hypoglycemia. Intravenous fructose was not converted to glucose.

1. **What is the cause of the fatigue, nausea, and light-headedness?**

2. **How is the lactic acidosis produced?**

3. **What other organ would be enlarged?**

CHAPTER 9: MINOR CARBOHYDRATE PATHWAYS: RIBOSE, FRUCTOSE, AND GALACTOSE

A 27-year-old black male has come to the clinic with complaints of fatigue and yellowing of his eyes and the palms of his hands. He has an elevated heart rate (HR 95, normal 60 to 90) and pallor around his mouth and in his nail beds. His liver is of normal size. His indirect bilirubin is elevated, and his hemoglobin is low (9.1 g/dL, normal 13.8 to 17.2 g/dL). He had been prescribed primaquine on his return home from an extended sales trip to Thailand for treatment of malaria that he had contracted there.

1. How does the pallor in his nail beds and around his mouth correlate with the yellow color in his eyes and the palms of his hands?

2. How are the symptoms in question 1 related to taking primaquine?

3. Why was his heart rate elevated?

CHAPTER 10: FATTY ACID AND TRIGLYCERIDE METABOLISM

A 4-month-old male was admitted to the hospital in a coma, and shortly after admission he went into cardiac arrest. He was successfully resuscitated. On examination, he was found to have cardiomegaly and hepatomegaly and was hypoglycemic, with a blood glucose of 15 mg/dL (normal 60 to 100 mg/dL). He had no acidosis or ketosis, but his blood ammonia was elevated (300 μg/dL; normal, <69 μg/dL). Further studies showed normal glucose, fructose, and galactose tolerance. A 10-hour fasting blood glucose was normal, but a 32-hour fast produced a drop to 66 mg/dL accompanied by a rise in serum triglycerides. The fast was ended at 32 hours due to the development of generalized seizures and cardiac arrest. He was resuscitated and given intravenous glucose. Liver and muscle biopsy showed accumulations of neutral fat.

1. Do the hepatomegaly and hypoglycemia indicate a glycogen storage disease?

2. What is the reason for the neutral fat accumulations in this patient's muscle and liver?

3. What could have caused the cardiac arrest and the associated seizures in this patient?

CHAPTER 11: METABOLISM OF STEROIDS AND OTHER LIPIDS

A 3-year-old child has hypertension and fluid retention. Laboratory studies show below normal serum cortisol, an increase in urine dehydroepiandrosterone, and an increase in serum ACTH. Although a genotype of XX was determined by cytologic analysis, the genitalia appear to be male.

1. What is the most likely cause of the hypertension and fluid retention?

2. Why does this genetically female child have male genitalia?

3. What tissues contain the biochemical abnormality in this patient?

CHAPTER 12: AMINO ACID AND HEME METABOLISM

An 8-month-old female is admitted to the emergency room with ataxia and episodes of screaming. She had become irritable shortly after being weaned to a mixed diet and demonstrated increasing vomiting. She was progressively lethargic, eventually developing a coma after a meal high in protein. Her liver function tests showed slightly elevated transaminases, and her blood ammonia was 290 to 700 μmol/L (normal 25 to 40 μmol/L). Her blood glutamine was also elevated, and blood pH was 7.5 (normal 7.35 to 7.45). Citrulline was not detectable in the blood, but orotic acid was elevated. Her condition improved on a low-protein diet.

1. The patient's elevated blood ammonia suggests a urea cycle defect. Based on the information available, which enzyme is most likely deficient?

2. How could elevated ammonia lead to the behavioral abnormalities seen in this patient?

3. How does hyperammonemia contribute to the elevated blood pH?

CHAPTER 13: INTEGRATION OF CARBOHYDRATE, FAT, AND AMINO ACID METABOLISM

A 29-year-old female medical student was admitted to the emergency room unconscious. Her blood pressure (lying down) was 90/45, pulse 125, respiratory rate 35. When she is raised to a sitting position, her systolic blood pressure drops to 40. Her heart sounds are normal. The emergency medical technician reported a fruity odor to her breath. Urinalysis shows the presence of glucose and ketones. Blood analysis gives a glucose measurement of 820 mg/dL, blood urea nitrogen (BUN) of 36 mg/dL (normal 8 to 23 mg/dL), pH of 7.25 (normal 7.35 to 7.45), bicarbonate of 10 mg/dL (normal 21 to 30 mg/dL), and K^+ of 5.5 mEq/L (normal 3.8 to 5.0 mEq/L). She was diagnosed with insulin-dependent diabetes mellitus at the age of 13 and has controlled it successfully with daily insulin injections of about 20 U/day. Her parents reported that she had been studying for final examinations for the past 4 days and had been alone in her room for most of that time. They did notice that she was extremely anxious about her marginal performance this semester and was afraid she might fail several of her courses. Treatment with regular insulin in isotonic saline and K^+ is successful, and she is released the next day.

1. Why was the patient's BUN elevated?

2. Explain the patient's blood pressure and heart rate symptoms, and give the reason for the sudden drop in systolic pressure upon sitting up.

3. Is the student's mental state relevant to her ketoacidosis? Explain why or why not.

4. Explain why her serum K^+ was elevated on admission, and why it was necessary to administer it in the saline drip along with her insulin.

CHAPTER 14: PURINE, PYRIMIDINE, AND SINGLE-CARBON METABOLISM

A 50-year-old male comes to your office with severe pain and swelling in his first metatarsophalangeal joint (MTP). He had celebrated his 50th birthday with a large steak dinner and a larger than normal amount of red wine. He normally limits his red meat intake because of a history of kidney stones that were determined to be uric acid stones. Urine analysis confirmed an elevated uric acid in his urine, with urate crystals present. On physical examination, he was febrile (38.3° C) and his MTP joint was warm and red. Blood analysis showed an increased erythrocyte sedimentation rate (ESR) and an elevation in his white blood cell count. An attack of gout was diagnosed, and he was treated with colchicine and NSAIDs for several days until the pain decreased. Long-term management with allopurinol was then prescribed.

1. Why was colchicine prescribed before allopurinol?

2. Why were all of his joints not affected?

3. How is his joint redness and warmth related to the white blood cell count and ESR?

CHAPTER 15: ORGANIZATION, SYNTHESIS, AND REPAIR OF DNA

A 25-year-old farm worker has just been diagnosed with malignant melanoma. She has been sensitive to sunlight all her life and has abundant freckles and bleached spots on areas of her body frequently exposed to the sun. There are additional skin abnormalities such as telangiectasias, erythema, and hypopigmentation. She is scheduled for removal of the melanoma, and increased protection from sunlight is prescribed.

1. What genetic disease does this patient have that predisposed her to malignant melanoma?

2. What normal component of skin protects DNA from UV irradiation? Where is it produced, and what is its location?

3. What is the most common form of skin cancer that is caused by UV radiation, and what are its characteristics?

CHAPTER 16: RNA TRANSCRIPTION AND CONTROL OF GENE EXPRESSION

A 2-year-old boy of Indian descent has been suffering an increasing number of infections. He was healthy at birth but has lost much of his appetite and his complexion has become pale. His parents have been supplementing his diet with iron, thinking he was anemic, but iron has not helped. Laboratory analysis of his blood reveals that his red blood cells contain hemoglobin A_2 and fetal hemoglobin, but no hemoglobin A. Cooley's anemia (homozygous β-thalassemia) is diagnosed, and the patient is scheduled for blood transfusions with deferoxamine therapy.

1. How can mutation at sites other than an exon disrupt the production of normal β-globin mRNA?

2. Some patients with Cooley's anemia develop a condition called hereditary persistence of fetal hemoglobin (HPFH) that alleviates the severity of the symptoms. What effect would HPFH have on the oxygen saturation curve?

3. How does deferoxamine help treat thalassemia patients who require regular blood transfusions?

CHAPTER 17: PROTEIN SYNTHESIS AND DEGRADATION

A Peace Corps worker in South America has reported to the clinic with a headache, sore throat, and fever. He is hoarse with a brassy cough. His posterior pharynx shows a "shaggy," gray membranous material. He reports that several days ago he had been cleaning out a hut that had been empty for a few months after the occupant had died of an infectious disease. A throat culture is positive for *Corynebacterium diphtheriae.*

1. **What other bacterial toxins have the same type of mechanism of action as the toxin produced by *Corynebacterium diphtheriae*, and what is the mechanism?**

2. **How could the patient have been infected when cleaning out the hut?**

3. **What treatment options are available to the patient?**

CHAPTER 18: RECOMBINANT DNA AND BIOTECHNOLOGY

A 3-year-old male is brought to the pediatrician because he has begun to stumble and has obvious difficulty running, jumping, and climbing stairs. His calf muscles have also become noticeably enlarged. Deletion scanning polymerase chain reaction (PCR) was used to confirm the diagnosis of Duchenne muscular dystrophy.

1. **What is the molecular basis for Duchenne muscular dystrophy?**

2. **Could his disease be predicted by symptoms demonstrated by his mother and father?**

3. **What is the function of dystrophin?**

CHAPTER 19: NUTRITION

A 13-month-old female of African descent was admitted to the hospital for growth failure. Her mother was concerned that she could not pull herself up to stand and her legs had become bowed. A dietary history showed that she was exclusively breast-fed and she refused all table food. Her mother rarely ate meat or green vegetables and avoided all dairy foods because of lactose intolerance. Her primary diet consisted of eggs, cornflakes, and potatoes. The patient was confined to home except for brief periods when she was taken outside heavily clothed. On physical examination, her height and weight were in the bottom fifth percentile. Radiographic findings indicated a widening of the epiphyseal plates.

1. **What dietary deficiency would explain these symptoms?**

2. **Why were the epiphyseal plates showing widening?**

3. **What other skeletal abnormalities would present in a patient with this disease?**

CHAPTER 20: TISSUE BIOCHEMISTRY

A 30-year-old male went to his family physician with the complaint that he is having increasing difficulty breathing (dyspnea). He works out in a gym at lunchtime and began to notice shortness of breath over a year ago, but now it occurs even at rest. Physical examination reveals a barrel-shaped chest with decreased breath sounds on both sides. CT imaging indicates a panacinar emphysema (cotton-candy appearance). α_1-Antitrypsin deficiency was diagnosed, and weekly injections of purified human α_1-antitrypsin were prescribed.

1. **Why is antitrypsin activity needed in the lungs, and where is it produced?**

2. **How is emphysema produced by cigarette smoking distinguished from α_1-antitrypsin deficiency?**

3. **How do the barrel-shaped chest and decreased breath sounds correlate with emphysema?**

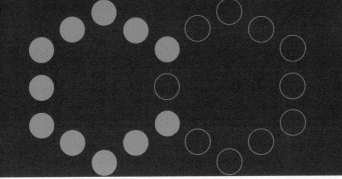

Case Study Answers

CHAPTER 1: ACID-BASE CONCEPTS

1. The suffix -osis denotes a process, usually an increase. In this patient, her acidosis is due to the process of excessive fat mobilization. Since the only point of control over fatty acid oxidation is at the point of hormone-sensitive lipase in adipose cells, all fatty acids released are oxidized by the liver at the maximum rate. The patient's anxiety over the biochemistry examination could have contributed in two ways: she may have forgotten to take her insulin, or the stress hormones, epinephrine, and glucocorticoids acted as insulin antagonists and raised her insulin requirement. The elevated blood sugar indicates that her body was not getting enough insulin, resulting in failure to suppress the mobilization of free fatty acids from her adipose tissue. Excess β-oxidation of these fatty acids led to the overproduction of CoA in her liver. The shunt pathway that disposes of the excess acetyl-CoA produces the ketone bodies acetoacetate and β-hydroxybutyrate, and raises the blood levels of these acidic metabolites.

2. Since the acidosis is being caused by the uncontrolled release of free fatty acids from adipose tissue, the most direct way to treat the acidosis is by administration of insulin. When the source of the ketone bodies is removed by suppression of fat mobilization, the normal buffering mechanisms provided by the renal and respiratory systems (in addition to the blood buffers [i.e., bicarbonate, phosphate, and hemoglobin]) will quickly restore the pH to the normal range. Because insulin causes up-regulation of the intracellular Na^+/K^+ATPase pump, it is important to coadminister the electrolyte potassium, since insulin will cause it to be removed quickly from the blood.

3. The equilibrium of the bicarbonate system is shifted toward the production of CO_2 from carbonic acid as the proton concentration rises. Therefore, ketoacidosis increases the respiration rate to eliminate CO_2 from the blood. As protons combine with bicarbonate to form carbonic acid, the concentration of bicarbonate in the blood falls. The increased pulse rate is related more indirectly to ketoacidosis, since it is due to a compensation for the drop in blood pressure, which in turn is due to a drop in blood volume. The blood volume is reduced in the untreated diabetic because of the polyuria precipitated by both increased spilling of glucose into the urine and the increased disposal of ketone bodies.

CHAPTER 2: STRUCTURE AND PROPERTIES OF BIOLOGIC MOLECULES

1. The presenting symptoms are consistent with classic hereditary galactosemia. Liver enlargement, lethargy, vomiting, jaundice, and failure to thrive all result from disruption of liver function due to the buildup of galactose 1-phosphate. This metabolite accumulates because the enzyme galactose-1-phosphate uridyltransferase (GALT) is genetically absent. The buildup of galactose 1-phosphate in the liver cell increases the amount of galactose that spills into the blood and urine. The elevated bilirubin (jaundice) is also due to liver cell damage from galactose 1-phosphate. Fructose is a reducing sugar, and it would appear in the urine of infants with hereditary fructose intolerance, but this infant tolerated both sucrose and fructose feedings. Sorbitol and galactitol are sugar alcohols, and because they lack an aldehyde group, they are not reducing sugars. Maltose is a disaccharide that is digested to glucose before it is absorbed from the gut.

2. Infants with galactosemia usually develop cataracts affecting the lens of the eye. Although red blood cells (RBCs) normally contain the GALT enzyme, the normal RBC count in this patient indicates that the RBCs are not affected when GALT is genetically deficient. Heart muscle, the optic nerve, and the CNS are sites of damage for many metabolic diseases, but not galactosemia.

3. The increase in serum galactose allows increased diffusion of galactose into the lens of the eye, where it is converted to galactitol by aldose reductase (this same enzyme converts glucose to sorbitol). The accumulation of this polyalcohol denatures the proteins in the lens, causing cataracts. If the patient is treated early with a lactose-free diet, the cataracts can be reversible.

CHAPTER 3: PROTEIN STRUCTURE AND FUNCTION

1. Prions are composed only of protein. Recombinant prions free of contamination from unidentified coinfectious agents can cause encephalopathy. Infectious agents normally are expected to contain a nucleic acid genome in order to replicate themselves. Prions do not replicate by genetic

means, but rather by altering the normally produced wild-type prion protein.

2. The infectious route for prions is by ingestion of infected tissue, such as brain tissue. The prion protein is protease resistant, allowing it to be absorbed intact from the digestive system. When the absorbed prions are distributed to the brain, they create amyloid fibrils by physical contact with normal wild-type prions that serve an as yet unknown function on the surface of neurons. The secondary structure in the wild-type prion protein (PrP) is converted from predominantly α-helical to β-pleated-sheet–rich structures (PrP^{Sc}). The β-sheet structure is the factor that confers protease resistance.

3. Prion infections are similar to hemoglobin cooperativity because they both involve the induction of a change in protein conformation through physical contact. When a subunit within hemoglobin binds oxygen, it undergoes a change in conformation and induces the same change in an adjacent subunit that is communicated through physical contact (breaking salt bridges). Similarly, when a prion protein comes into physical contact with a normal wild-type prion protein, it induces a new stable shape that includes rearrangement of its secondary structure. In both cases, a change in conformation occurs through physical contact.

CHAPTER 4: ENZYMES AND ENERGETICS

1. Simvastatin belongs to a group of inhibitors of cholesterol synthesis called "statins." They function as HMG-CoA reductase inhibitors and thus block the initial, and rate-determining, step in the cholesterol synthetic pathway. They were prescribed for this patient as an adjunct to a cholesterol-lowering diet.

2. The likely mechanism for all statin drugs is as a transition state analog. These are among the most potent enzyme inhibitors, since they work at very low concentrations. Transition state analogs have a structure that matches the substrate after it has undergone a structural change in the active site as it is converted to the product. Because they work at the active site, transition state analogs are competitive inhibitors.

3. Rhabdomyolysis induced by statin drugs is due to their effect on the synthesis of coenzyme Q (CoQ). The cholesterol pathway has isoprenoid intermediates that are used in the synthesis of the 10-unit isoprene hydrocarbon tail of CoQ. Inhibition of cholesterol synthesis thus also restricts the availability of isoprenoid units for CoQ synthesis as well as for prenylation of integral membrane proteins (see Chapter 5). Reduced CoQ concentrations lead to increased production of reactive O_2 intermediates (ROI) that cause free radical damage to cell components. A severely damaged muscle cell will leak its components, such as myoglobin, into the blood, producing myoglobinemia and myoglobinuria.

CHAPTER 5: MEMBRANES AND INTRACELLULAR SIGNAL TRANSDUCTION

1. This patient has cholera, a disease caused by *Vibrio cholerae*. This bacterium produces a toxin that induces the symptoms by interfering with electrolyte balance in the intestine through its action on the G_s protein in lumen cells. There is no inflammatory component to this disease; it is toxin-induced. The G_s protein can also be inactivated by the enterotoxin from enterotoxigenic *Escherichia coli*, the microorganism that produces traveler's diarrhea.

2. Cholera toxin binds tightly to G_{M1} ganglioside on the intestinal cell membrane. A toxin subunit enters the cytoplasm and triggers the ADP ribosylation of the G_s protein, permanently activating it. This stimulates transport of chloride into the intestinal lumen, resulting in a secretory diarrhea. Thus elevated cAMP in the intestinal lumen "equals" water and electrolyte secretion into the lumen.

3. Orthostatic hypotension can be caused by volume depletion. Reduction in blood volume reduces cardiac output through reduced preload. The reduced volume of blood in the heart chambers also produces less pressure to close the valves during contraction, thus reducing the heart sounds.

CHAPTER 6: GLYCOLYSIS AND PYRUVATE OXIDATION

1. The simultaneous appearance of lactate and pyruvate indicates an inability to metabolize pyruvate. If lactate alone were elevated, then a condition causing the accumulation of NADH, such as hypoxia or ethanol consumption, would be indicated. Inability to metabolize pyruvate can be caused by pyruvate carboxylase deficiency, but this is ruled out, since it would be accompanied by hypoglycemia (the blood glucose was normal). It could also be caused by a mitochondrial disease, but this is ruled out, since ragged red fibers are absent (ragged red fibers are characteristic of mitochondrial deficiency). The only remaining, and most likely, cause of elevated pyruvate is a deficiency in the pyruvate dehydrogenase complex or in the pyruvate dehydrogenase phosphatase enzyme that is needed to maintain the active form of the complex.

2. Anion gap refers to the anions in the serum other than bicarbonate and chloride that are needed to balance the sodium and potassium positive charge. Normally, the anion gap is accounted for by plasma proteins (normal = 16 mEq/L). However, when organic acids, such as lactate, accumulate in the blood, the normal buffering by bicarbonate causes a substitution of the organic acid for bicarbonate anion. This increase in anion gap is seen in various conditions, such as diabetes, that produce metabolic acidosis.

3. A deficiency of the pyruvate dehydrogenase complex (PDC) deprives the brain of its only source of energy, since it is totally reliant on glucose as an energy source except in conditions of extreme starvation (when it can use ketone bodies). Since the PDC connects pyruvate produced in glycolysis with the citric acid cycle and oxidative phosphorylation, any reduction in rate for this activity leads to a reduction in citric acid cycle activity. The brain can use amino acids that transaminate into citric acid cycle components, but each amino acid that enters the cycle must be matched by an acetyl-CoA from the PDC pathway. Deficiencies in PDC lead to developmental and degenerative abnormalities as shown by computed tomography or magnetic resonance imaging. Cerebral atrophy, ventricular dilation, and agenesis of the corpus callosum or medullary pyramids are occasionally associated with PDC deficiency.

CHAPTER 7: CITRIC ACID CYCLE, ELECTRON TRANSPORT CHAIN, AND OXIDATIVE PHOSPHORYLATION

1. Statin drugs are potent competitive inhibitors of HMG-CoA reductase, the rate-controlling step in cholesterol synthesis. The muscle aches (myalgia) would not be caused by lowering the rate of cholesterol synthesis, however, but by reduction in one of the precursors in the cholesterol synthesis pathway, namely, isoprene. This five-carbon hydrophobic unit is added to various biomolecules to help them dissolve in the lipid environment of membranes. In the case of coenzyme Q, 10 isoprene units are polymerized in a linear hydrophobic "tail" (see Fig. 7-3) attached to coenzyme Q. A reduction in the availability of isoprene due to the statin also reduces the amount of coenzyme Q in the electron transport chain, leading to a reduction in energy (ATP) output by the muscle mitochondria.

2. In severe cases in which patients are highly sensitive to the action of the statin, muscle fibers can sustain pathologic damage (myopathy) resulting in rhabdomyolysis with acute renal failure secondary to myoglobinuria. The myoglobinuria is caused by severe damage to the muscle fibers (rhabdomyolysis), allowing the cellular myoglobin to leak into the bloodstream and pass into the urine. In this case, the CPK was only slightly above normal, showing early but not pathologic signs. Myopathy is characterized by CPK values greater than 10 times normal. Another complication that can occur with statin drugs is liver damage, which is generally detected by elevations in serum transaminase enzymes. This patient's blood screen, which included serum transaminases, was normal.

3. The only known location and function for coenzyme Q is in the inner mitochondrial membrane, where it is a component of the electron transport chain.

CHAPTER 8: GLUCONEOGENESIS AND GLYCOGEN METABOLISM

1. The fatigue, nausea, and light-headedness are all symptoms of hypoglycemia. The effect of low blood sugar on the central nervous system (CNS) is usually mediated through the autonomic nervous system and can also lead to sweating, tremor, and palpitations. The effect of hypoglycemia on the CNS is referred to as neuroglycopenia.

2. The lactic acidosis is an indirect effect of an increase in pyruvate due to increased glycolysis. This patient has Von Gierke disease, a deficiency in glucose-6-phosphatase activity. Both glycogenolysis and gluconeogenesis in the liver produce glucose-6-phosphate (G6P) for conversion to glucose. However, glucose-6-phosphatase deficiency produces a marked increase in G6P in the cell. This pushes glycolysis to pyruvate, but the pyruvate is prevented from entering the citric acid cycle, since fatty acids are already producing large amounts of acetyl-CoA. The pyruvate is shunted into lactate, which then spills into the bloodstream.

3. Kidney tubules also become enlarged in this disease, for the same reason that the liver enlarges (i.e., stimulation of glycogen synthase by G6P). The renal tubules rely on glucose-6-phosphatase to release free glucose into the circulation, and when the G6P concentrations increase, glycogen synthase is stimulated to synthesize glycogen.

CHAPTER 9: MINOR CARBOHYDRATE PATHWAYS: RIBOSE, FRUCTOSE, AND GALACTOSE

1. The pallor is due to anemia. The blood is below normal for the hemoglobin value, and this reflects anemia. When anemia is due to accelerated hemolysis, hemoglobin is released into the circulation in amounts that overwhelm the ability of the liver to conjugate it so that it can be easily excreted. Instead, the unconjugated bilirubin, which is highly lipid soluble, becomes sequestered in the tissues, especially in fatty tissue such as the skin. Thus the yellow color, referred to as jaundice, is due to an elevation in bilirubin, specifically the unconjugated form of bilirubin measured as indirect bilirubin.

2. This patient is deficient in glucose-6-phosphate dehydrogenase (G6PD), an X-linked disorder seen in about 15% of American black males. Exposure of his red blood cells to primaquine has caused the hemolytic anemia. Primaquine creates active O_2 radicals that normally are neutralized by glutathione peroxidase. However, the activity of glutathione peroxidase is supported by NADPH produced in the pentose phosphate pathway. Thus a G6PD deficiency reduces the available NADPH and the ability of glutathione peroxidase to protect the red blood cell membrane from oxidative damage.

3. Patients with anemia are unable to transport enough O_2 to their tissues, leading to a compensatory increase in heart rate. This can be accompanied by a moderate degree of dyspnea as a further indication of reduced oxygenation of the blood.

CHAPTER 10: FATTY ACID AND TRIGLYCERIDE METABOLISM

1. This patient has a carnitine deficiency, which can also produce hepatomegaly and hypoglycemia. While glycogen storage diseases often present with hypoglycemia and hepatomegaly, only one produces cardiomegaly and is accompanied by cardiac failure. However, tissue biopsy would show glycogen accumulations within lysosomes, not fat accumulations. Also, Von Gierke's disease would have shown a fasting hypoglycemia, but it would have occurred within a few hours after the last meal rather than the 32-hour interval observed with this patient. In addition, a patient with Von Gierke disease will demonstrate both acidosis and ketosis, but this patient had neither.

2. The neutral fat accumulations are not normal components of muscle and liver tissue. They are due to the inability of fatty acids to be transported into mitochondria to undergo β-oxidation. The increased concentrations of free fatty acids are shunted into the pathway that forms triglycerides under these conditions, and the triglycerides aggregate into droplets. This would only occur under fasting conditions, when triglycerides are being mobilized from adipose tissue in a one-way route to the tissues.

3. Heart muscle is highly active and relies heavily on aerobic metabolism for its energy supply. Either glucose or free fatty acids are needed to support aerobic metabolism, and in this patient both are in short supply during fasting. This patient cannot manufacture glucose, because the energy supplied by free fatty acids is not available owing to the deficiency in carnitine. Likewise, the carnitine deficiency prevents the direct use of fatty acids by heart muscle. The greatly reduced energy supply to the heart can lead to the inability to conduct an excitatory impulse and to cardiac arrest. Although the brain does not rely on fatty acids for energy, the extreme hypoglycemia can explain the appearance of seizures.

CHAPTER 11: METABOLISM OF STEROIDS AND OTHER LIPIDS

1. This patient has a deficiency in 11β-hydroxylase activity. The resulting increase in deoxycorticosterone causes fluid retention due to sodium retention. The fluid retention is the cause of the hypertension.

2. The reduced secretion of cortisol has caused the pituitary to release increased amounts of ACTH as a signal to replace the deficit of cortisol. Since ACTH stimulates the desmolase enzyme that produces pregnenolone, the production of progesterone is also increased. This leads to an increase in the synthesis of testosterone, which causes the virilization of the genitalia.

3. The deficiency in 11β-hydroxylase activity affects the zona glomerulosa of the adrenal cortex, where 11-deoxycorticosterone is converted to corticosterone. It also affects the zona fasciculata of the adrenal cortex, where 11-deoxycortisol is converted to cortisol.

CHAPTER 12: AMINO ACID AND HEME METABOLISM

1. The most likely defect is ornithine transcarbamoylase. Any other downstream deficiency would cause an elevation in citrulline and ammonia, but citrulline is not present in the blood. Also, ornithine transcarbamoylase deficiencies are usually accompanied by an elevation in orotic acid, since the buildup of carbamoyl phosphate pushes the pyrimidine synthesis pathway.

2. Normal neurotransmission is disrupted by ammonia in several ways. Ammonia increases the transport of tryptophan across the blood-brain barrier, leading to an increase in the level of serotonin, which is the basis for anorexia in hyperammonemia. Chronic hyperammonemia is also associated with an increase in inhibitory neurotransmission due to down-regulation of glutamate receptors because extrasynaptic glutamate accumulates. This can lead to deterioration of intellectual function, decreased consciousness, and coma. Extracellular glutamate also results in activation of the N-methyl-D-aspartate (NMDA) receptor, causing the seizures in acute hyperammonemia.

3. Free ammonia can be excreted by the kidney through the deamination of glutamine by glutaminase and glutamate dehydrogenase. The ammonia released in the tubular cell diffuses into the tubular lumen, where it is trapped as the charged ammonium by reaction with protons. This pulls protons out of the blood, raising the pH. Further consumption of protons occurs when the α-ketoglutarate produced by glutamate dehydrogenase is converted to glucose via the gluconeogenic pathway.

CHAPTER 13: INTEGRATION OF CARBOHYDRATE, FAT, AND AMINO ACID METABOLISM

1. The elevated BUN represents the mobilization of amino acids for use by the liver to support gluconeogenesis. This occurs for the same reason that fatty acids are mobilized to such an extent that they spill into the ketogenic pathway to produce the acidic ketone bodies. The absence of insulin permits both of these processes to proceed at maximum rates. This is comparable to extended fasting when insulin levels have dropped and amino acids and fatty acids must be mobilized for the liver to produce glucose.

2. The below normal blood pressure is due to volume depletion. The appearance of glucose and ketones in the urine indicates that water is also being pulled out of the blood, since both these molecules bind water. The term diabetes refers to excessive urination. Blood pressure is a function of the cardiac output and the peripheral resistance. In this case, the lower blood volume has reduced the cardiac output, thereby lowering the blood pressure. The increased heart rate is a compensatory attempt to maintain the blood

pressure by increasing cardiac output. The drop in pressure when the patient rises to a sitting position is called orthostatic hypotension and is due to an inability to draw on blood normally pooled in the venous system and available to increase the cardiac output.

3. This patient has been under severe mental stress for several days. During this time, both epinephrine, the short-term stress hormone, and glucocorticoids, the long-term stress hormones, have been elevated. The effect of epinephrine is to mobilize free fatty acids, contributing to the ketoacidosis, and also to mobilize liver glycogen, contributing to an elevation in blood glucose. The glucocorticoids have an antiinsulin effect through their action to down-regulate IRS-1. Both hormones reduce the effect of the patient's insulin injections. It is unknown whether the student's stressful situation also may have caused her to neglect her daily insulin injections.

4. The serum K^+ concentration is affected in part by the activity of the Na^+/K^+-ATPase levels in the tissues. Insulin tends to up-regulate this membrane transporter; in the absence of insulin, it is down-regulated. This patient's serum K^+ was elevated, therefore, because its normal transport into the tissues was reduced. One of the greatest risks to a patient in ketoacidotic crisis is that the administration of insulin, accompanied by up-regulation of the transporter, will create a severe, although temporary, depression in the serum concentration of K^+. Coadministration of K^+ with insulin prevents this temporary depression.

CHAPTER 14: PURINE, PYRIMIDINE, AND SINGLE-CARBON METABOLISM

1. Colchicine does not treat the elevated uric acid, but it does interrupt the inflammatory response. Colchicine acts by blocking phagocytosis of the urate crystals by white blood cells, such as neutrophils. The sodium urate crystals are unique in that their needlelike structure punctures lysosomes, causing their digestive enzymes to be released into the cytoplasm. This also occurs in synovial tissue, causing destruction of that tissue. The tissue damage resulting from the action of the digestive enzymes develops a self-sustaining cycle of destruction as more white cells are recruited to the damaged area. Interrupting the phagocytic response interrupts and reduces the inflammatory process. The long-term treatment plan with allopurinol blocks the excessive uric acid formation and causes the purine degradation intermediates, hypoxanthine and xanthine, to increase. Neither of these intermediates has a tendency to form crystals and both are water soluble, thus allowing for their easy elimination by the kidney.

2. The joints in the extremities are affected by the formation of sodium urate crystals because they are colder than joints located centrally. The solubility of sodium urate is lower in the "colder" extremities and crystallizes more readily. The same concentration of sodium urate is present in all of the joints. Infants who have gout secondary either to von Gierke

disease (type I glycogen storage disease) or to Lesch-Nyhan syndrome will have "orange sand" in their diapers, since the urine, which is saturated with uric acid, drops to a temperature that permits uric acid crystallization.

3. The white blood cell count and increased ESR are both caused by the inflammatory process. The tissue damage caused by exposure to intracellular digestive enzymes stimulates an active inflammatory process that continues until the tissue damage is repaired. The joint redness and warmth are due to the local effect of autacoids that stimulate vasodilation.

CHAPTER 15: ORGANIZATION, SYNTHESIS, AND REPAIR OF DNA

1. The patient has xeroderma pigmentosum, a genetic disease caused by a deficiency in one of eight different excision repair enzymes (XPA through XPG). The skin abnormalities are all characteristic of this disease because the absence of repair inactivates normal genes and creates abnormal "clones" in the skin. Freckles and bleached spots are considered to arise as clones of these mutations.

2. The normal UV protection in the skin is the protein melanin, which is composed entirely of polymerized tyrosine. The tyrosine ring absorbs UV light and prevents it from reaching the nucleus. Melanin is contained in melanosomes that are transferred from the melanosomes which synthesize them to keratinocytes in the stratum basale and stratum spinosum. They are then localized distal (on the "sunny side") to the nucleus.

3. Basal cell carcinoma is the most common form of skin cancer caused by chronic exposure to UV light. It is a nonmetastatic cancer that infiltrates the deep tissues adjacent to its origin, usually sun-exposed areas of the body. It arises from the basal cell layer of the epidermis, from which it invades the underlying dermis.

CHAPTER 16: RNA TRANSCRIPTION AND CONTROL OF GENE EXPRESSION

1. Synthesis of the normal β-globin mRNA can be blocked by a mutation in the promoter, which would prevent RNA polymerase from binding, or by a mutation in a splice site, which would prevent functional mRNA from being translated.

2. The oxygen saturation curve in a patient with HPFH would be shifted to the left, indicating that it had a higher affinity for O_2. The allosteric effect of 2,3-BPG in the tissues would allow for sufficient unloading of O_2.

3. Deferoxamine (desferrioxamine) is a chelating agent that binds iron so that it can be eliminated from the body. Deferoxamine is needed because the anemic condition causes the gut to absorb more iron, which in Cooley's anemia is not needed. The additional iron added by the blood transfusions could easily lead to iron toxicity.

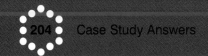

CHAPTER 17: PROTEIN SYNTHESIS AND DEGRADATION

1. Cholera toxin and pertussis toxin work through the same mechanism as diphtheria toxin, produced by *Corynebacterium diphtheriae*, but all have different targets. The mechanism is called ADP-ribosylation, in which the target protein is covalently modified through the attachment of an adenine diphosphoribose. The target protein for cholera is the G_s protein in intestinal mucosa, and for pertussis it is the G_i protein in the tissues of the respiratory tract.

2. The infectious disease that killed the previous occupant was *C. diphtheriae*. The pseudomembrane produced during advanced stages of the disease was coughed out into the environment, where it dried and turned to dust. The bacterium contained in this dust is stable in these conditions for several months.

3. The patient was treated with diphtheria antitoxin and erythromycin. The antitoxin is necessary to reduce the amount of active toxin, since it can continue to kill cells, and the antibiotic is to prevent the patient from being a carrier after recovery.

CHAPTER 18: RECOMBINANT DNA AND BIOTECHNOLOGY

1. Duchenne muscular dystrophy patients have deletions in their X chromosome large enough to remove one or more exons from the gene, producing a dysfunctional dystrophin protein. The missing exon is identified by use of primers for the most deletion-prone exons. The missing exon will be revealed by the absence of its DNA band on electrophoresis and blotting.

2. Duchenne muscular dystrophy is an X-linked disorder, and neither parent is necessarily affected. The father contributes only the Y chromosome, so the mother needs only one defective allele for the phenotype to appear in male offspring. With one normal allele in the mother, each son has a 50-50 chance of getting the disease.

3. Dystrophin helps link α-actinin and desmin intermediate filaments to the sarcolemma. It is one of several proteins that organize the myofilaments in skeletal muscle.

CHAPTER 19: NUTRITION

1. This patient is suffering from rickets resulting from a vitamin D (cholecalciferol) deficiency. She is not exposed to any significant amount of sunlight, and she is dependent on her mother for any dietary vitamin D. However, her mother's diet avoids the richest source of vitamin D—dairy products. Proper mineralization of bone requires adequate vitamin D, either from sun exposure or diet.

2. The epiphyseal plate has multiple zones of maturation terminating in Ca^{++} deposition (ossification) on the diaphyseal side. With normal Ca^{++} deposition, the calcification zone moves at the same rate as the zone of proliferation. However, with abnormal Ca^{++} deposition, the zone of calcification progresses more slowly, thus widening the distance to the proliferation zone and giving the appearance of a widening epiphyseal plate.

3. Rickets patients also show a flaring of the ribs where they meet cartilage, known as the rachitic rosary, as well as general flaring of the lower end of the rib cage itself (Harrison's groove).

CHAPTER 20: TISSUE BIOCHEMISTRY

1. Antitrypsin activity is needed in the lungs to neutralize the elastase released by neutrophils. α_1-Antitrypsin is produced in the liver and is a component of the serum proteins. It exists in balance with the elastase activity in the lungs, serving as a proteolytic shield. The specificity of action extends beyond trypsin to other serine proteases.

2. Emphysema produced by cigarettes is centrilobular, whereas emphysema produced by α_1-antitrypsin deficiency is more evenly distributed and is panacinar. This is consistent with the centrilobular deposition of particulate matter from smoke.

3. A barrel-shaped chest is created by chronic overinflation of the lungs. The reduced surface area due to erosion of the alveolar walls creates a less efficient gas exchange and reduces oxygenation of the blood. The decreased breath sounds are also due to overinflation of the lungs. The reduced surface area in the lungs leads to a reduction in resistance to air flow and less sound from turbulence.

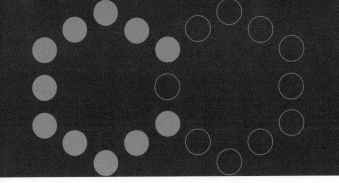

Index

Note: Page numbers followed by *b* indicate boxes, *f* indicate figures, and *t* indicate tables.